AF867839

Collaborative Emergency Medicine
for Veterinary Technicians

Collaborative Emergency Medicine for Veterinary Technicians

Edited by

Simone Conwell
VeG ER for Pets
Pikesville, MD
USA

WILEY

Copyright © 2027 by John Wiley & Sons, Inc. All rights reserved, including rights for text and data mining and training of artificial intelligence technologies or similar technologies.

Published by John Wiley & Sons, Inc., Hoboken, New Jersey.

No part of this publication may be reproduced, stored in a retrieval system, or transmitted in any form or by any means, electronic, mechanical, photocopying, recording, scanning, or otherwise, except as permitted under Section 107 or 108 of the 1976 United States Copyright Act, without either the prior written permission of the Publisher, or authorization through payment of the appropriate per-copy fee to the Copyright Clearance Center, Inc., 222 Rosewood Drive, Danvers, MA 01923, (978) 750–8400, fax (978) 750–4470, or on the web at www.copyright.com. Requests to the Publisher for permission should be addressed to the Permissions Department, John Wiley & Sons, Inc., 111 River Street, Hoboken, NJ 07030, (201) 748–6011, fax (201) 748–6008, or online at http://www.wiley.com/go/permission.

The manufacturer's authorized representative according to the EU General Product Safety Regulation is Wiley-VCH GmbH, Boschstr. 12, 69469 Weinheim, Germany, e-mail: Product_Safety@wiley.com.

Trademarks: Wiley and the Wiley logo are trademarks or registered trademarks of John Wiley & Sons, Inc. and/or its affiliates in the United States and other countries and may not be used without written permission. All other trademarks are the property of their respective owners. John Wiley & Sons, Inc. is not associated with any product or vendor mentioned in this book.

Limit of Liability/Disclaimer of Warranty: The contents of this work are intended to further general scientific research, understanding, and discussion only and are not intended and should not be relied upon as recommending or promoting scientific method, diagnosis, or treatment by physicians for any particular patient. In view of ongoing research, equipment modifications, changes in governmental regulations, and the constant flow of information relating to the use of medicines, equipment, and devices, the reader is urged to review and evaluate the information provided in the package insert or instructions for each medicine, equipment, or device for, among other things, any changes in the instructions or indication of usage and for added warnings and precautions. While the publisher and the authors have used their best efforts in preparing this work, including a review of the content of the work, neither the publisher nor the authors make any representations or warranties with respect to the accuracy or completeness of the contents of this work and specifically disclaim all warranties, including without limitation any implied warranties of merchantability or fitness for a particular purpose. No warranty may be created or extended by sales representatives, written sales materials or promotional statements for this work. The fact that an organization, website, or product is referred to in this work as a citation and/or potential source of further information does not mean that the publisher and authors endorse the information or services the organization, website, or product may provide or recommendations it may make. This work is sold with the understanding that the publisher is not engaged in rendering professional services. The advice and strategies contained herein may not be suitable for your situation. You should consult with a specialist where appropriate. Further, readers should be aware that websites listed in this work may have changed or disappeared between when this work was written and when it is read. Neither the publisher nor authors shall be liable for any loss of profit or any other commercial damages, including but not limited to special, incidental, consequential, or other damages.

For general information on our other products and services or for technical support, please contact our Customer Care Department within the United States at (800) 762–2974, outside the United States at (317) 572–3993 or fax (317) 572–4002.

Wiley also publishes its books in a variety of electronic formats. Some content that appears in print may not be available in electronic formats. For more information about Wiley products, visit our web site at www.wiley.com.

Library of Congress Cataloging-in-Publication Data applied for:

Hardback ISBN: 9781394293971

Cover Design: Wiley
Cover Images: Simone Conwell

Set in 9.5/12.5pt STIXTwoText by Straive, Pondicherry, India

Printed in Singapore
M131713210726

Contents

List of Contributors

Valerie Bogie
Insight Animal Behavior Services, USA
Valerie Bogie, LLC, USA
National Empowerment Center, USA
International Association of Veterinary Social Work, USA

and

MSSW, Veterinary Social Worker, USA

Julia Conny
VeG ER for Pets, Pikesville, MD, USA

and

Veterinary Emergency and Critical Care Society Member, USA

Simone Conwell
VeG ER for Pets, Pikesville, MD, USA

and

Veterinary Emergency and Critical Care Society Member, USA

Elizabeth Faux
VeG ER for Pets, Pikesville, MD, USA

and

Veterinary Emergency and Critical Care Society Member, USA

Fernanda Flynn-Galicia
Veterinary Technician Student, VeG ER for Pets, Brooklyn, NY, USA

Máriam Ordoñez
Veterinary Technician Student, Columbia MD, USA
VeG ER for Pets, Pikesville, MD, USA

and

Veterinary Emergency and Critical Care Society Member, USA

Ashley Salango
Practice Manager, Charm City Veterinary Hospital, Baltimore, MD, USA

Danielle Schuler
VeG ER for Pets, Pikesville, MD, USA

and

Veterinary Emergency and Critical Care Society Member, USA

Allison Snow
BluePearl Pet Hospital, Rockville, MD, USA

Talia Sundstrom
Regional Manager for Vetcor, Brandon, FL, USA

Puja Wright
BluePearl Pet Hospital, Rockville, MD, USA

Preface

Thoughts on Collaborative Veterinary Medicine

By Simone Conwell, RVT

I started working in veterinary medicine in 2008 as an assistant. Maryland did not have a lot of significant differences in what a registered technician and an assistant can do, and the "registered" was the only part of the title that was protected; technician was fine for everyone regardless of credentials. I have since gone on to be licensed in Maryland, and as I did so through an American Veterinary Medical Association (AVMA)-certified program, I can transfer my credentials to other states relatively easily (discounting the red tape). Maryland, as of October 2025, does allow for an alternative pathway to credentialing that still requires a degree, though credentials obtained that way cannot always transfer to other states (e.g. Tennessee). But this book isn't about that.

I have met an incredibly broad spectrum of people in vetmed. I've met doctors who were newly graduated and others who were approaching retirement. I've met doctors from other countries who were trying to learn how the US practices veterinary medicine and what from companion animal medicine they can bring home. I've met large animal vets. I've met boarded doctors. I've met a lot of students, both technicians and veterinarians. I've met a handful of veterinary social workers. I've met certified veterinary practice managers. And I have met a lot of receptionists, assistants, technicians, and vet tech specialists. Each one has an important role to play in our job, and no one role is more important than the other. I love my receptionists; former and current coworkers will tell you I should not be allowed to touch the phone because it breaks when I do (ask me about the time one asked if I wanted to send a text). And I love my assistants because they can figure out the e-collars. I will be the first in my hospital to admit I am absolutely terrible at bandages. Not just compared to the other technicians, I'm worse than a lot of the assistants. I tend to quick pets when I cut claws, so I don't do it very often. And that's all ok, because I don't need to be the best at everything.

We play to our strengths so often in vetmed. There's no reason why I can't set up my coworker for success by having all the bandaging supplies ready. So why should transfers and referrals be any different? I've heard many clients say their regular veterinarian told them to wait to get the radiographs/pain meds/bloodwork with us in the emergency room (ER), and they were annoyed that we would ask them for those records at all and that we charge significantly more. It became clearer to me when chatting with staff at general practices (GP) that they weren't considering that there are quite a few things they could do for their patients prior to transferring to the ER. They were worried we wouldn't think their x-rays were diagnostic for vomiting/diarrhea/heart disease/coughing, or that we would just repeat bloodwork immediately. And yes, sometimes we do have to repeat bloodwork, or at least verify the lack of platelets, but it's because we look for smaller trends than the every 3–6-month bloodwork a GP will run. The changes we're checking for are more immediate. And maybe we have to retake radiographs sometimes because something has changed.

But that doesn't mean we don't value records from our GP counterpart. At the same time, having worked with specialists and specialty technicians (and been one), I understand the frustration when ER doesn't place the sampling line or consider a potential treatment before doing things. I've been frustrated that an anemic patient was started on antibiotics before having blood drawn for North Carolina State University's tick tests, or that no one thought to pull blood from the anorexic shepherd that has cow patty diarrhea and has not eaten for 12 hours before they placed a nasogastric tube and started trickle feeding. That all comes from differences in how the disease is treated; ER is emergent and immediate, but specialty focuses on why and how to treat the root cause. We can learn from each other; I feel the best techs can see both points of view.

Which brings me to the assistants. Not every contributor is credentialed, and that was a deliberate choice on my part. I value the book learning from my associate's degree, don't get me wrong. I didn't realize how much I didn't know until I took the classes. But I was a knowledgeable assistant. My doctors pushed me to get the credentialing because they knew it would open more doors. But what about the people who are veterinary technician specialists (VTS) and wouldn't be recognized as a credentialed tech in another state because of how they obtained their credentials? Are they less knowledgeable, having passed the rigorous standards to obtain a VTS, than someone who became credentialed through an associate's degree just because they went through an alternative route? So, I asked some knowledgeable assistants to contribute because they are collaborating with their doctors, technicians, and receptionists on a day-to-day basis. And what's the point of being in medicine if we stop learning?

Abbreviations

AAHA: American Animal Hospital Association
AHDS: acute hemorrhagic diarrhea syndrome
CBC: complete blood count
CPR: cardiopulmonary resuscitation
DIC: disseminated intravascular coagulation
DKA: diabetic ketoacidosis
eDKA: euglycemic ketoacidosis
ER: emergency room
FP: frozen plasma
FFP: fresh frozen plasma
GDV: gastric dilatation and volvulus
GIFB: gastrointestinal foreign body
HHS: hyperosmolar hyperglycemic syndrome
IMHA: immune-mediated hemolytic anemia
IMTP: immune-mediated thrombocytopenia
IO: intraosseous
IV: intravenous
KCS: keratoconjunctivitis Sicca
kg: kilogram
ml: milliliter
mg: milligram
mOsm: milliosmole
PCV/TS: packed cell volume/total solids
POCUS: point of care ultrasound
PICC: peripherally inserted central catheter
pRBC: packed red blood cells
RAAS: renin-angiotensin-aldosterone system
rDVM: regular/referring doctor of veterinary medicine
RECOVER: Reassessment Campaign On Veterinary Resuscitation
SGLT2: Sodium-glucose cotransporter 2
U: units
UTO: urinary tract obstruction

Acknowledgments

Thanks to everyone who contributed to the following text, whether by writing a chapter, taking pictures and sending a text saying "put this in the book!" at 1 a.m., mentoring all of us, providing emotional support through our careers, and being flexible.

Thanks to the staff in GP who know vaccine schedules that some of us have forgotten and for doing dental cleanings and toenail trims.

Thanks to the urgent care staff who take some of the load from the GP and the ER, and kudos to any of you who stepped away from the ER for your own well-being.

Thanks to the specialty staff for being willing to focus on one specific area so we can all learn from you.

Thanks to the administrators for doing a thankless job and for caring enough to do it well. Social workers, we see you and thank you for just caring.

Thanks reception/CEC/CSRs everywhere for answering the phones and usually being the first person seen by our clients.

And to my fellow ECC people – thanks for being not quite right and thriving in chaos.

Part I

Back to Basics

1

What Defines Emergency?

Simone Conwell[1,2]

[1] *VeG ER for Pets, 1858 Reisterstown Road, Pikesville, MD, USA*
[2] *Veterinary Emergency and Critical Care Society Member, USA*

Le mot "triage" vient du "trier," comme sélectionner ou choisir, mais un plus comme séparer parce qu'on choisit quel patient est. le plus malade. C'est bien, n'est-ce pas? Non? Because you're expecting to read this in your native tongue. We have all heard the etymology of triage and understand what that means, but how do we apply it to our patients? What should we be looking for as a subtle sign of major illness? How do we know where exactly to send each patient if it's beyond what our hospital's capability is?

During the COVID-19 lockdown, at least in the United States, I believe everyone in veterinary medicine became used to seeing a red-to-green scale for how emergently a patient needed to be treated. It was always a little different, depending on which hospital had created the scale and what that area of the country tended to see, as well as whether it was from a specialty, emergency, urgent care, or general practice hospital. But they all looked something like this (Figure 1.1).

Where red is the most severe type of emergency, needing to be seen immediately, orange is slightly less severe, yellow is less severe than that, and green is the least severe and not a true emergency, though the owners may feel otherwise, and they should still be treated respectfully.

The truth is that the lines are not so clearly delineated between a critical, life-threatening emergency and one that has the potential to become critical. That is why it is so important to have an experienced technician, nurse, or assistant examine everything that comes into the hospital (Figure 1.2).

Some triage scales base the classifications on how long a patient can wait to be seen, which is probably more accurate than grouping each individual disease process as a specific level of urgency, as there is almost always some degree of nuance present. For example, anemia. A patient who is actively hemorrhaging due to trauma needs to be seen immediately so a compression bandage can be placed to stop the bleeding, while a patient known to have immune-mediated hemolytic anemia (IMHA) (see Chapter 10) and has pale gums but otherwise stable vitals should be seen soon, but can wait for at least some period of time, and a cat who is chronically anemic due to kidney failure that came in for vomiting because they are out of an antiemetic and has pale pink gums but otherwise completely normal vitals and is making biscuits in her carrier can wait for even longer. An inexperienced triage technician may look at the kidney cat and IMHA dog and decide they have the same level of urgency and should be seen almost as urgently as the patient who is bleeding out in the treatment area.

Figure 1.1 A simple color block triage scale provided by Simone Conwell, RVT, VTS (ECC).

Figure 1.2 A more accurate, blurred lines version of the block triage scale. *Source:* Provided by Simone Conwell, RVT, VTS (ECC).

There are always scenarios that present as a hard and fast "must be seen immediately." Any patient who is not breathing – and agonally breathing is not breathing – or gasping for air, has no heartbeat, is likely having heatstroke, is actively having a seizure, may have a broken spine, is laterally recumbent, or is a bearded dragon who ingested a lightning bug should be seen immediately (Knight 1999). The question "Do you want CPR (cardiopulmonary resuscitation) performed on your pet?" must be answered with a definitive yes or no for any patient that seems likely to go into respiratory arrest or is in cardiac arrest. But there is still more nuance within the CPR question, as open chest CPR can very easily occur during abdominal surgery, where the surgeon can go through the diaphragm to reach the heart. So while many owners and even many veterinary professionals would not initially consider open chest CPR, they may rethink it during a surgical code.

But what needs to go to the 24-hour emergency room (ER) or the specialty + ER hospital? Where do the vet urgent cares fit into this scale? I have seen a handful of these urgent care vets popping up around my area, and I applaud them. They can save clients' money and free up the ERs for more critical patients, and we can always take referrals from them. They can even do some procedures and refer them to a 24-hour facility for further care. So let's delve into where those dividing lines are. This text will focus on cats and dogs.

Primary care is the backbone of veterinary medicine. You guys vaccinate pets and provide flea, tick, and heartworm prevention; spay/neuter; investigate the little bumps that pop up out of nowhere; and take care of dental issues, so I never have to pick up a scaler again. I appreciate that so much. But what happens when you have a client who calls and says their pet has an emergency during the day? We understand in the field that sometimes your schedule is too tight, and you cannot see a long-term client because of that. So, we understand when you tell them to come to us for most things. But given the long wait times, what really needs to go to an ER immediately versus what could wait for a day or two to be seen with you?

- Acute lameness in a hind limb after running around outside
- Itchiness
- Reverse sneezing
- New, small bumps
- Pregnancy checks
- Removed a tick
- Most ear infections
- Broken teeth

Limping on the Hind Leg

I have had enough clients tell me that their regular veterinarian (rDVM) said that they should take orthopedic radiographs through the ER because we have a specialty for suspected cranial cruciate ligament (CCL) tears, and I do believe there is truly a misunderstanding with that one. The ER radiographs are going to be more expensive, and surgery is still probably going to redo them because the ER does not take ortho rads very often. It would be better for the client's wallet to have their rDVM take the radiographs with mild sedation there or wait until the surgical consult if the rDVM isn't comfortable taking this type of radiograph. It was my experience while I was in general practice that the surgery practices are very willing to do a lunch and learn about how to take appropriate radiographs for a suspected CCL tear, and if you send them enough bad radiographs, they may offer to do so without prompting. I suggest reaching out first if the team isn't comfortable with this type of radiograph. If this happens after hours, we are happy to see these patients and prescribe them pain medications, but during business hours, it isn't something the owners need to rush in immediately to be seen in the ER for, and they should understand that their rDVM can help guide them through this.

Itchiness

Parasite prevention should be a year-round habit, but many people think their pets can't get fleas in the winter, anecdotally speaking. The Companion Animal Parasite Council states on its website that fleas can survive in the winter and recommends year-round prevention as soon as possible. We in the ER still get phone calls routinely about people wanting to be seen because their pet has fleas. ERs do not generally carry significant amounts of flea prevention; they mostly carry nitenpyram to treat any adult fleas on hospitalized patients and for maggots (Budde 2023). That being said, if a patient is suffering from flea anemia that is so severe its gums are white, it probably needs a transfusion in addition to parasite control, and we in the ER would really like to see that patient sooner rather than later. Allergies are another common cause of itchiness, and that is a chronic condition that we in the ER are not generally set up to treat. If the skin is torn due to pruritus, we can, of course, prescribe antibiotics, but, overall, we recommend clients see their rDVM within a few days of seeing us for allergies.

Mange, whether demodectic or sarcoptic, was something I would see more often in the ER when I started in veterinary medicine in 2008. With the increase in medications in the isoxazoline family, we are seeing it less frequently. As most general practices carry something in this family on their shelves and ERs do not, this is something we are recommending for the rDVM to see instead of us.

Reverse Sneezing

Many clients, especially first-time dog owners, rush to the ER, saying their pet can't breathe because of reverse sneezing. While this misunderstanding is easily resolved, and we generally have a good laugh about it with the clients after their panic is over, it is not a great feeling when a triage for dyspnea is called while we're in the middle of a code. Discussing reverse sneezing with clients at first puppy appointments, asking if they're familiar with it, or playing videos about it in the waiting room/exam room while waiting for the doctor to come in would go a long way toward lowering everyone's heart rate.

New, Small Bumps

An unexpected bump can cause alarm for clients. Unless it is an abscess, the ER is probably not going to do much beyond an exam. Biopsy is the gold standard, and while we certainly can do that, if it's small, it is financially beneficial for the client to have that addressed at their rDVM. The rDVM will also be able to make accurate notes on size, shape, color, and growth progression. While we are again happy to see patients for these things, this is in the green category of the triage scale.

Pregnancy Checks

Seeing if a bitch that has tied is pregnant is not an emergency. Clients should expect, if they're breeding a patient, to maintain contact with a veterinarian who is well-versed in prenatal and neonatal care. While the ER is well equipped to manage pyometra, dystocia, neonate resuscitation, and hypocalcemia, we are generally handling the complications of pregnancy and parturition, not the breeding part. Again, our radiographs cost significantly more than at a general practice, and the client's money would be better spent with their rDVM. A bitch starting labor is also not a reason to come into the ER, and I believe people generally think they must go to the hospital because that's what happens in human medicine. Having in-depth conversations with owners in regard to the stages of labor and when to start being concerned, as well as giving them the number to the local ER in case they have questions when labor inevitably happens at 1:23 a.m., would help a lot of clients remain calm and may even prevent some anxious dogs from having complications during labor due to stress.

Ticks

Yes, they're creepy and crawly. They're vectors for complicated diseases. There is a myth about leaving the head in being a huge problem. They're another reason to advocate for year-round parasite prevention that will kill the tick before it can spread disease. But they aren't an emergency. If a client is having trouble getting the tick off after hours, the ER will remove it. But testing for tick-borne disease should be left to the rDVM. Most patient-side tests detect antibodies instead of antigens, meaning that they will detect an old infection instead of an active one (Myers 2024). Furthermore, it generally takes a few weeks for quantitative tests to be able to detect an active infection instead of an old one (CAPC n.d.). It's better for the client's wallet to wait for any testing after tick removal.

Ear Infections

Are ear infections frustrating? Yes. Can they require significant follow-up and long-term management? Also yes. Are they truly an emergency? Rarely. If the ear infection is so severe that the patient is actively bleeding, waiting until the rDVM has an appointment available is not the best course of action. Conversely, a hematoma that has not ruptured can most likely wait until the rDVM opens in the morning, particularly if it is small.

Teeth Problems

We in the ER cannot generally fix a tooth root abscess. We can prescribe antibiotics and pain medication. Most ERs also aren't set up to take dental radiographs to confirm if multiple teeth need to be addressed. It has been my experience across many ERs and hearing from clients when I was in general practice, that clients are generally shocked that the emergency vet could not fix the tooth root abscess, though I have never found a human hospital that was convenient for my dental emergencies when I am awake on the night shift. As complete oral health and assessment and treatment (COHAT) discussions have become more commonplace, it is worth starting to discuss 'dental emergencies' with clients at the same time as the teeth brushing conversations start. A broken jaw, electrical burn to the mouth, and perhaps broken teeth in a fight are things the ERs are equipped to handle, though the broken teeth really must be almost out for us to pull them. I have seen a handful of cases where the patient would not stop bleeding after oral surgery, and that is not a tooth problem but rather a hemorrhagic problem, and we would like to see those patients. Dental blocks are another thought; despite having done them frequently when I worked in general practice, I can count on one hand the number of times I have performed them in the ER (twice). Anyone who has had dental work knows how painful that can be; its best to leave extractions to those who will not have to look up landmarks for dental blocks.

Phone triage is hard. We understand and have had frantic owners describing something we were sure would need CPR when it arrived, and it was a broken toenail. But some of these things can wait a day or two to be seen and don't need to wait hours in the ER. Or they can go to urgent care, where most of the yellow triages can be seen.

Urgent cares can, without a doubt, handle simple cases of gastroenteritis, where a dog or cat has eaten something that doesn't agree with them. They can provide subcutaneous fluids and antiemetics and dispense more of these medications and probiotics to go home, and they warn the owners that if the patient vomits through the antiemetic, they should be seen again, as that is a concern for a gastrointestinal foreign body (GIFB). The urgent care can take radiographs and run bloodwork. They can suture up small lacerations, usually. They can see everything that is limping due to soft tissue injury, and maybe limping due to fractures, if there is someone comfortable with splinting the limb, if indicated. They can start the process of treating most blocked cats if a doctor or credentialed technician is comfortable doing the unblocking procedure (see Chapter 7). I have been lucky to have urgent cares near me that are staffed by people who used to be in the ER and wanted to not see everything and work the crazy hours, who are very capable of stabilizing patients enough to transport them to the 24-hour facility down the road. Some of them will even perform laparotomies for GIFB and gastric dilatation-volvulus (GDV) and then send them to the ER for 24-hour care.

The urgent cares can also handle ear infections, itchiness, and tick-covered pets. They are capable of performing CPR if they are the closest hospital to an unstable pet and then referring that patient on to a 24-hour ER. They can start diagnostics for heart failure in patients who fit the criteria. Urgent cares are not as uniform as ERs in terms of their ability to perform anesthetic procedures, and if an urgent care says they can only do the work-up for a foreign body but not actually cut, they should be believed, utilized, and valued as being able to start the case, and clients need to have clear expectations set from the start.

Urgent cares can also see potentially one of the most rewarding triages: vomit induction. If a cat or dog ingests a string, underwear, tampons, diapers, etc., the urgent care is just as easily able to induce vomiting and then reverse it and send that patient on their way. It is important to remember that inducing vomiting in a patient who has ingested zinc phosphide needs to be done outside, in a well-ventilated area, and the vomitus needs to be sealed due to the risk of phosphine gas production (CDC n.d.). Grape/raisin, nonsteroidal anti-inflammatory, and most other medications, including oclacitinib ingestion, should still come to the ER. The owners should call a poison control center dedicated to animals first and head to a 24-hour facility. The only exception should be if decontamination needs to happen immediately and the urgent care facility is significantly closer (<15 minutes travel time); then, they should continue on to a 24-hour facility.

Urgent cares are also capable of removing toys that are stuck on the lower jaw. Sometimes, it's not a toy but a dustbin handle. They can sedate these patients and either cut the toy or, hopefully, have enough relaxation to allow the handle to slide off (Image 1.1).

These examples seem like pretty clear-cut green/yellow triages and obvious ones that need to be seen sooner than the rDVM can sometimes accommodate without the lines being blurred. Sure, medication ingestion might require some nuance, but that is self-explanatory. But what about drug ingestion? Urgent care and rDVM can definitely see a typical marijuana ingestion, especially if the owners own up to it from the start and the pet (usually a dog, but there is always that one cat) has the typical startle response, can't hold its urine, is kind of ataxic, and just seems a little off in a way that makes perfect sense when the owner says they know Raven got into their stash. And with edibles becoming more common and some of them having xylitol present, most vets would say that it needs to go to a 24-hour facility just in case.

But what about a dog that ingests marijuana resin? We had that patient at my 24-hour hospital. Poison control told us this dog could feel the effects for 72 hours or longer. She was very ataxic, had no control of her bladder, was incredibly nauseous, and had a very dull/depressed mentation. If the patient has ingested marijuana before and been fine, the owner might not think to say resin was involved. Drug tests, if they are even run, do not show the level of exposure, just that there was potential exposure. I have heard from coworkers who lived in other places that dogs who ate synthetic marijuana or stronger versions of marijuana sometimes need a ventilator. So marijuana ingestion is one of those emergencies that can range from yellow to red.

What about other drugs, ones that are illegal? Even with marijuana being federally decriminalized in the United States, so many clients still think the veterinary staff is going to report them to authorities for their pet getting into their stash. In my experience, the only people who admit that their dog has been exposed to illicit drugs are (1) police whose working dog was exposed on the job, (2) rich people, or (3) very scary people who are a very specific subdivision of rich (Image 1.2).

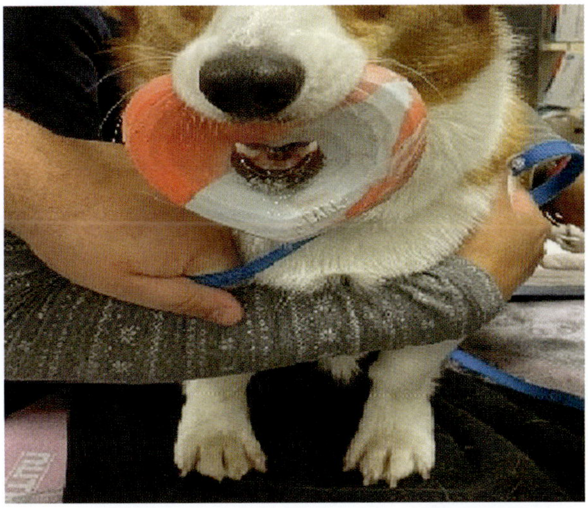

Image 1.1 A Corgi with a toy stuck on his bottom jaw. It was removed after he was given intravenous sedation and was able to be maneuvered off his jaw with minimal discomfort to him. The toy was thrown out at the owners request. *Source:* Photo courtesy of Simone Conwell, R.

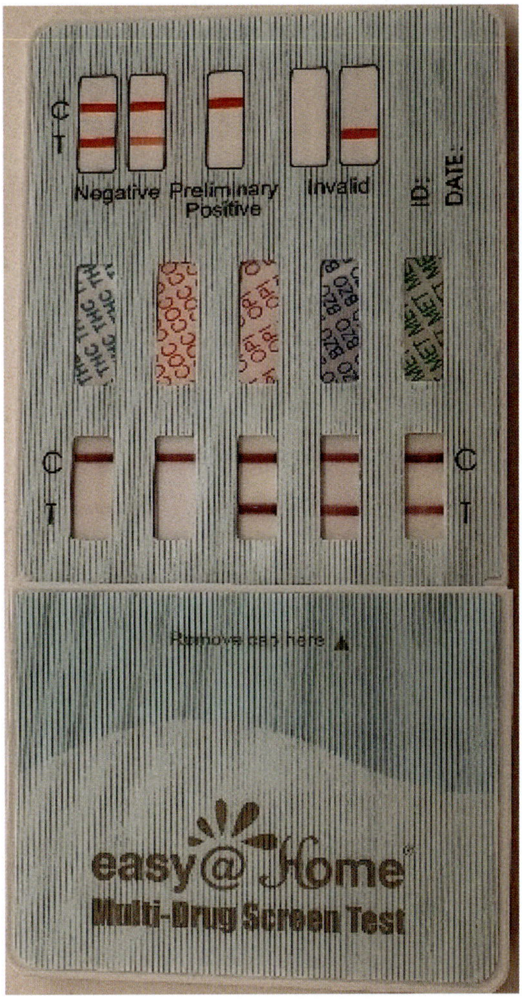

Image 1.2 A positive drug test for marijuana and cocaine. *Source:* Photo courtesy of Simone Conwell, RVT, VTS (ECC).

This client brought in an older lab-sized dog who was having significant trouble walking, muscle tremors, hypersalivation, and was significantly tachycardic on presentation. He also had an elevated temperature. The owner approved a full workup with bloodwork, radiographs, and urinalysis. Because everything had been so unremarkable, and because we were out of ideas, the doctor requested a drug test just in case. We ran it three times to confirm the results because the owner did not seem like the kind to lie about ingesting anything, and had been very conscientious and worried about the dog, was, in fact, in tears, worried about having to euthanize. The doctor had a delicate conversation, and we learned the partner was struggling with addiction and had been home alone before the dog's symptoms started, and there was suspicion that the partner was using again. This type of case requires significant compassion, as in addition to the stress over a beloved four-legged family member, we must remember that addiction hurts more than the user. This client did not need our judgment, our advice on leaving, or our disappointment. We needed to treat the pet, and we did that. Would an urgent care have carried out the drug tests and run one? Unknown. Drug tests do not always come up positive for known marijuana toxicity due to how animals metabolize it (Fitzgerald n.d.). We routinely leave it to the client to decide if they want the test run when they know marijuana exposure is possible because of the risk of false negatives. The cocaine-positive dog also brought up the question of how to treat cocaine toxicity, and it's unfortunately treated symptomatically (Khan n.d.). Enough time had passed that inducing emesis would likely not have helped, and the dog had been so nauseous that an antiemetic had already been given, rendering emesis induction difficult anyway. Would the outcome have been different if the owner had taken the dog to an urgent care or rDVM first? We can't know. We can't even know if the outcome would have been different at another ER, since not every ER is the same, just as not every rDVM and urgent care is the same. But this dog is an interesting case that could have presented to an rDVM or urgent care because he worsened as the time from ingestion increased. Initially, his owner said he was not walking too badly for an old lab, and he just seemed a little off. By the time we saw him (estimated about 4 hours after ingestion), he had progressed to a dog that was central to everyone's sight because he was so ill. He was ultimately able to go home, but there was a concern that he would not survive to discharge.

Ophthalmic Emergencies

I am convinced the only people in veterinary medicine who enjoy anything ophthalmic-related work in ophthalmology. Any eye issue is an emergency until proven otherwise. It might be something an rDVM can fit into their schedule if it's eye discharge in an older pug and they have had conversations with the owner previously that they believe their pug is at risk for developing keratoconjunctivitis sicca (KCS) (dry eye). Or it might be a traumatic proptosis and in need of a tarsorrhaphy or enucleation. Maybe there's hyphema, or an elderly cat is suddenly acting blind and, oh, by the way, his breath smells terribly uremic. Corneal ulcers can be superficial or deep, and waiting to address them can cause even more problems (Norkus 2019). I would also like to encourage rDVMs to see more ophthalmic emergencies when they are able because we in the ER do not have better medications unless there is an ophthalmology specialty attached to the ER. We are going to run the same eye tests (Schirmer, fluorescein, and tonometry) and fight with the tonometer as much to get it to work. If it is something unusual, we are equally likely to tell the owner to go to a specialist. If it is a long-term condition such as KCS, hypertension due to kidney failure, or glaucoma, we might diagnose them in the ER but will recommend all follow-up be with their rDVM or specialist (Images 1.3–1.5).

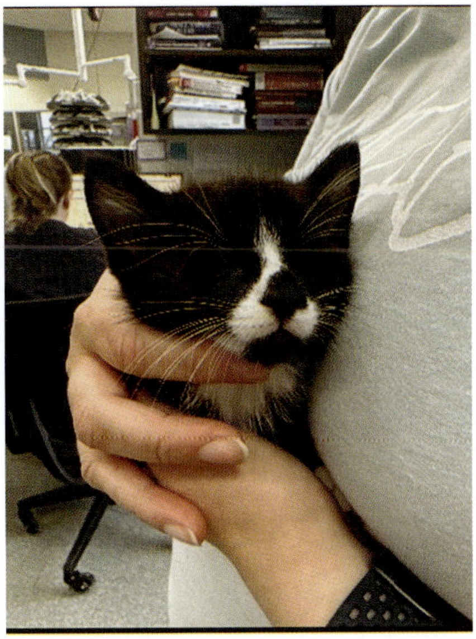

Image 1.3 Approximately 1 month old kitten with no eyes, possible due to infection. *Source:* Photo courtesy of Simone Conwell, RVT, VTS (ECC).

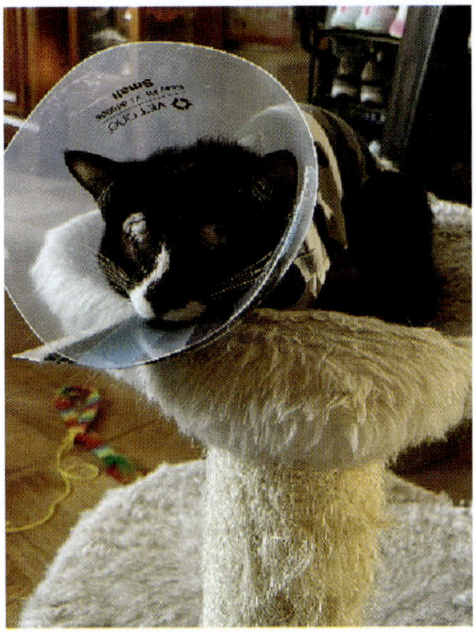

Image 1.4 The same kitten at 9 months of age in an Elizabethan collar following a neuter and tear duct removal due to constant drainage/risk of infection where the eyes should be. *Source:* Photo courtesy of Simone Conwell, RVT, VTS (ECC).

Seizures

Seizures are a frustrating disorder. They can have multiple causes, including but not limited to hypoglycemia, hypernatremia, hypocalcemia, liver shunts, toxicities, snake envenomation, heatstroke, canine distemper virus, and neoplasia, and there is even an idiopathic form (Norkus 2019). A seizure is certainly frightening for an owner and needs to be addressed. But – and stay with me on this – does it always need to be seen emergently? Potentially not. A first-time seizure in a dog or cat between 6 months and 5 years could be the first and only idiopathic seizure a pet will have (Norkus 2019). If that happens, we in the ER may advise those owners, particularly if they seem reluctant to come in,

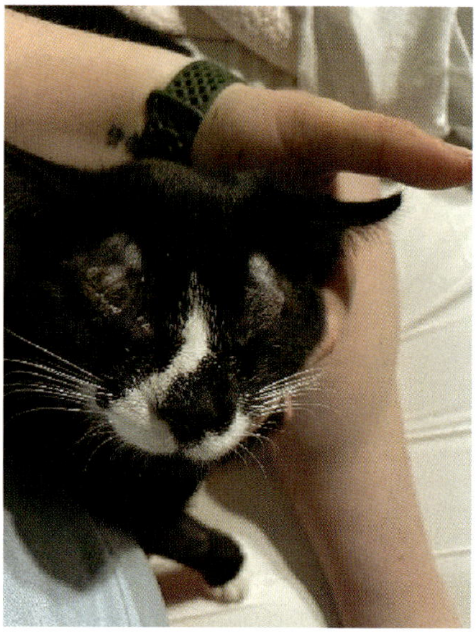

Image 1.5 The same kitten 13 days later after suture removal. *Source:* Photos courtesy of Simone Conwell, RVT, VTS (ECC).

that they can wait to see if they can get in with their rDVM in the next day or two, if there are no further seizures. If there are more than three seizures within a short period of time, we will recommend hospitalization and anticonvulsant medication to break the seizures. Metabolic seizures (hypoglycemia, hypernatremia, and hypocalcemia) need to have a cause identified and need to be addressed by an ER or urgent care. Hypocalcemia is often seen in nursing bitches and queens experiencing inadequate calcium intake and are typically able to be discharged relatively soon after presentation, with the understanding that the puppies or kittens need to be weaned or bottle fed after that (Norkus 2019). Meanwhile, hypernatremia can require days of hospitalization to correct a chronic change (Randels-Thorp 2017). Hypoglycemia may be a relatively easy fix in a toy breed that is not being fed with appropriate frequency, but an insulin overdose may require more interventions. Liver shunts often require specialty to find the shunt and require a boarded surgeon to correct it (Norkus 2019). Canine distemper requires hospitalization and aggressive treatment, and still, the dog may not survive (Silverstein 2023). Toxicities, snake envenomation, and heatstroke should be hospitalized and treated supportively. Seizures caused by a neoplasm need magnetic resonance imaging (MRI) to identify the seizure and neurosurgery if it is possible to remove it (Silverstein 2023).

Overall, it is not wrong to tell a client with a pet experiencing a seizure to seek emergency care rather than waiting to be seen. If the client seems likely to want advanced imaging, it is worth recommending that they locate an ER with a neurology specialty for transfer. Owners should anticipate that the imaging will be expensive; patients are anesthetized for an MRI because they cannot move, and the machines are loud. Owners should understand that anesthesia is non-negotiable for an MRI, given that even humans find it difficult to have head MRIs due to the enclosed space, sound, and face cage to keep their head in place.

Trauma

Trauma can mean different things to different people. A broken and bleeding nail on an otherwise healthy dog is not emergent, though owners occasionally beg to differ. A dog that has been shot definitely should be taken to the nearest ER for pain management. I have seen dogs hit by cars that were fine and dogs that were almost cut in half by the impact. There are different levels of shock involved due to the compensatory mechanisms bodies experience when the initial trauma occurs (Norkus 2019). Compensatory shock is characterized by activation of the renin-angiotensin-aldosterone system (RAAS) and neuroendocrine response, resulting in constriction of the peripheral blood vessels and splenic contraction to shunt blood back to the more critical organs: the heart, lungs, and brain (Norkus 2019). Vital signs may be normal to slightly tachycardic and slightly pale or, conversely, injected mucous membranes (Norkus 2019). The splenic contraction typically results in a normal packed cell volume despite significant hemorrhage (Norkus 2019). Tissues start to become hypoxic due to inflammatory cytokines (Norkus 2019). Because the signs of compensatory shock may be so close to normal parameters, it is understandable that owners may misinterpret them and believe their dog is fine only to discover it is in decompensatory shock a short while later (Norkus 2019). It is therefore advisable for all patients who have experienced some sort of trauma to seek care soon after, and preferably at an urgent care or ER, to verify that they are not at risk of decompensating.

Urogenital Emergencies

Urinary tract infections (UTIs), though annoying, can be treated by the rDVM. A sterilely obtained sample sent off for culture is the best way to ensure antimicrobial stewardship, and pain medications and broad-spectrum antibiotics should be started while waiting for the results of the culture. Multidrug-resistant (MDR) UTIs are on the rise, which is concerning for both human and animal medicine, given that *Escherichia coli* is a very common cause of UTIs in dogs, and thus they can become a reservoir for such resistant bacteria (Sevilla 2024). However, there is a condition that clients frequently mistake for a UTI that is much more life-threatening: the urethral obstruction in male cats. Please see Chapter 8 for a more in-depth look at urethral obstructions in male cats and treating them. But for the purpose of phone triage, any male cat that is in and out of the litter box should be evaluated as soon as possible to rule out a urethral obstruction.

Pyometra is likely among the first emergencies many in the field think of when reproductive emergencies are mentioned. A pyometra is an infection of the uterus and occurs within 1–3 months of an estrus cycle (Norkus 2019). Because the cervix is open during estrus, it is easy for bacteria to enter the uterus and become trapped when estrus ends (Norkus 2019). From there, the pyometra may be classified as open (visible discharge from the vagina) or closed (no discharge visible), and a closed pyometra is more difficult for owners to recognize and thus may cause a delay in treatment (Norkus 2019). It has been my experience that many owners believe their pet is pregnant and is experiencing dystocia when they come in. An abdominal point-of-care ultrasound (POCUS) will show otherwise. The main treatment in the United States is an ovariohysterectomy (OVH). This is something that can be done by most rDVMs as they do perform OVH procedures more frequently than their urgent care and ER counterparts; the difference is the amount of pus involved. Because the risk of sepsis is not insignificant, pyometra surgery should be performed as soon as the patient is stable enough to tolerate anesthesia (Norkus 2019).

Prostatitis can be a cause of male dogs struggling to urinate. It may require castration to correct it if it is benign, antibiotics if bacterial prostatitis or a prostatic abscess, or a consultation with oncology if prostatic carcinoma is suspected (Norkus 2019). Other causes of difficulty urinating in intact male dogs may include bladder stones, some of which may be lodged in the urethra (Norkus 2019). A cystotomy is needed to remove the stones. It is possible to attempt to retropulse the stones back into the bladder with the use of a red rubber catheter and sterile saline; the bladder may also be drained this way. This is another emergency that could go to the rDVM or urgent care as well as the ER; it just depends on the time of day and how comfortable the rDVM and staff are performing a cystotomy if necessary.

Vomiting and Diarrhea

I had a coworker point out that humans often self-treat for vomiting and diarrhea because we generally can make it to the bathroom or sink and are not leaving feces and vomit on the floor, regarding how owners tend to view vomiting and diarrhea in our patients, which was a fair point in my opinion. While cat owners – and I say this as a cat owner myself – might ignore occasional vomiting as a "hairball" or "just something cats do," dog owners seem less lackadaisical about their pet vomiting. So when does it need to go to the ER versus waiting for the rDVM to open? Unfortunately, there is probably not any hard-and-fast rule for that. Pancreatitis is a common cause of gastrointestinal distress in canines and can range from mild to severe. Likewise, acute hemorrhagic diarrhea syndrome (AHDS) (see Chapter 12) can turn deadly fast. GIFB (Chapter 17) may also cause vomiting. But there are more benign causes, such as a new treat that just didn't agree with that patient, or maybe there was an abrupt diet change. These simpler cases can be treated easily with supportive care at an rDVM, and even the more concerning causes of vomiting and diarrhea can generally be started at the rDVM before transferring. Then we move into the more orange-red, infectious causes for vomiting and diarrhea, particularly in young puppies and kittens: parvovirus (Norkus 2019).

Parvovirus in puppies and panleukopenia in kittens (a parvovirus) typically present in under-vaccinated animals and are characterized by vomiting and diarrhea, often described as having a specific "parvo smell" (Norkus 2019; Silverstein 2023). Both diseases need aggressive treatment and stabilization for the best chances of survival (Silverstein 2023). There have been outpatient protocols for treating canine parvovirus (CPV), but I am unaware of any such studies related to panleukopenia (Venn 2017). Panleukopenia recovery generally takes longer than that of CPV and has an approximately 51% survival rate (Silverstein 2023). CPV has more recent literature on it, possibly because dog owners are more likely to visit the vet than cat owners (Bir 2020). CPV also has a newer treatment, a monoclonal antibody developed by Elanco (Larson 2024). The monoclonal antibody has been shown to improve survival rates in puppies with CPV when administered soon after a positive test (Larson 2024). Even though these patients are ideally hospitalized at an ER facility, it is possible that an rDVM will diagnose, start bloodwork, and place an intravenous catheter in these patients prior to transferring. If the rDVM is in an area that has a high enough rate of CPV, it could be worthwhile to invest in the monoclonal antibody and administer it prior to transfer to the ER in order to give these puppies the best chance of survival. Where I live in Maryland, it is not necessarily something I would expect most rDVMs to carry because while we do see CPV regularly, it is something we can go weeks or months without seeing. However, states like Texas see CPV much more frequently, according to Elanco's (n.d.) ParvoTrack tool, and have over 2200 reported cases for 2025. It might make sense for the rDVMs in Texas to keep updated on current treatment for CPV, both in and outpatient, to try to mitigate this disease.

The next emergencies are going to always be ones that should be evaluated by the ER, whether they are attached to a specialty or not. Basic stabilization may need to be done at an rDVM or urgent care if they are closer, or the owner did not realize how critical their pet was prior to a visit. On the color triage scale, these patients are dark orange/red and black. I did not include black in the first images because it is always patients who are actively dying, and it is a hard and fast color with no nuance.

Respiratory Distress

Cats and dogs may experience respiratory distress for a plethora of reasons. A dog may get a ball caught in her throat while playing and be unable to breathe around it. A cat may experience a severe asthma attack. Another dog might be stung by a bee in the throat, and the tissue is now swollen. Cats and dogs do experience heart failure (Silverstein 2023). These patients will all require oxygen, though the amount of time they need it may vary. For example, if the dog choking on the ball is able to be quickly sedated and the ball dislodged, it is possible that the dog will not need oxygen for very long at all. The other patients will require the underlying disease to be treated in order to no longer be oxygen dependent (Silverstein 2023).

Heatstroke

Heatstroke can have many devastating effects on the body if the temperature becomes high enough for long enough, including seizures, organ dysfunction, brain damage, arrhythmias, and disseminated intravascular coagulation (DIC) (Norkus 2019). It is treated by cooling the body and constant monitoring (Norkus 2019). Cooling too quickly can throw the body into hypothermia and require rewarming (Zager 2023). If there is no option but for the owners to drive a significant distance, the pet should be wetted down with room temperature water and the air conditioning in the car on high to give them the best chance of survival (Zager 2023).

Collapse

This is a very frightening time for owners, and unfortunately, whether their pet recovers depends on the cause of the collapse. If a pet is experiencing syncopal episodes related to heart disease, treatment may help prolong life (Silverstein 2023). If the collapse is due to severe anemia, the cause of the anemia will determine if the patient survives despite blood transfusions. Cats with underlying heart disease may not show symptoms and acutely arrest (Silverstein 2023). All veterinary personnel should be familiar with the most current RECOVER guidelines for worst-case scenarios where CPR needs to be performed. Instructors for RECOVER workshops may be found at https://recoverinitiative.org/find-an-instructor/ and searched by country and state.

Kirby's Rule of 20

Why would anyone who works in emergency and critical care suggest that some of these emergencies be seen by an rDVM or an urgent care? Is it only because of money? No, of course not. It's for a few reasons. I know our rDVM colleagues are booked out in advance. I don't want them to see patients who are beyond their capabilities, but I want them to feel like they can see certain cases that are categorized as emergent if they have the time. I want their technicians and assistants to feel utilized and that their knowledge isn't limited to vaccine schedules because they are the ones who will be involved in managing chronic diseases. They have established relationships with owners, and trust is there. It has been a long time since I worked in primary care, but I had clients who asked for me specifically. I am willing to bet there are others currently in primary care who have that happen now, and they care for those pets significantly and deserve to be involved in their emergency care, whether it's through updates or preparing them to transfer to the ER.

I don't recall from which lecture I saved a particular slide of Kirby's Rule of 20, but I keep it on my desktop as a reminder (Newfield 2021). This checklist is to remind us that our patients may be present for one particular problem, but that they are an entire living being and have needs (Box 1.1).

Box 1.1 Kirby's Rule of 20.

1. Oxygenation/ventilation	11. Renal function/urine output
2. Cardiac function/rhythm	12. Nutrition
3. Mentation/intracranial pressure	13. Immune status/WBC/antibiotics
4. Blood pressure/perfusion	14. Coagulation
5. RBC/hemoglobin	15. GI motility
6. Fluid balance	16. Drug metabolism
7. Oncotic pull	17. Pain control
8. Albumin	18. Bandage/wound care
9. Acid–base balance	19. Nursing care/mobility/catheter care
10. Electrolytes	20. Tender Loving Care

Most of these will be addressed by the ER. But the tender loving care starts at the rDVM, who makes sure that their patients know who to call in an emergency.

Works Cited

Bir, C.O. (2020). Familiarity and use of veterinary services by US resident dog and cat owners. *Animals (Basel)* 10 (3): 483. https://doi.org/10.3390/ani10.30483.

Budde, J.A. (2023). *Plumb's Veterinary Drug Handbook*. Randels-Thorp is Ames, Iowa: Wiley-Blackwell.

Center for Disease Control (CDC). (n.d.). Occupational Phosphine Gas Poisoning at Veterinary Hospitals from Dogs that Ingested Zinc Phosphide — Michigan, Iowa, and Washington, 2006–2011. Retrieved from www.cdc.gov: www.cdc.gov/mmwr/preview/mmwrhtml/mm6116a3.htm

Companion Animal Parasite Council (CAPC). (n.d.). CAPC Guidelines. Retrieved from capcvet.org: capcvet.org/guidelines

Elanco. (n.d.). ParvoTrack. Retrieved from https://yourpetandyou.elanco.com/us/campaign/stop-parvo

Fitzgerald, A. Z. (n.d.). Detecting and quantifying marijuana metabolites in serum and urine of 19 dogs affected by marijuana toxicity. *Journal of Veterinary Diagnostic Investigation*, 33(5), pp.1002–1007. https://doi.org/10.1177/10406387211027227

Khan, S. (n.d.). Toxicities from Illicit and Abused Drugs. Retrieved from Merck Veterinary Manual: www.merckvetmanual.com/toxicology/toxicities-from-human-drugs/toxicities-from-illicit-and-abused-drugs?query=cocaine

Knight, M.G. (1999). FIrefly toxicosis in lizards. *Journal of Chemical Ecology* 25 (9): 1981–1986:https://doi.org/10.1023/A:10.1072303515.

Larson, L.M. (2024). Early administration of canine parvovirus monoclonal antibody prevented mortality after experimental challenge. *Journal of the American Veterinary Medical Association* 262 (4): 506–512. https://doi.org/10.2460/javma.23.09.0541.

Myers, S. S. (2024, December). Diagnostic testing for tick-borne diseases: recommendations and interpretation of results. *Today's Veterinary Practice*. Retrieved from https://todaysveterinarypractice.com/parasitology/diagnostic-testing-for-tick-borne-diseases-recommendations-and-interpretation-of-results/

Newfield, A. (2021). Critical Veterinary Patient Don't Forget Kirby's Rule of 20. Retrieved from vetgirlontherun.com: https://vetgirlontherun.com/critical-veterinary-patient-dont-forget-kirbys-rule-of-20-vetgirl-veterinary-continuing-education-blog/

Norkus, C. (2019). *Veterinary Technician's Manual for Small Animal Emergency and Critical Care*. Hoboken: John Wiley & Sons, Inc.

Randels-Thorp, A.A. (2017). *Acid-Base and Electrolyte Handbook for Veterinary Technicians*. John Wiley & Sons, Inc.

Sevilla, E.O. (2024). *Multidrug Resistance in Pathogenic Escherichia coli Isolates from Urinary Tract Infections in Dogs*. Spain: Frontiers in Veterinary Science https://doi.org/10.3389/fvets.2024.1325072.

Silverstein, D.A. (2023). *Small Animal Critical Care Medicine*, 3e. St. Louis, MO: Elsevier.

Venn, E.P. (2017). Evaluation of an outpatient protocol in the treatment of canine parvoviral enteritis. *Journal of Veterinary Emergency and Critical Care* 27 (1): 52–65. https://doi.org/10.1111/vec.12561.

Zager, E. (2023). Heatstroke in dogs: a life-threatening emergency. VetGirlontheRun.

2

Bloodwork Basics

Simone Conwell[1,2]

[1] *VeG ER for Pets, 1858 Reisterstown Road, Pikesville, MD, USA*
[2] *Veterinary Emergency and Critical Care Society Member, USA*

Complete blood count (CBC), chemistry and electrolytes (chem/lytes), and blood glucose (BG). What are we as technicians and assistants supposed to do with these values when they're abnormal? Do we ignore them? It's not our job to interpret results. We cannot diagnose patients based on bloodwork. But why should we not understand them? It will further our knowledge of when and where to draw blood on a patient, if they can afford to have significant blood draws, and when to be concerned about infection – both to our other patients and to that particular patient if there is concern for immunocompromise.

CBC

The CBC explores the red and white blood cells and quantifies them. It can indicate types of anemia, dehydration, infection, and whether there are adequate platelets (Himelman 2022).

Red Blood Cells

If the red blood cell (RBC) count is increased, this can be indicative of polycythemia (Norkus 2019). The hematocrit (HCT) and hemoglobin concentration (HGB) will also be increased (Norkus 2019). The overall total volume of RBC is increased in polycythemic patients, which increases blood viscosity, which increases cardiac workload and hinders microcirculation, which leads to an increased thrombosis risk, hypoxia, and can even cause neurologic complications (Norkus 2019). Causes of polycythemia can be primary or secondary, depending on whether they depend on erythropoietin levels (Norkus 2019). However, there can also be a *relative* polycythemia due to dehydration, fluid loss, or diuretics (Norkus 2019). Examples of fluid loss include profuse vomiting and diarrhea or excessive urination. Splenic contraction after an injury, where the spleen shrinks to release stored red blood cells in a compensatory mechanism, will cause an increase in the total circulating RBC but not the total volume (Himelman 2022). It is also important to note that Greyhounds, as usual, are outliers in that they appear to be polycythemic, but this is their normal state (Zaldívar-López et al. 2011).

Packed cell volume (PCV) and HCT are often used interchangeably to express the measurement of RBC mass, but they are different ways of measurement (eCornell). The HCT is a calculated value displayed by hematology machines and is subject to mechanical error (eCornell). The PCV is a direct measurement read after centrifuging blood in a hematocrit tube using a chart (Cornell University School of Veterinary Medicine 2025a) (Images 2.1 and 2.2).

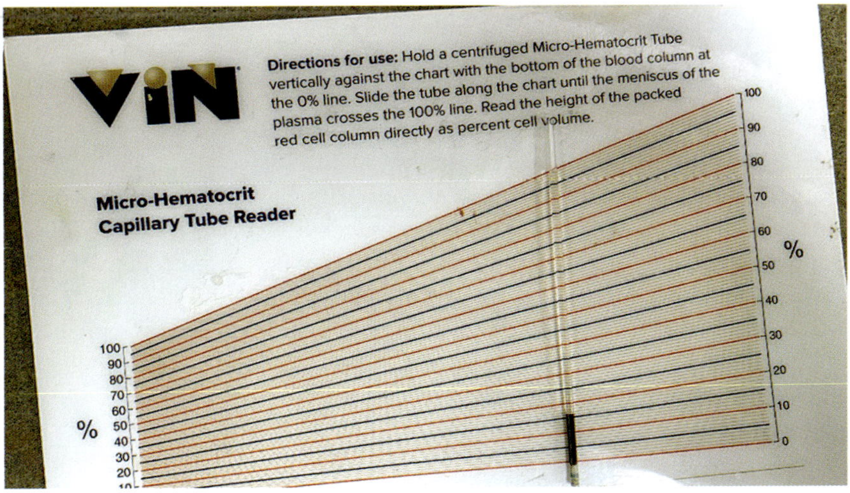

Image 2.1 Picture of a PCV tube against the chart. *Source:* Photo courtesy of Simone Conwell, RVT, VTS (ECC).

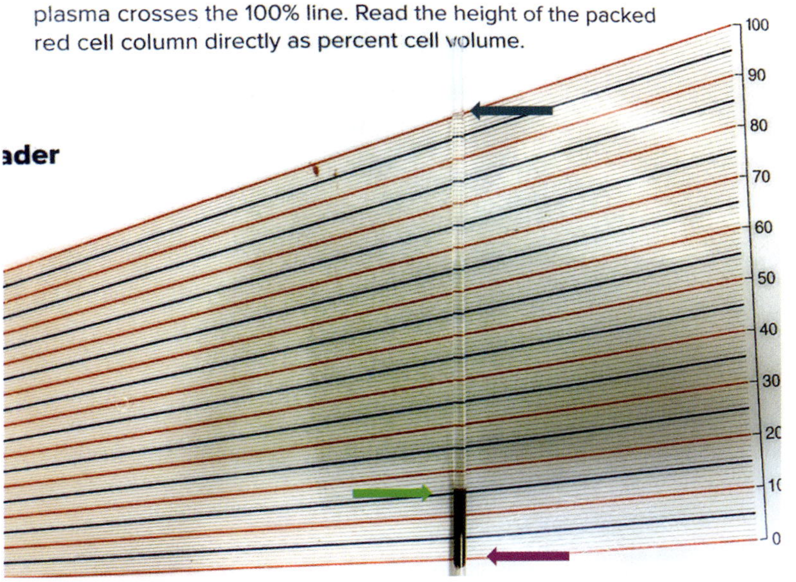

Image 2.2 How to read a PCV tube. The purple arrow shows where the top of the clay is lined up with the 0%, as that is where the RBC line starts. The green arrow indicates where the PCV is actually read, as a percentage where the RBC ends. The blue arrow is where the total solids end and lines up with 100% when reading a PCV tube. Photo courtesy of Simone Conwell, RVT, VTS (ECC).

A decrease in RBC, PCV, and/or HCT can be classified as anemia (Himelman 2022). There can be artificial causes of anemia, such as excess ethylenediaminetetraacetic acid (EDTA), the chelating agent in lavender top tubes used for CBC (Himelman 2022). This is why it is important to be sure that blood tubes are filled appropriately. Hemorrhage will, of course, cause anemia, whether it is due to a penetrating wound or a more insidious hemangiosarcoma on the spleen (Himelman 2022). Other common causes of anemia include liver disease, bone marrow suppression, chronic renal failure (CRF), neoplasia, and immune-mediated disorders (Himelman 2022). Having one disease as a cause of anemia does not preclude having another (Himelman 2022).

Regenerative anemias will have an increased reticulocyte count and nucleated RBC as well as an increased mean corpuscular volume (MCV), which is a measurement of the size of the RBC (Himelman 2022). Causes of regenerative anemia include trauma, surgery, and internal bleeding like hemangioblastoma (Himelman 2022). Non-regenerative anemias have a normal MCV, no nucleated RBC, and tend to have a low-normal reticulocyte count (Himelman 2022). It is important to remember that patients coming in for tachypnea could be anemic or hypotensive, either due to the root cause of anemia or a comorbidity (Himelman 2022). If the anemia is chronic (like with CRF cats), it is possible for the owner to have slowly acclimated to tachypnea caused by anemia. This is where annual or biannual bloodwork will uncover potential problems before they are emergent.

White Blood Cells (WBCs)

After the COVID-19 pandemic, most people probably know that neutrophilia is an increased WBC and indicative of infection, but it can also be due to inflammation, stress (stress leukogram in cats, anyone?), steroid use, and granulocytic anemia (Himelman 2022). Neutropenia, or decreased WBC, can indicate chemotherapy use, increased destruction due to immune-mediated processes, infection, and sepsis (Himelman 2022). Looking at the different types of WBCs will give more indication as to what is causing the changes.

Bands

Band cells are immature neutrophils. Their presence indicates that more WBC are needed and can be caused by severe inflammation, such as in systemic inflammatory response syndrome (SIRS), sepsis, infection, and neoplasia (Himelman 2022). Generally, they are seen during severe illness (Himelman 2022).

Left Shift

I would occasionally hear my doctors describe a CBC as having a left shift. A left shift occurs when there are immature neutrophils present; that is, a larger number of band neutrophils are present than would be expected in a healthy pet (Cornell University School of Veterinary Medicine 2025b).

Lymphocytes

A lymphocytosis may be due to age, recent vaccines, chronic inflammation/infection (herpes virus in cats), hypoadrenocorticism, or lymphoid neoplasia (Himelman 2022). Lymphopenia is seen with steroid use, protein-losing enteropathies, chylous effusions, immunosuppression, and with stress – the stress leukogram in cats (Himelman 2022). Other causes of a stress leukogram include hyperadrenocorticism, where excessive corticosteroids are produced, and endogenous stress in chronically ill animals (Cornell University College of Veterinary Medicine 2025).

Eosinophils

An eosinophilia is most commonly associated with allergies or a hypersensitivity, but it can also indicate hypoadrenocorticism, infection (including parasites and fungi), hypereosinophilic syndrome in cats, and neoplasia (Himelman 2022). Eosinopenia is not indicative of anything.

Monocytes

Monocytosis is most associated with inflammation and infection or neoplasia, or all three in one (Himelman 2022). This is because monocytes are the janitors of the body and phagocytose cellular debris left from inflammation or infection, antigens destroyed by lymphocytes, and any general foreign substance (Norkus 2019).

Basophilia

Back in the olden days, when I did manual differentials for every patient, I was told basophils were the creation of bored pathologists, and they were probably lies due to how infrequently they were seen. They are the rarest blood leukocyte in most healthy animals, explaining why they are rarely seen (Mau et al. 2025). Basophilia, though rare, is associated with hypersensitivity, parasitic infections, and most commonly, neoplasia (Himelman 2022) (Image 2.3).

Platelets

I am not going to go through the clotting cascade. Platelets, also called thrombocytes, are essential in primary hemostasis – the formation of platelet aggregates and platelet plugs (Silverstein 2023). Common causes of thrombocytosis are inflammation and infection, trauma, surgery such as a splenectomy, steroids, exercise, chemotherapeutic rebound, and neoplasia (Himelman 2022). It may be seen in dogs with septic peritonitis (Silverstein 2023). Very severe cases of thrombocytosis may indicate an increased risk of a thromboembolic event (Himelman 2022).

Thrombocytopenia is more commonly seen in my experience. With cats in particular, we often see platelet clumping (Himelman 2022). Usually, we attribute it to a slow blood draw, though due diligence should always be done, and a blood smear made, and a manual platelet count performed to be sure there is clumping. Other causes of thrombocytopenia include immune-mediated thrombocytopenia (IMTP) (see Chapter 11), increased consumption such as occurs during disseminated intravascular coagulation (DIC), decreased production, neoplasia, sequestration, and infection (Himelman 2022). Spontaneous hemorrhage is clinically visible at platelet counts under 30,000 platelets/μl (Norkus 2019). Signs of thrombocytopenia can include petechia and ecchymosis (Silverstein 2023).

Charles King Cavalier Spaniels (CKCS) in particular are often referred to internal medicine services for thrombocytopenia and no clinical signs. A blood smear will often show macrothrombocytes; that is, abnormally large platelets (Himelman 2022). It is present in approximately 50% of CKCS and does not affect their ability to clot (Cowan 2004) (Image 2.4).

Hematology

3/8/24	11:05 PM	
TEST	RESULT	REFERENCE VALUE
RBC	**6.18**	**6.54 – 12.20 M/μL**
Hematocrit	**26.9**	**30.3 – 52.3 %**
Hemoglobin	**9.2**	**9.8 – 16.2 g/dL**
MCV	43.5	35.9 – 53.1 fL
MCH	14.9	11.8 – 17.3 pg
MCHC	34.2	28.1 – 35.8 g/dL
RDW	18.8	15.0 – 27.0 %
% Reticulocytes	0.1	%
Reticulocytes	3.7	3.0 – 50.0 K/μL
Reticulocyte Hemoglobin	17.9	13.2 – 20.8 pg
WBC	11.73	2.87 – 17.02 K/μL
% Neutrophils	91.0	%
% Lymphocytes	6.6	%
% Monocytes	1.6	%
% Eosinophils	0.7	%
% Basophils	0.1	%
Neutrophils	**10.67**	**2.30 – 10.29 K/μL**
Lymphocytes	**0.78**	**0.92 – 6.88 K/μL**
Monocytes	0.19	0.05 – 0.67 K/μL
Eosinophils	**0.08**	**0.17 – 1.57 K/μL**
Basophils	0.01	0.01 – 0.26 K/μL
Platelets	401	151 – 600 K/μL
MPV	15.7	11.4 – 21.6 fL
Plateletcrit	0.63	0.17 – 0.86 %

RBC Run

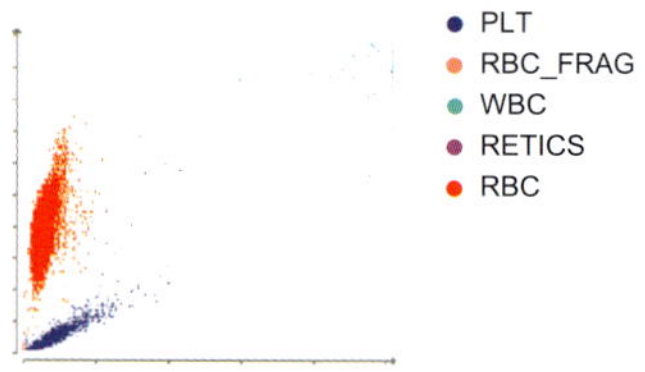

Download

WBC Run

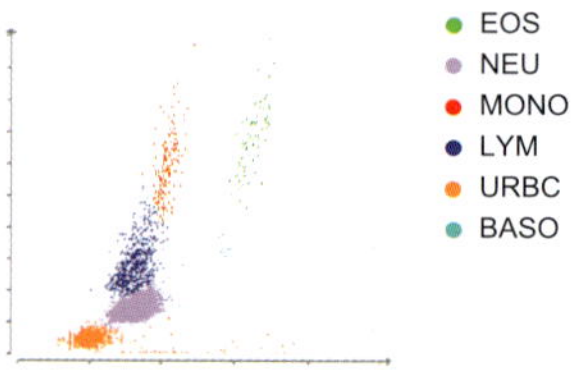

Download

Anemia without reticulocytosis - Likely non-regenerative anemia; consider pre-regenerative anemia.

Lymphopenia - Likely stress leukogram (glucocorticoid response).

Image 2.3 CBC results from a cat with small cell GI lymphoma being treated with prednisolone and chlorambucil, premedicated with trazodone and gabapentin prior to visit and blood draw due to temperament. RBC and hematocrit are low, indicative of anemia, but without reticulocytes, indicating it is likely non-regenerative. He had received his last dose of chlorambucil only a 4 days prior and was not at the nadir (lowest WBC), but looking at the different white blood cells, he had mild neutrophilia and lymphopenia, indicative of a stress leukogram. The stress leukogram was likely due to his chronic steroid use. *Source:* Photos courtesy of Simone Conwell, RVT, VTS (ECC).

Chemistry

We in vetmed often refer to chem panels and lytes in one breath as if they are always run together. That is not the case for every blood panel. And while everything is important on the panels, they have different levels of importance depending on the pet's life stage. Furthermore, we can add

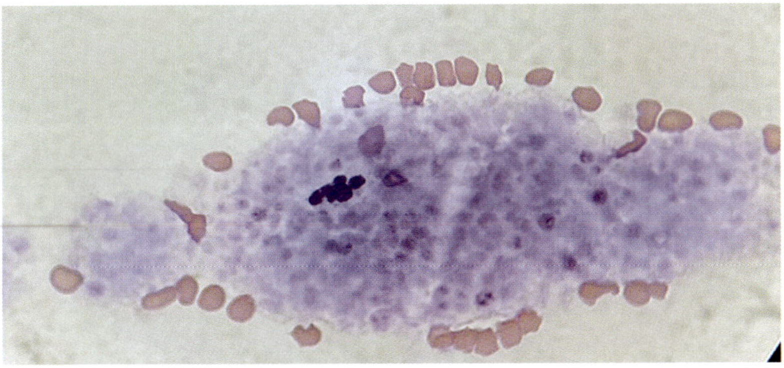

Image 2.4 A very large clump of platelets under microscope. *Source:* Photo courtesy of Simone Conwell, RVT, VTS (ECC).

other tests to the chemistry and lytes panels that often get grouped in with them because they are run on the same machine. For most purposes, the chem panel reflects the health and functionality of the abdominal organs.

Liver Enzymes

The liver values refer to alkaline phosphatase (ALP), gamma-glutamyl transferase (GGT), total bilirubin (tbil), alanine transferase (ALT), aspartate aminotransferase (AST), and amylase. Overall, a decrease in any of these values is not clinically significant (Himelman 2022). The liver metabolizes carbohydrates, fats, and proteins in addition to synthesizing clotting factors, metabolizing hormones, and biotransformation, including the metabolism of drugs and toxins (Drobtaz 2012). Elevations in cholesterol, ALP, and GGT may be indicative of infection, toxin ingestion, phenobarbital or long-term steroid use, neoplasia, pancreatitis, biliary disease, hyperadrenocorticism, diabetes, and hepatic lipidosis (Himelman 2022). Tbil may also be increased with those diseases, but is often commonly seen with hemolysis, such as in immune-mediated hemolytic anemia (IMHA, see Chapter 11), RBC destruction from Heinz bodies in cats, sepsis in cats, and as an artifact due to hemolysis and lipemia (Himelman 2022).

ALT and AST are leakage enzymes that are more specific to liver damage (Himelman 2022). They will increase for the same reasons ALP will; however, they will be more highly increased with acute liver injury (Himelman 2022). Additionally, cats with hyperthyroidism often have increases in ALT, as do other inflammatory conditions. Muscle injury and ischemia will cause ALT and AST to rise, and chemistries will show increased creatine kinase (CK) as well (Himelman 2022).

Amylase elevations may indicate pancreatitis, chronic renal failure (CRF), gastrointestinal (GI), or liver disease, and lipase elevations may additionally be seen with steroids and peritonitis (Himelman 2022).

It is important to remember that a serious infection that affects the liver is leptospirosis, which is zoonotic (Silverstein 2023). If liver values are extremely elevated, there is concern that the clotting times may be affected, and caution should be used during venipuncture (Himelman 2022).

Kidney Values

We often refer to the blood urea nitrogen (BUN) and creatinine (creat) values in tandem, but we can learn different information from each one. An increase in BUN may be prerenal and indicate dehydration, a high-protein diet, GI bleed, hypoadrenocorticism, and tissue catabolism (Himelman 2022). It can also indicate renal disease, whether that is an infection such as pyelonephritis, non-steroidal anti-inflammatory drug (NSAID) ingestion, or CRF, as well as postrenal disease such as urethral obstruction (Chapter 8), as well as a uroabdomen (Himelman 2022). Decreased BUN may indicate severe liver dysfunction, low protein intake, hypoadrenocorticism, and severe polyuria/polydipsia due to diabetes, hyperadrenocorticism, hyperthyroidism, and steroid or diuretic use (Himelman 2022).

Creat elevations have the same prerenal causes as BUN, excluding high-protein diets and GI bleeds, and the same renal and postrenal causes (Himelman 2022). Cephalosporin use can artificially increase creat, and myositis and trauma will increase creat without increasing BUN (Himelman 2022). Decreased creat is seen with marked muscle atrophy (Himelman 2022).

I remember the first time I heard of symmetric dimethylglarginine (SDMA) testing in 2015. This was a potentially exciting new test for me on a personal level because I am very much a cat person, and my childhood cat growing up had CRF. It is more precise for estimating glomerular filtration rate (GFR) and more sensitive than creat in assessing renal function in humans, and allows for earlier detection of CRF in cats (Hall et al. 2014). Unlike creat, it is not influenced by muscle atrophy and increases with a 40% reduction in GFR instead of 75% like creat (Himelman 2022).

SDMA, BUN, creat, and urine specific gravity should all be used together to determine why there is kidney dysfunction.

Blood Protein and Albumin

Albumin is the most abundant protein in the body; it is imperative for maintaining fluid balance and protein transport (Silverstein 2023). Causes of hyperalbuminemia are dehydration or artifact, and it is not considered clinically significant. Hypoalbumenia is seen in malabsorption/malnutrition, liver disease, protein-losing enteropathies, high-protein effusions, and hypoadrenocorticism (Himelman 2022).

Hyperglobulinemia is often seen in dehydration and with chronic infections such as feline infectious peritonitis (FIP) and with neoplastic disorders. Hypoglobulinemia occurs with blood loss and protein-losing enteropathies (Himelman 2022).

Glucose

Glucose is one of those values that everyone thinks is straightforward initially. Hyperglycemia can be due to diabetes, and beyond that, diabetic ketoacidosis (DKA) or hyperosmolar hyperglycemic syndrome (HHS), or steroids, pancreatitis, stress in cats, paraneoplastic syndromes, and acromegaly in cats (Himelman 2022). Chapter 9 will focus on diabetes and the associated complications. Hypoglycemia is seen with young animals who haven't eaten frequent enough meals, sepsis, liver failure, hypoadrenocorticism, insulin excess (overdose), xylitol ingestion, diabetes insipidus, and delay in running the sample, and can be seen on the alphatrak with hemoconcentration (Himelman 2022). Hypoglycemia as an indicator of sepsis is perhaps overlooked at a regular veterinarian (rDVM), as it is often viewed as a machine error or a delay in the sample being run, while hyperglycemia may be inaccurately diagnosed as diabetes when it is a stressed kitty or a value over 600 mmol/dl, which indicates HHS.

Lytes

The most common electrolytes run are sodium (Na), potassium (K), chloride (Cl), and calcium (Ca). Hypernatremia can be deadly due to cerebral dehydration caused by water shift and the formation of idiogenic osmoles (Ueda 2022). Causes of hypernatremia can be GI loss, diuresis in diabetics, CRF patients, and those on diuretics; pure water loss due to fever/panting, diabetes insipidus, water deprivation, and sodium excess caused by things like hyperaldosteronism or salt-water or paintball ingestion (Himelman 2022). Unless it is confirmable that the patient ingested a large amount of salt (acute change), the sodium must be dropped gradually to prevent death (Ueda 2022). Hyponatremia can also be caused by GI losses, including whipworms, as well as hypoadrenocorticism, diabetes, blood loss, hypoaldosteronism, effusions, and edema, as well as being secondary to hyperlipidemia, hyperproteinemia, and hyperglycemia (Himelman 2022). Like hypernatremia, care must be taken to correct hyponatremia slowly or quickly, depending on whether the changes are chronic or acute (Randels-Thorp 2017).

Causes for changes to chloride are the same as sodium, with the exception of hyperchloremia due to potassium bromide therapy for seizures. Bromide occupies the same family on the periodic table of elements and sometimes can cause a pseudohyperchloremia (Himelman 2022).

Hyperkalemia, or elevations in potassium, can become deadly due to their creation of dangerous arrhythmias (Randels-Thorp 2017). Causes include decreased excretion, such as in CRF, medications, metabolic acidosis, effusions, and urethral obstructions (Himelman 2022). Hypokalemia is often seen with patients experiencing GI losses, renal losses, diabetic ketoacidosis, and with diuretic use (Himelman 2022). Correction of hyperkalemia should be swift, and calcium gluconate should be given to stabilize the heart when appropriate (Randels-Thorp 2017). If the hypokalemia is severe, a central line should be considered (Himelman 2022).

Hypercalcemia is often seen with neoplasia, but can also be present in hyperparathyroidism, hypoadrenocorticism, CRF, infectious disease, and cholecalciferol and vitamin D toxicosis (Himelman 2022). Treating the underlying cause or providing supportive care is how hypercalcemia is managed. Hypocalcemia is commonly seen with eclampsia in animals that have recently whelped and should be corrected with intravenous calcium gluconate before moving to an oral form (Budde 2023). Other causes for hypocalcemia include CRF, hypoparathyroidism, hyperadrenocorticism, malabsorption, and, interestingly, anticoagulants in stored blood products (Himelman 2022).

Electrolyte imbalances may also be indicative of an Addisonian crisis. There will often be hyperkalemia, hypercalcemia, hypoglycemia, and hyponatremia (Randels-Thorp 2017). This needs to be managed appropriately with steroids, as Addison's is characterized by insufficient steroid production, including aldosterone, which maintains electrolyte and fluid balance (Randels-Thorp 2017). The disruption to the electrolyte and fluid balance also affects the renin–angiotensin–aldosterone system (RAAS), which affects blood pressure. So if a patient presents in an Addisonian crisis, a large volume of fluids will not correct the blood pressure – the underlying disease must be treated (Image 2.5).

Other Tests

It is common to use in-house tests for parvovirus, heartworm disease and tickborne illnesses, feline immunodeficiency virus, feline leukemia, and leptospirosis. These tests often rely on enzyme-linked immunosorbent assay technology and give answers in minutes. Other types of patient – or cage – side tests include rapid immunomigration tests. Both these types of tests bind to a specific antibody or antigen and have been evaluated against the microscopic agglutination test (MAT) and give results much quicker than polymerase chain reaction (PCR), where the DNA or RNA is replicated and tested directly (Idexx Lepto n.d.; Zoetis n.d.). While these tests are convenient and usually correct, it is important to follow diagnostic algorithms for each disease (Image 2.6).

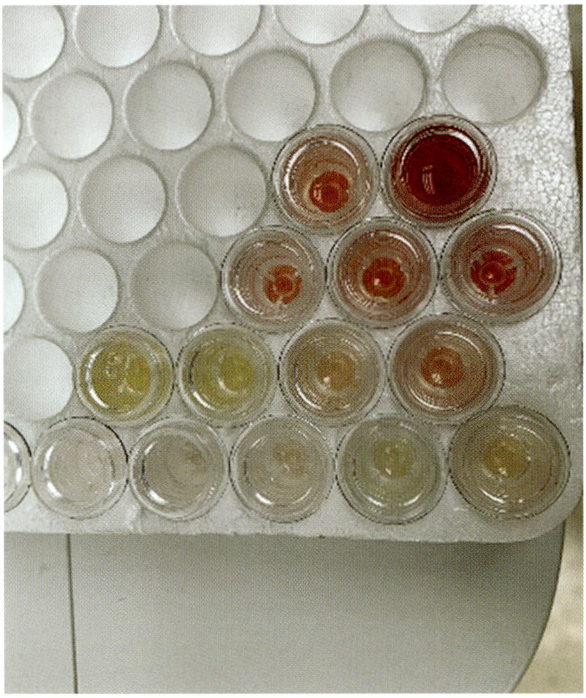

Image 2.5 Spun plasma samples in a variety of colors. How lipemic, hemolyzed, or icteric a sample is may skew chemistry results. *Source:* Photo courtesy of Simone Conwell, RVT, VTS (ECC).

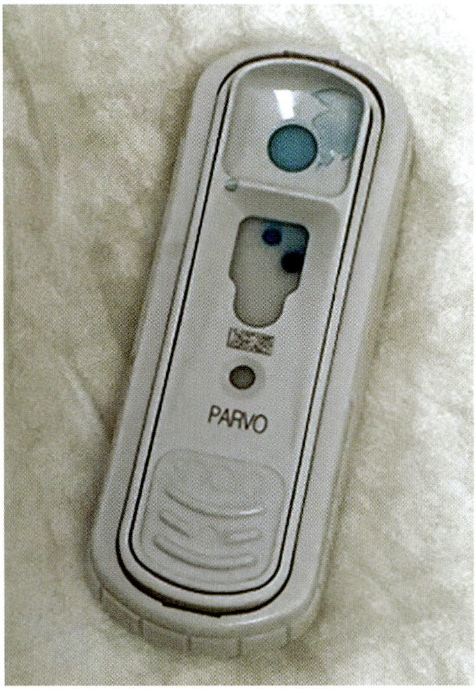

Image 2.6 A positive parvovirus SNAP test, a type of enzyme linked immunoassay (ELISA) test. *Source:* Photo courtesy of Simone Conwell, RVT, VTS (ECC).

Works Cited

Budde, J.A. (2023). *Plumb's Veterinary Drug Handbook*. Wiley-Blackwell.

Cornell University College of Veterinary Medicine. (2025). Leukogram Patterns. Retrieved from eclinpath.com: https://eclinpath.com/hematology/leukogram-changes/leukogram-patterns/

Cornell University School of Veterinary Medicine. (2025a). Hematocrit. Retrieved from eclinpath.com: https://eclinpath.com/hematology/tests/hematocrit

Cornell University School of Veterinary Medicine. (2025b). Left Shift. Retrieved from eclinapth.com: https://eclinpath.com/hematology/morphologic-features/white-blood-cells/left-shift/

Cowan, S.B. (2004). Giant platelet disorder in the Cavalier King Charles spaniel. *Experimental Hematology* 32 (4): 344–350. https://doi.org/10.1016/j.2004.01.008.

Drobtaz, K.M. (2012). *Manual of Small Animal Emergency and Critical Care Medicine*. Iowa: WIley-Blackwell.

Hall, J.Y., Yerramilli, M., Obare, E. et al. (2014). Comparison of serum concentrations of symmetric dimethylarginine and creatinine as kidney function biomarkers in cats with chronic kidney disease. *Journal of Veterinary Internal Medicine* 28: 1676–1683. https://doi.org/10.1111/jvim.12445.

Himelman, J. (2022). Bloodwork Interpretation for the Veterinary Technician. Cornell Nursing Series.

Idexx. (n.d.). Lepto Research Paper. Retrieved from www.idexx.com: www.idexx.com/files/lepto-research-paper.pdf

Mau, A.K., Keller, S.M., and Kol, A. (2025). A clinical and hematologic approach to basophilia in dogs, cats, and horses. *Veterinary Clinical Pathology* 54: 24–34. https://doi.org/10.1111/vcp.13404.

Norkus, C. (2019). *Veterinary Technician's Manual for Small Animal Emergency and Critical Care*. Hoboken: John Wiley & Sons, Inc.

Randels-Thorp, A.A. (2017). *Acid-Base and Electrolyte Handbook for Veterinary Technicians*. Ames, Iowa: John Wiley & Sons, Inc.

Silverstein, D.A. (2023). *Small Animal Critical Care Medicine*, 3e. St. Louis, MO: Elsevier.

Ueda, Y. (2022). Management of Sodium Disorders. International Veterinary Emergency and Critical Care Symposium.

Zaldívar-López, S., Marín, L.M., Iazbik, M.C. et al. (2011). Clinical pathology of Greyhounds and other sighthounds. *Veterinary Clinical Pathology* 40 (4): 414–425. https://doi.org/10.1111/j.1939-165X.2011.00360.x.

Zoetis. (n.d.). WITNESS Lepto Technical Bulletin. Retrieved from www.zoetisus.com: www.zoetisus.com/content_assets/docs/Diagnostics/technical-papers/WITNESS-lepto-technical-bulletin-WIT-00115.pdf

3

Fluid Therapy Basics

Elizabeth Faux[1,2]

[1] *VeG ER for Pets, 1858 Reisterstown Road, Pikesville, MD, USA*
[2] *Veterinary Emergency and Critical Care Society Member, USA*

Understanding fluid therapy and how to monitor patients on fluids is an integral skill in emergency medicine. Throughout this chapter, we will discuss various aspects of fluid therapy and the intensive patient monitoring that goes along with it. Fluid therapy is a broad topic, so this chapter will cover the basics to get you started. However, further research and dedication to keeping up with the latest consensus statements are needed to further your knowledge in this area. In the emergency department (ER), the majority of our patients will require fluid therapy of some kind, and fluids are one of the most important medications that you will administer. It is important, moving forward, that we adopt this thought process and treat fluids like medications. They can treat a wide variety of conditions, but they come with very serious side effects. Thorough patient monitoring is vital whenever we are administering fluids to our patients.

When discussing fluid therapy, it is important to understand a few key principles. We will begin our discussion with the first concept(s) to understand: fluid dynamics and identifying fluid compartments. The bodies of our canine and feline patients are made up of 60–70% water. This is also known as total body water (TBW). Many fluids within the body contain water and contribute to TBW: saliva, blood, cerebrospinal fluid, etc. This TBW is distributed throughout the body into different compartments: the intracellular fluid compartment (ICF) and the extracellular fluid compartment (ECF) (Wereszczak 2023).

The intracellular compartment represents about ⅔ of the TBW (~66%). The ICF is composed of the fluid within the cells. This fluid maintains the shape and basic function of the cells. The ECF represents the remaining ⅓ of the TBW, equal to ~33%, and can be further divided into the intravascular and interstitial subcompartments. The intravascular compartment contains all the body fluid within the blood (blood + plasma) and lymphatic vessels. The interstitial compartment contains all the body fluid surrounding the cells (AAHA 2024; Wereszczak 2023).

The fluids contained in the compartments of the body are composed of various solutes. Solutes are present in a variety of sizes and shapes and can be electrically charged. Ions are the charged particles and are the most abundant of the solutes. Cations are ions with a positive charge. The most common cation in the ECF is sodium (Na^+). The most common cation in the ICF is potassium (K^+). These two cations play major roles in supporting membrane potential and cell function. Anions are negatively charged ions. The most common anion in the ECF is chloride (Cl^-). The most common anion in the ICF is hydrogen phosphate (HPO_4^{2-}). Because of the charge that each of these ions carries, they can conduct a current in a solution and are generally referred to as electrolytes (Wereszczak 2023).

The next important concept to understand is osmolality. This is the measure of solute concentration within body fluids. The higher the concentration of solutes, the higher the osmolality and vice versa. Osmolality is an important concept because it governs the movement of fluids through the body and is closely maintained via hormone-regulated feedback loops. When the body detects a change in osmolality in the blood, hormones are released that stimulate thirst or water excretion, depending on the change. Water moves freely between the ICF and ECF according to changes in osmolality. Electrolytes are the largest catalysts of these fluid shifts. Other molecules, such as proteins, can also cause changes in osmolality (Mathews 2017).

Now that we understand fluid distribution and movement through the body, we should clarify some common conditions: dehydration versus hypovolemia. Being that this is a chapter on fluids, these terms are related but NOT interchangeable. Dehydration refers to a loss of TBW from all compartments (intracellular and extracellular). Hypovolemia refers to a volume deficit in the intravascular space. Now that we have covered these basic fluid concepts, we can move into discussing patient assessment and building a fluid prescription (Mathews 2017).

A thorough history is vital in establishing a baseline of fluid needs for every ER patient. The process of obtaining a history begins when the owner calls in to the hospital and continues when they arrive. When an owner calls into the clinic, it is important to keep the phone call brief and get as much information as possible efficiently. At times, an owner can have a rather emotional response to what they are witnessing with their pets. In these cases, ask them to pause and ask for a one-sentence description of what they are seeing. At this point, I will advise them to immediately come to the hospital. We have this luxury in emergency medicine. However, this is not likely to be the case when you are in GP or specialty where your schedule is largely appointment-based. As always, when faced with an emergency, do the best you can and get creative when you must. Once I am sure that the owner and pet are as safe as they can be and on their way to the clinic, I will prepare the receiving area of the hospital. Any more on this would be beyond the scope of this chapter, but we will cover more of this in stabilizing the emergent patient.

Once the owner arrives, I will spend some more time getting a thorough history and obtaining patient vitals, all of which can heavily inform fluid prescription later during treatment. A thorough patient history can include obtaining answers to any/all of the following questions:

Was there trauma? Any visible wounds or blood? Has the patient been eating or drinking normally? Has there been any vomiting or diarrhea? If so, for how long?

At the same time that I am obtaining a history, I am obtaining patients vital signs and doing a brief physical exam. A simple TPR can tell a lot about a patient's hydration status and, coupled with the history and brief physical exam, can give enough information to create an initial fluid prescription. Some common physical exam findings seen with fluid loss/dehydration are decreased skin turgor, dry mucous membranes, tachycardia, sunken eyes, dry corneas, altered pulse pressure, and decreased body temperature. The assessment of skin turgor depends on fat and elastin, so age and body condition can create challenges (AAHA 2024). A decrease in body temperature can be an indicator of poor perfusion (AAHA 2024). As discussed earlier, it will be beneficial to attempt to differentiate between the hydration status and volume status. Patients who are presenting dehydrated (inadequate fluid distribution in all compartments) can still have normal blood pressure and circulating volume (AAHA 2024). Serial assessment of these patients is crucial, along with evaluation of continued losses and quick intervention. Patients who present with suspected hypovolemia can be hypotensive from fluid loss in the intravascular space, but can be euhydrated (normal hydration). Obtaining an accurate patient weight will give a good starting point and can be used to compare to serial weights as you reassess your patient's hydration (Mathews 2017).

This is likely when the doctor will start communicating some orders for very altered and critical patients. The patient may even be deteriorating in front of you if the fluid loss is so significant. We will need to obtain diagnostics to determine the degree of derangement. This can be especially challenging in the severely dehydrated or hypovolemic patient. Establishing venous access needs to be a priority so that fluids can run concurrently with performing diagnostics. An intravenous catheter (IV) is the "gold standard," but not always possible. Intraosseous (IO), subcutaneous (SC), and enteral routes can also be chosen for rapid fluid administration; however, all of these techniques come along with significant downsides (Mathews 2017). IO catheters can be technically challenging, and most hospitals do not carry the supplies and are not meant to be long-term solutions. Subcutaneous fluids allow for a large volume of fluids to be given; however, this is still not enough to cover significant and ongoing losses. Enteral fluids, or oral administration, depend on the animal being able to physically drink and take in enough to account for ongoing losses. Common sites of IV catheterization are the right and left cephalic veins, medial and lateral saphenous, and left and right dorsal pedal (Norkus 2019). However, the dorsal pedal placement can be painful for the patient. Whichever route you choose, establish IV access as quickly as possible and continue to obtain some diagnostics. I am not a proponent of the adage of "go big or go home" for IV catheters. I believe in thinking critically about each patient and placing the appropriate gauge catheter for that individual, taking into consideration fluid therapy, projected length of hospital stay, etc. For example, if I have a gastric dilatation volvulus (GDV/Bloat) come in, I know that we will be giving multiple fluid boluses. I will place the largest short catheter I can in this patient. Placing long catheters may be tempting, as these patients are most often large. However, a long catheter will make administering boluses challenging, and we need to replace fluid quickly. We will go into more detail about this later in the chapter. Another example is if I have a stable feline patient that is getting a few days of IV fluid therapy following lily ingestion, I will place a smaller short catheter. This kitty will likely only need fluids and some IV medication administration. It will be more comfortable for the patient and just as stable as a larger catheter (Norkus 2019).

I will use a fresh catheter to obtain a blood sample at placement only. I will not continue sampling from a catheter once it is in use. After catheter placement, obtain blood as part of a minimum database. This is a great opportunity for you to anticipate what is needed and begin getting some of these diagnostics completed before even being asked. A minimum database is the minimum diagnostics that are needed in each scenario, which will provide enough information to determine a differential diagnosis. The diagnostics included in this minimum database are as follows:

Blood pressure: A systolic blood pressure can be obtained by a Doppler machine. Blood pressure will show if the patient is hypotensive or hypertensive. In significant or ongoing fluid losses, the patient will likely be hypotensive. A Doppler (systolic) blood pressure <60 mmHg is considered hypotensive. If you have an electronic multiparameter machine, this could obtain an oscillometric blood pressure and give you the systolic pressure/diastolic pressure and mean arterial pressure (MAP). I use caution with oscillometric readings as they can be quite inaccurate. Regardless of the machine you have available, be sure to obtain serial values and make adjustments to treatment plans based on trends.

Test name	Description and considerations	Interpretations
Complete blood count (CBC)	• Evaluation of red and white blood cells includes hematocrit (red blood cell level)	• ↑ in hematocrit (HCT) can indicate dehydration • ↓ in HCT can indicate anemia, acute hemorrhage, or hypovolemia
Packed cell volume (PCV) + total solids (TS)	• A PCV/TS should always be run in combo with a CBC • PCV should directly correlate to the HCT on CBC	• ↑ in PCV can indicate dehydration • ↓ in PCV can indicate blood loss, hypovolemia, or chronic disease (anemia)
Chemistry (Chem) and electrolytes (Lytes)	• Includes enzymes for internal organ function (liver/kidney), proteins, and electrolytes	• Elevations in renal values (BUN, Crea, Phos) can be seen with severe dehydration • Changes to electrolyte balance, such as K^+ elevations (blocked cats)
Blood glucose (BG)	• This value should be included in most in-house kits. There is also a very practical and efficient cage-side glucometer	• ↑ of glucose, as in diabetes mellitus, can cause an increase in urinary losses
Urine specific gravity (USG)	• Obtain this value as part of a full urinalysis	• USG can become extremely concentrated (>1.030) in volume loss with normal renal function
Blood lactate (Lac)	• Indication of tissue perfusion • Measure of byproduct (lactate) of anaerobic metabolism	• ↑ lactate indicates that there is inadequate tissue perfusion (resulting in a shift to anaerobic metabolism)
Blood gas analysis	• Assessment of acid–base status and perfusion status	• Severe dehydration can lead to poor tissue perfusion, which can affect the patient at a cellular level, resulting in anaerobic metabolism and lactic acid build-up. Over time, this can progress into metabolic acidosis • A special machine is required to run this test
Ultrasound: aFAST/tFAST	• Useful diagnostic tool to look at the thorax and abdomen to determine any underlying causes for the patient's presenting status	

Source: Cornell University College of Veterinary Medicine (2025a, b).

Now that we have obtained some useful information on the patient, we can begin developing the fluid prescription. The calculations to determine losses and fluid rates for canines and felines are many and varied (AAHA 2024). First, we will discuss the difference between crystalloid and colloid fluids. Then we will discuss the different types of crystalloids, which we will classify in terms of tonicity. The tonicity of a fluid is the ability of the fluid to alter the cell volume by changing its water content (Maldonado 2023).

Crystalloid Fluids

Crystalloid fluids contain water and electrolytes (Na^+, Cl^-, K^+, and HCO_3^-). There are many commercially available fluids; it is best to become familiar with what you have in your hospital. Crystalloids are made up of solutes that can dissolve in water and pass through vessel walls and distribute throughout the body's compartments. These fluids have an osmolality similar to plasma (AAHA 2024). Because of this, they can mimic plasma when administered and help maintain fluid balance and hydration. Crystalloids remain in the intravascular space for a fairly short time. They are quickly redistributed to the tissues and cells; only a small amount remains in the intravascular space after ~1 hour (AAHA 2024).

Colloid Fluids

Colloids contain larger particles that remain in the intravascular space for longer periods, which is helpful in intravascular volume expansion. They exert osmotic pressure, which causes a fluid shift from the interstitial space to the intravascular space. Colloids can be natural (plasma) or synthetic (hydroxyethyl starch). Synthetic colloids can be controversial in veterinary medicine, but remain the preference for some. Always exercise caution when administering them (AAHA 2024).

Isotonic Fluids

Isotonic fluids are crystalloids with a similar composition to extracellular fluid, allowing for the efficient movement of water and electrolytes across cell membranes. We reach for these fluids when we want to replace fluids, maintain hydration, or restore fluid balance. There are several commercially available fluid types to choose from. We will review some of the common types that we commonly keep in the ER. Lactated Ringers solution (LRS) is a common fluid used in fluid resuscitation. LRS contains a mixture of electrolytes and lactate, which serves as a buffer. Plasmalyte is another type of fluid that we will reach for. This crystalloid is also used for fluid resuscitation. Plasmalyte contains electrolytes in water plus lactate (buffer), which is formulated to mimic plasma in the body. Notably, 0.9% (full-strength) sodium chloride is another type of fluid that is formulated with water and sodium chloride salt. Sodium chloride is used in a variety of ways around the ER. We use it for fluid resuscitation, flushing catheters to maintain patency, and for diluting medications. Finally, we have 5% dextrose in water (D5W), which can be classified as isotonic or hypotonic (once in circulation). We reach for this fluid to dilute some medications and to provide fluid resuscitation in cases of free water loss (AAHA 2024).

Hypertonic Fluids

Hypertonic fluids are those that are formulated with a larger concentration of solutes compared to body fluid. These fluids exert an osmotic effect, promoting the movement of fluid out of the intracellular space and into the intravascular space. This effect temporarily supports intravascular circulating volume and can also be used in cases of head trauma. Hypertonic saline is an example of this type of fluid. Hypertonic saline can be formulated with concentrations from 3% to 27%.

This fluid should be administered slowly over 10 minutes to avoid adverse reactions such as bradycardia and vasodilation. It is also important to administer crystalloids in addition to hypertonic saline to support intravascular volume so that you do not cause additional dehydration and decreased tissue perfusion in an already sick patient (AAHA 2024).

Hypotonic Fluids

Hypotonic fluids are those that are formulated with a smaller concentration of solutes compared to body fluids. In other words, hypotonic fluids have a lower osmolarity than body fluids. When given intravenously, hypotonic fluids can cause a shift of water from the extracellular space into the intracellular space. When using this fluid, it is important to maintain close patient monitoring (serial weights and vitals) as it can cause cells to swell as water moves intracellularly. Thus, hypotonic fluids are given only in specific situations when promoting intracellular hydration or lowering intracellular solutes is the goal. Diabetic ketoacidosis (DKA) or hyperglycemic hyperosmolar syndrome (HHS) are examples of one of these specific situations. In ER, you will commonly find 0.45% (half-strength) saline as a hypotonic fluid (AAHA 2024).

Now that we have reviewed the types of fluids that are commonly found in the ER. We can review how to create a fluid prescription. Several factors will influence which fluid we choose, such as patient hydration status, weight, vital signs, and ongoing losses (vomiting, diarrhea, and panting). First, we should put together the history that we obtained when the patient presented and the hydration assessment. Hydration assessment should be completed during the physical exam and is documented in the medical record as a % value. Below, you will find a helpful chart to reference when assessing your patients.

Dehydration percent (%)	Physical exam findings[a]
<3%	Normal physical exam
3–5%	Mild dehydration, normal physical exam, recent history of fluid loss (vomiting, diarrhea)
6–8%	Moderate dehydration, tacky mucous membranes Mucus Membranes (MM), slight prolonged capillary refill time Capillary Refill Time (CRT)
8–10%	Severe dehydration, dry MM, prolonged CRT, increased skin turgor
11–15%	Life-threatening dehydration, shock present, changes in mentation

[a] Adapted from Norkus (2023).

At this point, we have compiled all the information on our patient to create a custom fluid therapy plan: patient weight, percent dehydration, and an estimation of ongoing losses. The next portion of this chapter is an interactive guide to creating a fluid plan. This will include some practice questions – the answers are included at the end of this chapter … so no reading ahead!!

Steps to building a fluid plan for your patient

1) Assess your patient
   a) Physical exam
   b) Hydration assessment
   c) Temperature, Pulse, Respirations (TPR) and body weight
   d) Blood pressure

2) Assess ongoing losses
   a) Drooling
   b) Excessive panting
   c) Vomiting and diarrhea
3) Calculate the fluid plan using the resources below
   a) Calculate any boluses if indicated
   b) Calculate rehydration (fluid deficit) over 12–24 hours
   c) After 1–24 hours, calculate the maintenance rate

Important Fluid Calculations[a]

Fluid bolus	
Canine	15–20 ml/kg
Feline	5–10 ml/kg
Shock bolus	
Canine	90 ml/kg
Feline	40–50 ml/kg
Rehydration	Fluid deficit (L) = body weight (kg) × %dehydration (as a decimal)
Maintenance	
universal/RER	$[\text{BW (kg)}^{0.75} \times 30] + 70 = \text{ml/d}$
Canine	$132 \times \text{BW (kg)}^{0.75}$
Feline	$80 \times \text{BW (kg)}^{0.75}$

[a] Adapted from AAHA (2024); Norkus (2023), and Wereszczak (2019).

If your patient is moderately (>5%) dehydrated or worse, then administering a fluid bolus can be helpful in supporting circulating volume while you are getting other treatments started. A bolus is a larger volume of fluid administered over a short time. The typical bolus calculation for canines is 15–20 ml/kg and for felines is 5–10 ml/kg. We can repeat these boluses one to two times to support blood pressure and circulating fluid volume in our emergent patients. For those patients who are even more critical, we would calculate a "shock" fluid bolus. These "shock" bolus volumes are administered in aliquots. This allows for time to reassess the patient before giving the next bolus and altering the fluid plan as soon as a response can be observed (increase in blood pressure, improved mentation, etc.). Close monitoring is strictly necessary, as it is easy to give too much and fluid overload the patient, which could be life-threatening. This includes rechecks for improvement in blood pressure, vital checks for normalizing vital signs, and recheck body weights. An increase in body weight of 1 kg can indicate ~1 l in resuscitation.

Example Fluid Plan

Tater Tot: 8 kg, 6% dehydrated, rehydrate over 12 hours

$$8\ \text{kg} \times 0.06 = 0.48 \times 1000 = 480\ \text{ml}$$

$$480\ \text{ml} / 12\ \text{hours} = 40\ \text{ml} / \text{hr}$$

After 12 hours, calculate the maintenance rate and adjust accordingly.
New weight: 8.5 kg after 12 hours

$$\left[8.5(\text{kg})^{0.75} \times 30\right] + 70 = \text{ml} / \text{d}$$

$$219.34\ \text{ml} / \text{d} = 9\ \text{ml} / \text{hr}$$

Practice Problems

1 Calculate a fluid bolus for the following patient: 8 kg canine and administer via fluid pump over 30 minutes.

2 Calculate the fluid deficit for the following patient: 15 kg canine, 8% dehydrated. Then calculate the rate to replace this volume over 24 hours.

3 Calculate a fluid bolus for the following patient: 2.5 kg feline and administer via fluid pump over 20 minutes.

4 Calculate the fluid deficit for the following patient: 6 kg feline, 6% dehydrated. Then calculate the rate to replace this volume over 12 hours.

5 Calculate the full fluid plan (fluid deficit for rehydration + maintenance) for the following patient:

   10 kg canine, 8% dehydrated

6 Calculate the full fluid plan (fluid deficit for rehydration + maintenance) for the following patient

   4 kg feline, 10% dehydrated

7 Develop a full fluid plan for the following patient

   50 kg canine, 5% dehydrated, blood pressure at admission 50 mmHg, rehydrate over 24 hours.

Fluid type	Fluid name	Cation(s)	Anion(s)	Lactate	Extras
Isotonic	**Lactated Ringers Solution (LRS)** • Fluid resuscitation Correcting electrolyte abnormalities	• Na^+ • K^+ • Ca^{2+}	• Cl^-	• Contains lactate, metabolized to bicarbonate in the liver, which helps to regulate pH	• Does not contain magnesium • Composition varies among manufacturers

(Continued)

Fluid type	Fluid name	Cation(s)	Anion(s)	Lactate	Extras
Isotonic	**Plasmalyte** • Fluid resuscitation • Similar to plasma electrolyte composition	• Na^+ • Ca^{2+} • Mg^{2+}	• Cl^-	• Contains lactate • Metabolized to bicarbonate in the liver, which helps to regulate pH • Buffering capabilities, maintains acid–base balance	
Isotonic	**0.9% Sodium chloride (NaCl)** • Fluid resuscitation • Intravenous hydration • Medication dilution	• Na^+	• Cl^-	—	—
Isotonic	**5% Dextrose in water (D5W)** • 5% dextrose (5 g dextrose/100 ml water) • Source of free water for hydration	—	—	—	• Isotonic but becomes hypotonic when metabolized by the body
Hypotonic	**0.45% Sodium chloride (NaCl)** • Used in specific cases with higher concentrations of solutes (DKA) • Increase cellular hydration	• Na^+	• Cl^-	—	• Promotes water shift from the extracellular space to the intracellular space via osmosis
Hypertonic	**Hypertonic saline solution** • 3–23.4% concentration • Contain higher concentrations of solutes that exert an osmotic effect, shifting water out of the cells into the intravascular space	• Na^+	• Cl^-	—	• **4–7 ml/kg (k9) and 3–4 ml/kg (fel)** • Indicated in the treatment of hyponatremia, cerebral edema, and shock

Answers to Practice Problems

1 Calculate a fluid bolus for the following patient: 8 kg canine and administer, via fluid pump over 30 minutes.

Canine bolus calculation: 15–20 ml/kg
8 kg × 20 ml/kg = 160 ml total
Administer over 30 minutes
Fluid pump rate = 160 ml (bolus total) × 2 (factor of time/desired delivery)[1] = 320 ml/hr (rate)
Fluid pump volume to be infused (VTBI) = 160 ml (total volume of fluid to deliver)

2 Calculate the fluid deficit for the following patient: 15 kg canine, 8% dehydrated. Then calculate the rate to replace this volume over 24 hours.

Fluid deficit (L) = body weight (kg) × %dehydration (as a decimal)
15 kg × 0.08 = 1.2 l deficit (1.2 ml × 1000 = 1200)
1200 ml/24 hours = 50 ml/hr for 24 hours

3 Calculate a fluid bolus for the following patient: 2.5 kg feline and administer via fluid pump over 20 minutes.

Feline bolus calculation: 5–10 ml/kg
2.5 kg × 5 ml/kg = 12.5 ml total
Administer over 20 minutes
Fluid pump rate = 12.5 ml (bolus total) × 3 (factor of time/desired delivery) = 37.5 ml/hr (rate)
Fluid pump volume to be infused (VTBI) = 12.5 ml (total volume of fluid to deliver)

4 Calculate the fluid deficit for the following patient: 6 kg feline, 6% dehydrated. Then calculate the rate to replace this volume over 12 hours.

Fluid deficit (L) = body weight (kg) × %dehydration (as a decimal)
6 kg × 0.06 = 0.36 deficit in liters (0.36 ml × 1000 = 360 ml)
360 ml/12 hours = 30 ml/hr for 12 hours

5 Calculate the full fluid plan (fluid deficit for rehydration + maintenance) for the following patient

10 kg canine, 8% dehydrated
10 kg × 0.08 = 0.8 deficit in liters (0.8 ml × 1000 = 800 ml)
800 ml/24 hours = 33 ml/hr for 24 hours
Recheck weight at 24 hours = 12 kg
$[12(\text{kg})^{0.75} \times 30] + 70$ = ml/d = 263 ml/d = 11 ml/hr (± depending on continued losses and patient vitals)

1 30 minute delivery = multiply by 2 (delivers volume over ½ hour), 15 minute delivery = multiply by 4 (delivers over ¼ hour).

6 Calculate the full fluid plan (fluid deficit for rehydration + maintenance) for the following patient:

4 kg feline, 10% dehydrated

4 kg feline, 10% dehydrated
4 kg × 0.1 = 0.4 deficit in liters (0.4 ml × 1000 = 400 ml)
400 ml/24 hours = 16 ml/hr for 24 hours
Recheck weight at 24 hours = 4.5 kg
$[4.5(\text{kg})^{0.75} \times 30] + 70$ = ml/d = 162 ml/d = 7 ml/hr (± depending on continued losses and patient vitals)

7 Develop a full fluid plan for the following patient

50 kg Canine, 5% dehydrated, blood pressure at admission 50 mmHg, rehydrate over 24 hours.

First, due to low blood pressure, consider a 20 ml/kg fluid bolus to start
50 kg × 20 ml/kg = 1000 ml
Administer over 20 minutes with pressure bag – fluid pumps will not deliver this fast
Recheck BP – 70 mmHg consider a repeat 20 ml/kg bolus
Recheck BP – 120 mmHg

Because we administered the fluid boluses – we can consider utilizing the maintenance rate instead of the replacement rate as this animal is only 5% dehydrated and we can control/prevent any ongoing losses
$[50(\text{kg})^{0.75} \times 30] + 70$ = ml/d = 634 ml/d = 26 ml/hr (± depending on continued losses and patient vitals)

** Please note that each individual patient may require more or less fluids than the maintenance calculation dictates. Remember that each patient is different and continue to monitor for any changes/improvements in monitored parameters.

Works Cited

American Animal Hopsital Association. (2024). 2024 AAHA Fluid Therapy Guidelines for Dogs and Cats. Retrieved from www.aaha.org: www.aaha.org/resources/2024-aaha-fluid-therapy-guidelines-for-dogs-and-cats

Cornell University College of Veterinary Medicine. (2025a). Chemistry. Retrieved from Eclinpath: eclinpath.com/chemistry

Cornell University College of Veterinary Medicine. (2025b). Hemogram Baics. Retrieved from eclinpath.com: https://eclinpath.com/hematology/hemogram-basics/

Maldonado, K. A. (2023). Biochemistry, hypertonicity. StatPearls, https://www.ncbi.nlm.nih.gov/books/NBK541095/

Mathews, K. (2017). *Veterinary Emergency and Critical Care Manual*. Guelph: LifeLearn Inc.

Norkus, C. (2019). *Veterinary Technician's Manual for Small Animal Emergency and Critical Care*. Hoboken: John Wiley & Sons, Inc.

Wereszczak, L. (2023). Fluid therapy in critical care: finding the balance: proceedings of the veterinary technician multidisciplinary systems review. International Veterinary Emergency and Critical Care Symposium. Aurora.

Part II

Preparing to Transfer

4

Transferring With Catheters

Simone Conwell[1,2]

[1] *VeG ER for Pets, 1858 Reisterstown Road, Pikesville, MD, USA*
[2] *Veterinary Emergency and Critical Care Society Member, USA*

I started in a practice that did emergency medicine and general practice in 2008. I did that for 2 years before getting burned out, did some research in a lab, and then went back to general practice (GP) and stayed there for 10 years before returning exclusively to emergency medicine. During my time in GP, I worked with doctors, techs, and assistants who never did emergency medicine and had no desire to ever try it. I also worked with others who had burned out like me. And I got to experience our local ER and specialty practices coming to speak to us, usually about cardiopulmonary resuscitation (CPR) and radiographic positioning for lameness. And now I'm on the other side of those lectures, where I'm the one going to the GP to speak, usually about CPR. Inevitably, there are specific cases the staff wants to talk through. And they have questions about the pictures in my lectures, about the unconventional catheter placements in some of my photos. Especially when they notice they are not all 18-gauge catheters. Speaking to one GP that sits in a fun little triangle where, depending on the day, it may take their clients the same amount of time to reach three different ERs (including my own), I suggested that they either (a) leave in the catheters if a patient they're referring has one, (b) place a catheter if they haven't, or (c) place a second, bigger catheter in the back leg so I can turn it into a sampling line. The veterinarian who was present for that lecture has been in the field about the same amount of time as I have, and he was as shocked about the idea that he could do some of the workup and catheter placement as his staff was. So this chapter will discuss catheter selection with regard to transferring to the ER.

In 2008, the prevalent saying was "go big or go home" in regard to catheter size. But to paraphrase Jurassic Park, just because we can doesn't mean that we should. Is it ideal for a large-bore catheter? Absolutely. Does a 5-kg cat need an 18 g catheter in the cephalic vein? No. Absolutely not. Are there times that a catheter needs to be big? Absolutely. But, especially after having experienced having to be poked repeatedly for multiple catheters in the hospital myself, I want to remind everyone to consider the patient's size, normal health, and current medical conditions that require hospitalization. For example, we know that patients with disorders that make them more prone to bleeding, like immune-mediated thrombocytopenia (IMTP), would do better with a smaller catheter to minimize vascular damage and hemorrhage. An elderly cat with kidney disease might have high blood pressure that makes the vein seem artificially robust, only to blow as soon as a needle touches it. Maybe a newly diagnosed epileptic Jack Russell terrier has had three seizures in four hours, and the owner wants to admit it for overnight care to break the seizure cycle. That dog isn't going to be on fluids overnight. Does he really need a 20 g catheter when he's small, and it really

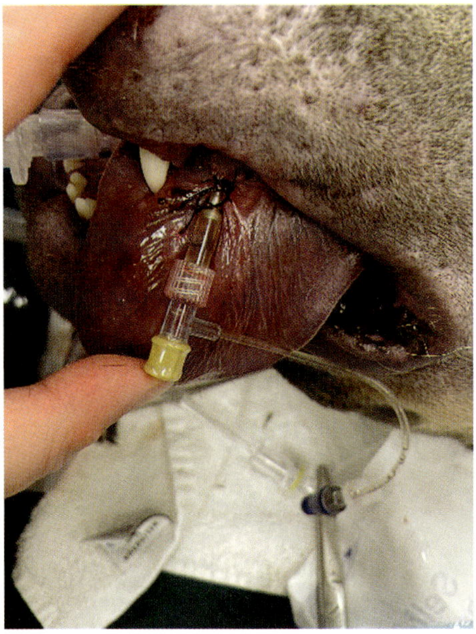

Image 4.1 A sublingual catheter placed in a bulldog during cardiopulmonary resuscitation due to difficult venous access (heatstroke, obese). *Source:* Photo courtesy of Simone Conwell, RVT, VTS (ECC).

looks like a 22 g catheter would be a better fit? Alternatively, a large cat with flea anemia needs a blood transfusion, and a 20 g catheter looks like it might be possible. Should a 22 g be the default, or should you go for that 20 g? There's a newly diagnosed diabetic that is suspected to be in diabetic ketoacidosis (DKA) and is going to the ER for further care. Should you place a hind limb catheter in addition to the front? (Image 4.1).

The answer to all of these questions is generally, it depends. If your IMTP patient is a large dog, a 24 g intravenous catheter (IVC) is not appropriate. But maybe you'd normally reach for an 18 g IVC. Instead, a 20 g IVC would still allow for component therapy and would allow for sufficient fluids to be administered without further risk of thrombophlebitis (Yasuda 2021). Perhaps that kidney cat's veins are so fragile that a 24 g IVC is the only thing anyone in the practice is comfortable placing. The Jack Russell is intact, so his skin is tougher than anticipated, and that 22 g keeps burring and barely goes through the skin, so you opt for a 20 g instead. When you look at the DKA's hind legs, you realize that you've never placed a catheter in one and aren't sure how to secure it. Or if you should go medial or lateral. Then there are comorbidities. Is there trauma to the limb? Is there hypotension secondary to hypovolemic shock because the patient has been vomiting all night? Is the patient just a difficult stick? (Images 4.2 and 4.3).

Difficult vascular access (DVA) is a known concept in human medicine, even if there are multiple definitions, and there are often specialized teams and equipment (Lee et al. 2021). This concept exists in veterinary medicine, but not in the literature, and is often referred to as the "two poke rule," which is very common at most hospitals, where if someone cannot achieve venous access after two pokes, they switch out. Human medicine has had incidence and risk factors studied, but veterinary medicine has not, and while ultrasound-guided catheterization and intraosseous catheterization are more accessible now, they are still not as commonly used as in human medicine (Lee et al. 2021). Human medicine has scoring systems for pediatrics and adults, known as difficult intravenous access (DIVA), and is useful in identifying patients at risk for DVA (Lee et al. 2021). Factors that contribute to DVA, aside from age, include dehydration, hypotension, metabolic disorders, cardiovascular disease, scarring from recurrent catheterization, and obesity (Lee et al. 2021).

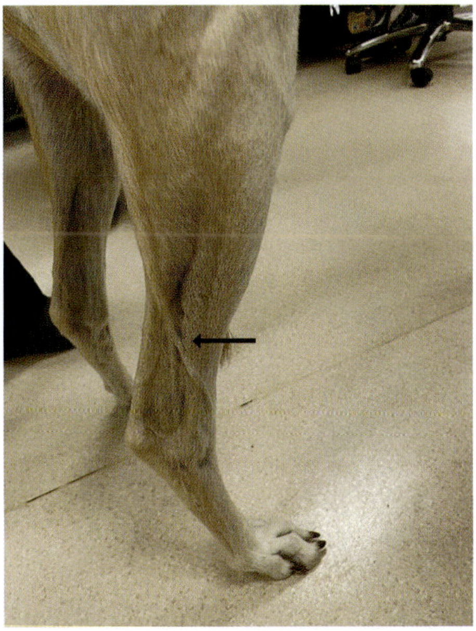

Image 4.2 Lateral saphenous (black arrow) vein on a dog. *Source:* Photos courtesy of Simone Conwell, RVT, VTS (ECC).

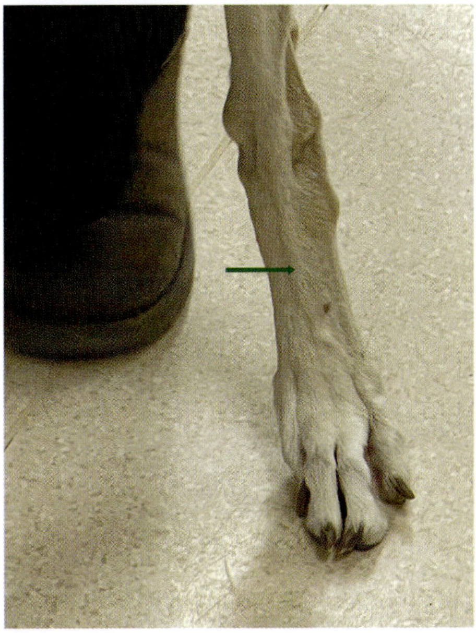

Image 4.3 Pedal vein (green arrow) on a dog. *Source:* Photos courtesy of Simone Conwell, RVT, VTS (ECC).

As a human who is known to be a DVA, with scar tissue from recurrent catheterization, I can anecdotally say nurses grimace every time they have to place a catheter in me, and it's not uncommon for them to request an ultrasound or someone from the vascular access team to place it because they cannot find a vein. Our patients living with chronic disorders likely have similar issues with catheter placement and venipuncture in general, but ultrasound-guided catheterization is not as common in veterinary medicine. Another consideration is that while short, small-diameter catheters decrease the risk of thrombophlebitis, short, large-gauge catheters enable rapid fluid administration (Lee et al. 2021). Long catheters cause a proportional increase in resistance due to physics, particularly in small-bore catheters (Lee et al. 2021). There are always ways around these complications, such as venous cutdown, including poking the skin with a larger needle to create a small relief hole (this is an alternative to a full cutdown, but it is a type of cutdown) to facilitate catheter placement (Lee et al. 2021).

The most common place for a peripheral catheter is the cephalic or accessory vein in the front leg. But saphenous veins are also viable options, as are pedal veins, corpus cavernosum, aural, and jugular veins if the cephalic is just not possible or the patient is very young. Sublingual is also possible if the patient is anesthetized or having CPR performed, and it is easy to access the tongue. Intraosseous (IO) catheters may be placed in the ER, usually during CPR, but in neonatal puppies and kittens, using a needle when venous access is not possible is a very viable method (Images 4.4 and 4.5).

When do transfers need multiple catheters? If there is a chance they are getting multiple medications that have compatibility issues or are highly osmolar. Patients who are likely to get a high number of blood draws would also benefit from a secondary catheter that can be turned into a sampling catheter. Types of disease processes that should automatically have multiple catheters include GDV, DKA, insulin overdoses, hypo- and hypernatremic patients, xylitol ingestion, septic patients, hemoabdomens, and potentially renal failure patients. These patients generally need fluids, sometimes large volumes, which circles back to the original question: what size is appropriate? This is where some physics gets involved. The Hagen-Poiseuille equation is used to calculate flow rates and is:

$$\text{Flow Rate} = \frac{(P_1 - P_2)\Pi R^4}{8 \times \text{Length} \times \text{Viscosity}}$$

Summarized, flow depends on the catheter's radius and should exponentially increase as the catheter radius increases (Hughes 2000). So bigger catheters have higher flow rates, unquestionably. This

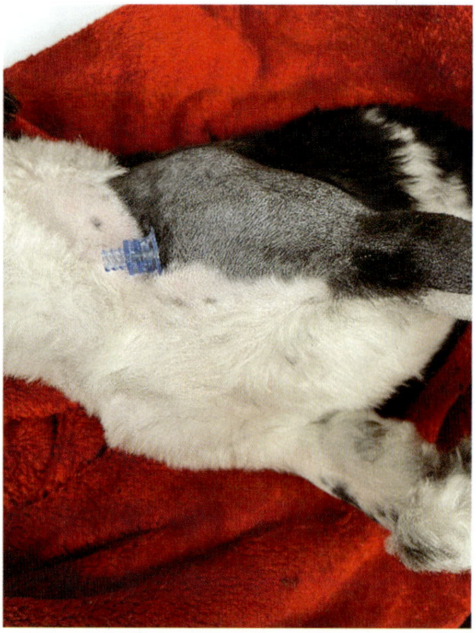

Image 4.4 An IO catheter placed with an IO gun during CPR. *Source:* Photo courtesy of Alli Opishinski, CVT.

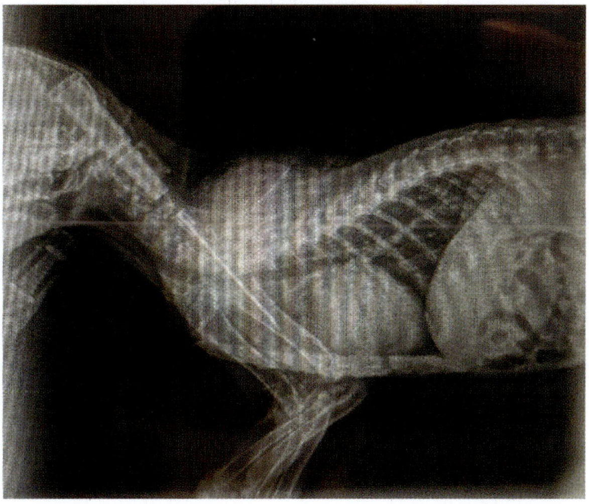

Image 4.5 Radiographic confirmation of a needle as an IO catheter in a neonate kitten. *Source:* Photo courtesy of Simone Conwell, RVT, VTS (ECC) (B).

means a 24g IV catheter can deliver a max flow rate of 1200 milliliters/hour (ml/hr), a 22g max flow rate is 2160 ml/hr, a 20g max flow rate is 4500 ml/hr, and an 18g is 5280 ml/hr (IEM n.d., Hughes 2000). These four sizes are the most common ones I have come across, so we will only discuss them for this part. Now consider the patients most likely to have a 22g catheter: cats. No cat needs 2L of fluids in an hour. That is a recipe for fluid overload. In fact, the total shock dose for a cat is 60 ml/kilogram (kg). In order for a total shock dose for a cat to be 2160 ml, the cat would have to weigh 36 kg (snow leopard size). As we start with lower volumes of fluid instead of doing a full shock bolus, needing an 18g IV in a cat becomes even more unnecessary. So, placing a 22g, or a 20g if the patient's lean body weight is on the larger size, in a cat or cat-sized dog is very reasonable. Total shock bolus for a dog is about 90 ml/kg, but again, we start with lower doses for fluid resuscitation.

For our giant dog breeds, placing an 18g or larger IV catheter is ideal because they will need higher rates and volumes of fluid most of the time. Being able to flow faster is ideal for crystalloid fluids. That being said, if the patient is so dry and hypotensive that the veins are flat and there is a significant risk of venous trauma or the vein blowing, size down. The catheter can always be replaced after the volume status has been partially corrected.

Going back to flow rates, the viscosity of the fluid being infused will decrease the flow rate. This is important for our colloids. Natural colloids are blood and blood component therapy, including pRBC, plasma, and albumin. Because colloids are more viscous, a larger catheter is ideal when administering them. Therefore, patients with hemoabdomens or anemic patients ideally need at least a 20g IV catheter to avoid lysing the blood (Yagi 2016). With cats, sometimes a 20g catheter is just not going to happen, and allowances such as decreasing the rate or diluting the blood product with normal saline can be made (Hughes 2000).

When to Stop

If placing a catheter is causing your patient so much stress that they might experience cardiopulmonary arrest, it is time to stop, pause, and re-evaluate the approach. Is the patient in respiratory distress and turning cyanotic whenever any restraint is attempted? Can medications like butorphanol be given to calm them down? If the patient is in congestive heart failure, can furosemide be administered? Is the patient incredibly painful due to a fracture and is now experiencing anticipatory pain? Give a pure mu-opioid like hydromorphone or methadone in the muscle and let them sit while that absorbs. Patience is a virtue. If, despite having completed all these steps, you are still struggling to get an IV into the patient, perhaps it is time to consider a central line, unless it is contraindicated by comorbidities (coagulation issues and head trauma). If that is the case, and a transfer is imminent, please let the hospital that will be taking the case know this patient does not have a catheter due to XYZ reasons, and the decision was made to preserve the remaining veins for them rather than cause trauma. Being in the ER, I would much rather hear that than go to check one of the less commonly used veins and discover it had been poked multiple times and is now unusable.

Works Cited

Hughes, D.B. (2000). Emergency vascular access. *Emergency Surgical Procedures* 30 (3): 491–507.

IEM Education Project Team. (n.d.). IV Catheters and Flow Rates. Retrieved from International Emergency Medicine Education Project: https://iem-student.org/2018/08/06/iv-catheters-and-flow-rates/

Lee, J.A., Guieu, L.S., Bussieres, G., and Smith, C.K. (2021). Advanced vascular access in small animal emergency and critical care. *Frontiers in Veterinary Science* https://doi.org/10.3389/fvets.2021.703595.

Yagi, K.A. (2016). *Manual of Veterinary Transfusion Medicine and Blood Banking*. Ames, Iowa: Wiley Blackwell.

Yasuda, H.Y. (2021). Occurrence and incidence rate of peripheral intravascular catheter related phlebitis and complications in critically ill patients: a prospective cohort study. *Journal of Intensive Care* https://doi.org/10.1186/s40560-020-005180-4.

5

Stabilizing the Emergent Patient

Elizabeth Faux[1,2]

[1] *VeG ER for Pets, 1858 Reisterstown Road, Pikesville, MD, USA*
[2] *Veterinary Emergency and Critical Care Society Member, USA*

Day in and day out, animals of all shapes and sizes walk, or are carried, into veterinary emergency hospitals. How can you possibly prepare for and treat all these patients? Throughout this chapter and the next, we will discuss just that. First, we will dive into how planning, preparation, and creativity can give you all the tools to treat even the most critical patient. Then we will discuss the basics of fluid therapy in the next chapter, expanding on many of the principles discussed here. Stabilizing an emergent patient can be very overwhelming. I hope this chapter conveys that you likely already possess all the knowledge and skills to save your patient's life and give it the best chance of survival.

First, let's define a few things: planning and preparation, as these are two of the most important steps in stabilizing the emergent patient. Planning can be defined as the process of thinking through the actions needed to achieve a desired result. Preparation is the action of putting these plans in motion to achieve the same desired result. In this case, the desired result is to treat as many animals as possible safely and effectively, especially in an emergency situation. If you think about it, your hospital probably already has protocols based on planning and preparation for various functions. For example, you may have a plan for how to safely get into surgery or how to treat an isolation patient. If your practice already has a plan for emergent patients, you should consider periodic reviews and revisions to meet your needs more effectively. Every plan and protocol needs to be re-evaluated to stay current and effective. My experience is that when I have a new idea, I present as many research-driven facts as I can to support that and show the value to our clients and patients when presenting to leadership. And I always make a PowerPoint (I LOVE a PowerPoint) with all the details. After you set up a plan or update your current protocol, you should begin mapping out how this would look in your hospital. I have had the privilege of working in many emergency hospitals throughout my career, and one thing remains the same in all of them: we have a designated area where we always treat our sickest patients. This is usually a spot closest to the door so that we have the least amount of space to travel before treatment can begin. If you do not have a designated spot already, pick a spot in your hospital and make sure that the whole team knows where it is. The second constant in all my practices is that each area is well stocked with things that we may need. You do not want to have to run to another room or area of the hospital to grab items to treat your patient. This could be whole tables with drawer space or simply a box that can be carried to the patient. It doesn't matter how fancy it all is; it matters how well you can use it and communicate with your team (Figure 5.1).

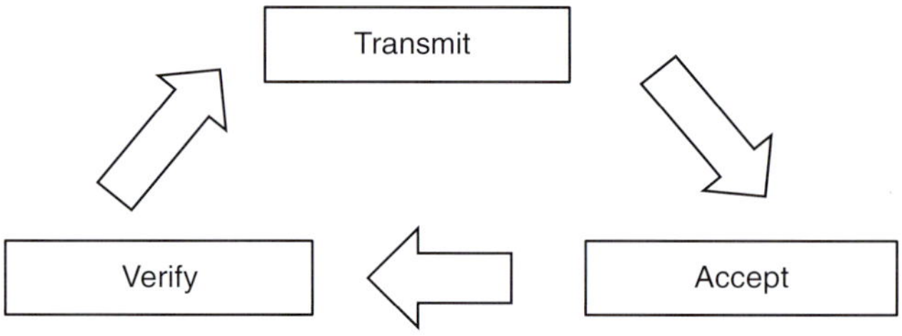

Figure 5.1 Figure courtesy of Elizabeth Faux, RVT, VTS (ECC).

Communication is the next most important factor in any emergent situation. It is best to take a circular approach to communication. "Closed Loop Communication" is a perfect example of this (see diagram). Closed-loop communication consists of three parts: (1) A transmitter initiates a communication directly to an intended receiver, using their name; (2) the receiver acknowledges the communication with a verbal confirmation and will ask for clarification if necessary; and (3) the original transmitter confirms that the communication has been received and understood, closing the loop (Salik and Ashurst 2023). You are most likely to utilize closed-loop communication in an arrest scenario: the doctor gives orders for drugs, intubation, etc., a team member acknowledges, and the doctor confirms closing the loop. It would sound like this:

DOCTOR: Beth, please intubate and begin breathing for our patient.
BETH: I will intubate now ... the patient has been intubated with a 5fr ET tube, starting respirations now.
DOCTOR: Understood, thank you.

This is an extreme example, but I would suspect that you are already using closed-loop communication in your hospital, and you may not even know it. Another example would be if an owner calls in with a possible emergency. The receptionist or tech on the phone would then initiate a closed loop to the rest of the team. It would sound like this:

RECEPTIONIST/TECH: I just spoke with Mr. Smith, he is bringing Fluffy right in, he says he cannot wake him up and he is not doing well.
TECH/DOCTOR TEAM: Thank you, how far out is he? We will begin setting up for him in exam room 2, please put him and Fluffy right in as soon as he arrives.
RECEPTIONIST/TECH: Understood, I will do that. ETA was about 15 minutes when we got off the phone.

This second scenario highlights a very important advantage in planning and preparation for treating emergent patients, phone calls, and triage. Owners may not be able to call in to the clinic every time that there is an emergency. However, we can make a habit of using this to our advantage when they do by creating a quick plan and prep as seen above. A well-trained receptionist or technician can get vital information from a quick phone call. It is very important to practice scenarios during downtime to become more confident and efficient. It will be imperative to get as much information as possible and then get the owner off the phone so that they can focus on getting into the clinic quickly and safely. There are often heightened emotions when an owner calls with an emergency. It is important to make the owners feel heard, even if you suspect this may not be a true emergency. It is often easier to de-escalate an anxious owner when you have assessed the patient and taken vitals, which are normal. Until the owner and patient are in the hospital, assume that the owner is conveying information accurately and prepare for the worst.

Once the patient arrives, the real fun begins! You should begin your assessment of the patient from the moment that it is brought through the door. As you progress through your initial exam and collect the vitals, you will use most of your senses. First is sight, what do you see? Within the first few seconds, you should be able to complete a quick visual assessment. Do you see any obvious wounds? Is the patient having difficulty breathing? Can you visualize the color of the skin and/or gums from a distance? You should count the respirations for your vitals check at this time. The more information you can gain without touching the patient, the better. Next is sound. Is the animal vocalizing? Do you hear any abnormal breath or heart sounds as you auscultate the chest? Next is touch, can you readily palpate a pulse? The pulse rate is most easily obtained by palpating the femoral pulse, and I like to palpate this while I am auscultating the chest to ensure that the beats are matching. If they were not, this would indicate that the animal has pulse deficits, which indicates several larger issues, such as cardiac disease, arrhythmias, or severe dehydration/hypovolemia, progressing to shock. Is the patient cold or warm? Finally, there is smell, and yes, you will use this sense quite a bit. Can you smell ketones on a diabetic patient? Can you smell feces or urine? Can you smell blood? (Image 5.1)

The next step is to obtain vitals on your patient. I would like to pause to note that this is all being presented in a step-by-step manner, but all these initial patient observations and assessments should be happening simultaneously. These patients can deteriorate in seconds, sometimes before our very eyes. We must complete our assessment and communicate what we find to the doctor as quickly and efficiently as possible so that we can determine which diagnostics and treatments are needed – these will also need to happen quickly, but we will get to that in a bit. First, vitals! You may already be familiar with the process of obtaining a "TPR," or temperature, pulse, and respirations, or in simpler terms, getting patient vitals. However, this is so much more than that. The following vital signs should be included in all initial patient assessments: mentation, temperature (temp), heart rate (HR) and pulse, respiratory rate (RR) and respiratory character, mucus membrane color (MMC) and character, capillary refill time (CRT), blood pressure (BP), and pain score (Norkus 2019). We can also give an honorable mention to electrocardiogram (EKG) and

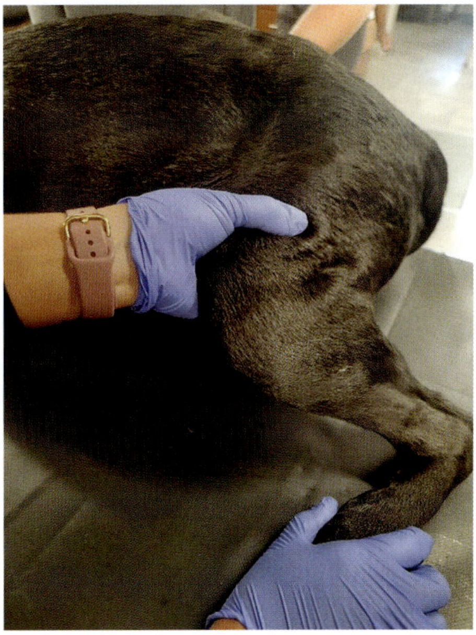

Image 5.1 Palpating femoral pulse. *Source:* Photo courtesy of Elizabeth Faux, RVT, VTS (ECC).

point-of-care ultrasound (POCUS). If your practice has these capabilities, it can give a lot of information about the structure and function of the heart and internal organs (Norkus 2019).

Mentation can be assessed as the patient is entering the clinic or as you are approaching the animal. Mentation can be characterized in many ways, including anxiety, aggression, lethargy, dullness, coma, and seizures. The Modified Glasgow Coma Score can assist in determining the degree of change in mental status. This scale assesses a number of patient parameters and generates a score; the higher the score, the better the outcome.

Normal Vitals in Cats and Dogs

Temperature

Patient temperature is obtained via a rectal thermometer. This is the most accurate method. There are new scanning and ear thermometers; however, the scan function is not very accurate for our fur-covered patients, and an ear thermometer puts your hands directly toward the sharp end of our patients – the mouth. Although the ear thermometers can be effective for healthy and friendly animals. In a reactive or painful patient, you could get an axillary temperature. This is not a very accurate measure due to the patient's fur. If you opt for this method, you should add 1–2 °F to represent a more accurate value. Hypothermia, low body temperature, can present alongside several conditions with numerous presenting complaints such as shock, renal disease, hypothyroidism, hypovolemia, cardiac disease, and poor perfusion. There are two terms that we can use to characterize an elevated body temperature in our canine and feline patients: hyperthermia and pyrexia. Both terms refer to elevated body temperature but indicate differing underlying conditions. Pyrexia, fever, is an elevation of the body's core temperature, which is closely controlled by the thermoregulatory center in the hypothalamus. This elevation in body temperature is triggered by a physiological process secondary to infection, inflammation, or malignancy. In contrast, hyperthermia is an elevation in core body temperature from an outside source, not regulated by the hypothalamus (Balli 2023). The most common example of this is heat stroke, originating from an environmental source. Regardless of the change in body temperature, immediate support should be given to the patient. Gentle warming via a circulating water blanket, warm blankets, or thermal blankets should be given to hypothermic patients (Norkus 2019). Active cooling should be initiated quickly, in cases of hyperthermia only, via room-temperature water baths and fans. Active cooling should be stopped once the core body temperature has reached 103 degrees fahrenheit. Ice is not recommended in active cooling measures; however, if you are using it, ensure that it is not touching the patient. Regardless of the measures taken, you should monitor the temperature often and adjust the warming/cooling plan as needed (Mathews 2017).

Heart Rate

Next up are heart rate and pulse. There can be some variation for giant (lower rate) and toy breeds and puppies (higher than the range). Bradycardia, or a low heart rate, and tachycardia, or an elevated heart rate, can tell us a great deal of information. Bradycardia can be caused by hypothermia, hyperkalemia (elevated serum potassium levels), medications or toxins, hypothyroidism, progressive stages of shock, respiratory diseases, or central nervous system abnormalities. Tachycardia can be caused by pain, hypovolemia, hypotension, hypoxemia (low blood oxygen levels), hypoxia (low tissue oxygen levels), hypercapnia (elevated carbon dioxide levels), cardiac disease, and hyperthermia (Mathews 2017). Ideally, you will obtain the heart rate via a stethoscope at the same time you palpate the femoral pulse. If you do not palpate a pulse beat for each heartbeat, it is an indicator of pulse deficits, which can indicate if an arrhythmia is present.

This would be a good indication to then get an EKG and a POCUS exam to obtain additional information about the character of the arrhythmia present and if there are any structural or blood flow abnormalities.

Respiratory Rate

Respiratory rate or character can often be assessed simultaneously as you assess the heart rate and pulse. Oxygen delivery to tissues is a critical byproduct of normal respiration in our patients. Therefore, **any**, even small, deviations from normal patterns should be reported and investigated. Deviations from the normal can be defined by abnormal rate and rhythm. Counting respirations is only part of assessing the respiratory system. Characterizing the breathing is the next step. Apnea is the absence of any breathing pattern and can be caused by airway obstruction, medications, muscle paralysis, severe hypothermia, and central nervous system disease or abnormalities (Mathews 2017). This would require initial intervention with immediate intubation and likely other resuscitation efforts. I will refer to the beginning of this chapter when we discussed having an area of the hospital or a crash box stocked with the necessary items for a code. Dyspnea is difficulty breathing and can be further characterized by whether there is inspiratory or expiratory effort. Dyspnea can be caused by anxiety, pain, airflow obstruction, chest wall problems, pleural space disease, or cardiac disease (Mathews 2017). Tachypnea is an increased respiratory rate (>40 bpm). Tachypnea can result from pain, anxiety, hyperthermia, respiratory acidosis, respiratory insufficiency, medications, pleural space disease, hypovolemia, and anemia (Norkus 2019). Many of these animals will likely benefit from oxygen supplementation to help stabilize the patient and facilitate diagnostics and treatments. This can be achieved via an oxygen line and mask providing flow-by or in an oxygen chamber. When using an oxygen mask, use a flow rate of 2 l/min; anything more will be irritating to the patient. If you have no oxygen chamber, you can create one by covering the front of a kennel with see-through cling wrap; just ensure to leave a small ventilation area so that the patient does not overheat (Norkus 2019). This same concept can be applied to an e-collar – cover with plastic wrap, feeding oxygen into the enclosed space. Both methods can contribute to overheating and patient anxiety and, therefore, should be used only when all other options are unavailable. These animals often respond poorly to restraint and treatment. Minimize handling and consider giving a small dose of a partial mu opioid, such as butorphanol, to relieve anxiety (0.1–0.3 mg/kg IM) (Budde 2023).

Capillary Refill Time (CRT)

Capillary refill time and MMC are the next parameters to assess. CRT is a good assessment of peripheral perfusion. Prolonged CRT (>2 seconds) may indicate compromise in perfusion (blood/oxygen delivery to tissues and vital organs) and may be caused by hypotension, hypothermia, or hypovolemia. Rapid CRT may be seen in early sepsis (Mathews 2017). The mucous membrane color in a normal healthy animal should be pink. Feline mucous membranes can appear a little lighter, but can still be in the normal range. Any color other than pink/light pink is considered abnormal. MM color can also be an indicator of perfusion. Pale mucous membranes can indicate blood loss, hypovolemia, hypothermia, or pain. Injected (red) mucous membranes can indicate fever, hyperthermia, or sepsis. Cyanotic (blue/purple) mucous membranes can indicate dangerously low oxygen levels. A pulse oximetry (SpO_2) machine can further confirm decreased oxygen concentration. Icterus (yellow-orange MM) can result from hepatic (liver) abnormalities. Some of these would include hemolysis, liver disease, toxicity, or sepsis. Brown MM color can be seen in acetaminophen toxicity caused by methemoglobinemia (Mathews 2017).

Blood Pressure (BP)

Blood pressure is a critical and often missed vital sign in our emergent patients. Hypotension (low blood pressure) can indicate hypovolemia, shock, and cardiac abnormalities. Hypertension (elevated BP) can indicate anxiety, pain, and various systemic causes. BP can be obtained on a multiparameter machine or a Doppler machine. The Doppler is my personal favorite as I find it to be more accurate. The benefit is that the multiparameter machine can give you systolic/diastolic (MAP), while the Doppler can only provide the systolic pressure. In my experience, it is important to focus not only on the number that you get, but also on the trend. Blood pressure should be reassessed at regular intervals, and treatment adjusted accordingly at each interval.

Pain is another vital sign that is often overlooked or not assessed at all. It is important if you note pain in your patient to communicate this and note where so that all team members can take care when handling the patient. Pain can be categorized into mild, moderate, severe, or excruciating (Mathews 2017). Various pain scales are recognized in veterinary medicine. These are valuable defined scales that can assist in quantifying pain in our patients. Colorado State University (CSU) has developed pain scales for canines, felines, and horses. They offer free printouts that can be displayed around your hospital for ease of reference. They may be found at https://vetmedbiosci.colostate.edu/vth/services/anesthesia/animal-pain-scales/(Colorado State University James L. Voss Veterinary Teaching Hospital, 2025). The Glasgow pain scale is another, albeit much longer, pain scale. Various free forms of this scale are available online. Once you build confidence using this scale, it is an easy process to integrate into your physical exam and patient assessment (Royal Canin, 2025).

After completing your patient assessment, it is time to get treatment and diagnostics started. Again, all of these assessments and treatments are meant to happen simultaneously, and you will have your whole team to help you perform multiple treatments at once. Communication is key! While all our patients will present in different ways, many of the initial interventions will be similar. First, obtain venous access. This should be achieved without compromising or stressing the patient. Place the intravenous catheter (IVC) that best suits the patient. If you need to give multiple boluses or blood products, place a larger bore catheter (20–18G IVC). If you will only be running fluids and giving occasional IV medications, then you can place a smaller gauge IVC (24–22G). The adage, "go big or go home," is not always necessary, especially with emergent and critical patients, as an excessively large catheter can be a source of inflammation and infection if not cared for properly. In some cases, you can even consider multiple catheters. Common sites of catheter placement are cephalic (preferred), saphenous (lateral/medial), jugular, and dorsal pedal. The latter two are only to be used in emergent situations when all other options are exhausted. Dorsal pedal catheters can be painful, and jugular catheters are not ideal unless sterilely placed. While establishing venous access, provide any additional support that may be needed, such as heat support or oxygen therapy. On occasion, you may need to do things in a stepwise fashion if the treatments are stressful for the patient. If the patient has been assessed as dehydrated or hypovolemic, then you can begin fluid therapy at this time. The doctor would take the initial assessment of the patient and create a fluid plan. This may include boluses or maintenance rates. Whatever the fluid plan, the patient will need to be reassessed at regular and frequent intervals, and the fluids adjusted accordingly. A full "TPR" and blood pressure should be included in this reassessment. We will discuss fluid therapy in depth in the next chapter.

Concurrently with beginning treatments, a minimum database of diagnostics can help to determine a diagnosis for the patient. I will always obtain and hold blood when I place an IVC, as long as it does not compromise the patient or the catheter. This is something very simple that can save time later. As you learn more about treating emergent patients, you will learn to anticipate what the doctor is going to ask for. The minimum database for most patients is the minimum diagnostic bloodwork needed to reach a differential diagnosis. The complete blood count (CBC) indicates any changes in the red and white blood cells. Every CBC should be accompanied by a packed cell volume. The PCV is the fastest method to determine the red blood cell component of blood. Low PCV% can indicate blood loss or anemia. Elevated PCV levels can indicate dehydration. The CBC and PCV give a lot of information; however, the most important areas to look for changes are listed below:

Reading	Association	Why is this useful
Hematocrit (HCT)	Machine calculated value. The product of the mean cell volume (MCV) and the red blood cell count [HCT (%) = (MCV × RBC) ÷ 10]	Assessing anemia and blood loss
Hemoglobin Concentration (HGB)	Measured HGB on red blood cells (oxygen carrying capacity)	Assessment of oxygen delivery to tissues
Red Blood Cell (RBC) Count	the concentration of red cells in the whole blood (red blood cells + plasma components)	Assessing anemia or blood loss
Reticulocyte Count	This value represents young erythrocytes (RBCs) with no nucleus.	The presence of these cells in increasing numbers can indicate a response from the bone marrow to anemia. This would indicate a regenerative anemia
White Blood Cell (WBC) Count	this is the total number of WBCs (leukocytes) in the circulating blood	Assessment of infection or inflammation
Neutrophils	(segmented/mature) immune cells which circulate in the blood for a short time, then migrate out into the tissues	Assessment of infection or inflammation
"Band" Neutrophils	(immature) immune cells. Their presence in a blood sample is referred to as a "left shift".	can indicate a bone marrow response to infection or inflammation
Lymphocytes	WBCs produced in the lymphoid tissue as opposed to the bone marrow.	These cells circulate for a long time, and changes in the blood concentration of lymphocytes indicate redistribution rather than loss

(Continued)

Reading	Association	Why is this useful
Moncytes	These are large immune cells that are produced in the bone marrow. They migrate into the tissues.	Assessment of inflammation or stress response
Eosinophils	WBCs produced in the bone marrow and then migrate into the tissues. They can survive for several days.	Increased numbers can be attributed to parasitic infections and allergic responses.
Basophils	WBCs produced in the bone marrow.	These cells can be involved in parasitic infections.

Source: Cornell University College of Veterinary Medicine (2025a, b).

A serum biochemical profile (chemistry) should also be obtained as part of a minimum database. There are several different in-house testing options available. Even more options for chemistry tests are available, including a variety of combinations to suit every need. Along with the doctor, you will select the best chemistry option for your patient that requires the least amount of blood. The contents of a basic chemistry profile are listed below:

Reading	Organ/association	Why is this useful
Total protein (TP)	All proteins	Total concentration of all serum proteins
Albumin (Alb)	Protein synthesized in the liver	Amino acid formation for cellular function
Globulin (Glob)	All non-albumin proteins	Produced in inflammatory response
Blood urea nitrogen (BUN)	Renal value	Indicator of glomerular filtration rate (GFR)
Creatinine (Crea)	Renal value	Indicator of glomerular filtration rate (GFR)
Alanine aminotransferase (ALT)	Hepatic value	Indicator of hepatic injury
Alkaline phosphatase (ALP)	Hepatic value	Indicator of gallbladder function/ bile file
Total bilirubin (TBIL)	Hepatic value	Indicator of hepatic function
Amylase	Pancreas	Pancreatic function
Lipase	Pancreas	Pancreatic function
Glucose	Carbohydrate	Indicator of energy metabolism
Sodium (Na^+)	Electrolyte	Indicates changes in fluid distribution. Part of Na^+:K^+ pump
Potassium (K^+)	Electrolyte	Major intracellular cation. Major role in resting cellular membrane potential. Part of Na^+:K^+ pump
Chloride (Cl^-)	Electrolyte	Major extracellular anion. Major role in osmolality and acid–base balance

Source: Cornell University College of Veterinary Medicine (2025a, b).

I like to make a habit of "stalking" the blood machines so that I can see the results as soon as they are complete. This way, I can see important values and prepare treatments based on these changes. For example, is the blood glucose low? Then I can prepare a dextrose bolus (0.5 ml/kg, diluted 1:2 with saline) and let the doctor know that it is ready if they want it administered (Budde 2023). Blood glucose is not only available as part of pre-made chemistry panels, but there are cage-side point-of-care machines that give you results in mere seconds. It is a good idea to invest in a few of these for your hospital so that you can have results and add treatments that much faster. There is also a point-of-care machine available for blood lactate. Normal blood lactate for canines and felines is <2.5 mmol/l. This is a value that we rely on heavily in emergency medicine (Norkus 2019). Blood lactate is an indication of tissue perfusion (oxygen delivery). When there is a significant reduction in tissue oxygen delivery, the result is a shift to anaerobic metabolism. Lactate is a byproduct of anaerobic metabolism and therefore can indicate the degree of derangement and is a loose indicator of prognosis – the higher the lactate, the worse the outcome may be. Lactate should be checked serially over several hours and following treatments. A correction of blood lactate with treatment, over time, is a positive indicator for your patient (Norkus 2019).

There are a few other blood values that may be considered depending on the individual patient. Blood gas and activated clotting factors can give valuable information for a critical case and efficiently inform our treatment plan. Blood gas is another test that indicates if there is impaired tissue oxygen delivery and if anaerobic metabolism is present. Ideally, this is run on an arterial sample; however, this can be very technically difficult. A venous blood gas can be just as effective and is much faster and less stressful for our patients. Activated clotting times (ACT) are a quick test of the coagulation status of the patient. Before you consider more advanced nursing procedures, such as nasal oxygen, a central line, or a feeding tube, this can be valuable information to have, as you do not want to induce more blood loss if your patient is deficient in clotting factors (coagulopathic). ACT can also be an indicator (among other clinical signs) of potential systemic inflammatory response, such as disseminated intravascular coagulation (DIC).

Now that we have obtained all of the lab work, we can focus on other diagnostics. It is worth noting that at any point during initial stabilization, if there is additional treatment needed, that should be the focus. You will continue to monitor your patient's vitals, including pain and blood pressure, so you may need to pause diagnostics to administer fluid boluses if your patient is still hypotensive. Do not neglect administering pain medication. Unless we need to assess the neurologic status of our patient, think of a dog with a spinal injury, then we may need to consider holding pain medication only until after the assessment. You are your patient's main advocate, so you will work closely with the rest of the care team and the doctor to keep the patient as comfortable and stress-free as possible during treatment. As we continue to assess our patient, we can get other diagnostics such as radiographs, abdominal ultrasound, or cardiac ultrasound. Radiographs can give a picture of internal organ structures and indicate if there are any abnormalities present, such as a mass or a foreign body. Radiographs should be taken in three views and should be collimated specifically for the region you wish to view. For example, if you are looking at the abdomen, then a right lateral, left lateral, and ventral dorsal view should be taken. Ensure that proper pain medication and/or sedation have been administered before radiographs or ultrasound to aid in positioning, patient comfort, and staff safety. Abdominal and thoracic ultrasound can show the detailed structure of the organs, including any masses or changes. It can also show if there is any third-spacing (free fluid) present in the chest or abdominal cavity. Tapping this fluid can be a helpful diagnostic tool. A simple "centesis" kit can be put together and kept with your other emergency supplies. An example of a centesis kit would include the following:

- Butterfly catheters (various sizes)
- Long IVC (size 20–18G)

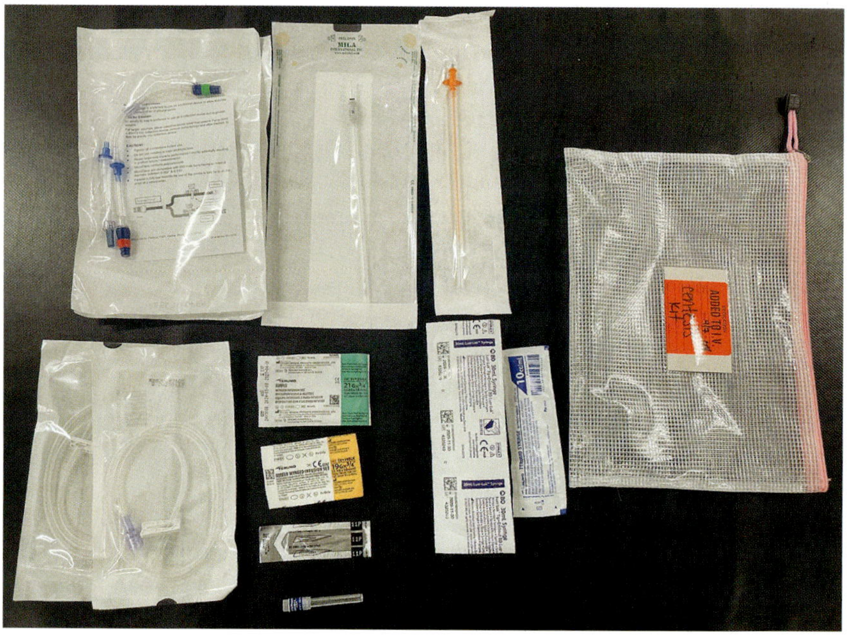

Image 5.2 Sample of the contents of a centesis kit. *Source:* Photo courtesy of Elizabeth Faux, RVT, VTS (ECC).

- Syringes (various sizes)
- Sterile gloves
- Chlorhex and alcohol scrub to sterilely prep
- Tubes to collect samples (white top tube and purple top tube) (Image 5.2)

You are well on your way to stabilizing your emergent patient. Now we will review a few of the most common emergencies that we see and apply what we have learned. What follows are examples of some of the most common emergencies that you may see and how you can approach them.

Trauma

Some of the common trauma cases that we see are patients who have been hit by a car (HBC), or a fall from a tall area (high-rise), or even gunshot wounds (GSW).

- First and foremost, assess the patient and take note of any obvious wounds and determine if pain medication and/or oxygen are necessary.
- While one team member works on obtaining vitals and administering oxygen if needed, you can place an IVC and obtain some blood to hold.
- If there is hemorrhage or large wounds, place a very light wrap over them of cast padding, cling, and vet wrap until the doctor can sedate the patient and explore the wound. For example, if an HBC has a large abdominal or thoracic wound, place a wrap over it to avoid additional contamination.
- This patient will likely have some level of shock and altered oxygen saturation to tissues, so checking pressure and administering fluids as quickly as possible is paramount.

- As these patients are often very painful, you can consider a constant rate of infusion (CRI) of pain medication. Fentanyl is a great option for this (2–5 mcg/kg/hr). Below is an example of a fentanyl CRI for a 20 kg dog running at 3 mcg/kg/hr (fentanyl concentration: 50 mcg/ml).

$$\frac{3\text{mcg} \times 20\text{kg}}{\text{hour}(\text{hr})} = \frac{60\text{mcg}}{\text{hr}} \quad \frac{60\text{mcg} \times 1\text{ml}}{50\text{mcg}} = \frac{1.2\text{mlfentanyl}}{\text{hr}}$$

- Radiographs will be needed to assess any trauma and discover any trauma injuries that cannot be initially observed. For example, there can be changes to the chest that are only observed with radiographs.
- Once all these diagnostics and initial treatments are complete, you will need to continue to monitor this patient and administer IVF, pain medication, and IV antibiotics if indicated. A soft, cushy kennel should be set up in the main hospital area so that close observation can be continued. Most trauma cases are at a high risk of decompensating, and some changes to the lungs do not "declare" themselves for a few days. Hourly vital checks, or a minimum of respiratory checks, will be needed, and full vitals and blood pressure are needed every 4–6 hours, depending on the individual patient.

Gastric Dilatation Volvulus (GDV)

GDV is one of the most common and most critical emergencies that you may see. The majority of large-breed dog owners are knowledgeable about this condition and can act quickly. However, some are not familiar, and the condition can present in many different ways, so you must act quickly when there is ANY level of suspicion for GDV. This condition is 100% fatal if immediate intervention is not pursued and surgery is not completed quickly. More information on this subject can be found in Chapter 16.

- IV access, oxygen supplementation, and pain medication should be the first treatments completed if you suspect GDV. (Fentanyl is a great choice here because it works great and can be a CRI as part of your anesthetic plan later.) This is a case where you should "go big or go home" with your catheter placement. A minimum of 20 G is ideal as you will likely be administering multiple fluid boluses to compensate for any shock states present. I prefer two IVCs in these patients, so two team members working on IVC and another on vitals and fluids would be ideal. If there are not that many people to help. One team member can be on IVCs, and the other can assist. Oxygen supplementation (50–150 ml/kg/min), in the form of flow-by via tube or a mask, is usually well tolerated by the patient. Oxygen is extremely important in these cases due to decreased oxygen delivery to tissues (Norkus 2019).
- As soon as an IVC is placed, get a fluid bolus going. Typically, 1 l of fluids (Plasmalyte or similar) per large dog is reasonable. I don't even put it on a pump; I will often use a pressure bag for these first boluses. The rotation of the GDV is cutting off the perfusion to the hind end of the patient, so they are often already exhibiting signs of shock or are close to it, so re-establishing that perfusion will set you and the patient up for success (Norkus 2019).
- While you place your IVC, you should have obtained some blood to run. A CBC and chemistry profile is ideal. While you are waiting on that to come back, you can get a PCV, a BG, and a lactate. The lactate will likely be elevated, so this can help guide fluid therapy (Norkus 2019).
- You will need to obtain a blood pressure reading to see if you need additional fluids or even medications to support blood pressure before surgery. If your patient is hypotensive before

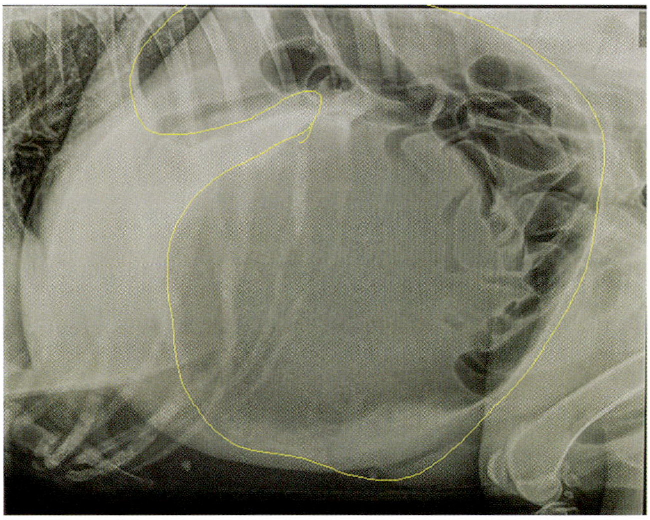

Image 5.3 Photo of a radiograph of a GDV with the "smurf hat" outlined in yellow. *Source:* Photo courtesy of Elizabeth Faux, RVT, VTS (ECC).

surgery, this will only worsen under anesthesia, so a plan should be made to begin correcting this before surgery. If necessary, a vasopressor (norepinephrine or dopamine CRI) should be prepped or started.

- If the patient is "stable" enough, a single right lateral radiograph can confirm a GDV. You will be looking for a "double bubble" or "smurf hat" (see photo below) of the stomach on X-ray (Norkus 2019).
- Prep the OR and get into surgery. The treatments that you have performed until now are just a "band-aid." This patient needs surgery now, so prep the OR and anesthetize the patient (Image 5.3).

Acute Abdomen

Acute abdomen is a broad term that can indicate several underlying conditions. For this chapter, we will restrict this to encompass a hemoabdomen and septic abdomen (ruptured foreign body). These cases can be challenging to correctly identify as well. These patients come in so sick that it is often difficult to stabilize them, let alone determine the diagnosis.

- First IV access. We need to obtain blood and have IV access to administer IVF and pain medication. While one team member is working on this, another can be obtaining vitals and administering oxygen. These patients are so compromised due to significant blood loss or becoming septic that their oxygen delivery to tissues is compromised.
- Obtain a blood pressure and assist the doctor in a POCUS abdominal and thoracic exam. Bolus IV fluids based on the blood pressure results.
- If there is free fluid present in the abdomen, obtain a sample. This sample can be compared to a peripheral PCV if it is blood. This can indicate if active hemorrhage is present. A lower PCV in the abdominal fluid versus the peripheral sample indicates slow or "controlled" hemorrhage. If the PCV is higher in the abdominal sample versus the peripheral sample, then the hemorrhage is active, and the patient will decompensate quickly. You may need to consider administering a blood product to this patient. If it is not blood, a blood glucose can be run on this fluid and a peripheral sample as well. If the BG in the abdominal fluid is higher than that of the peripheral

blood sample, this can indicate sepsis, as the bacteria from the septic abdomen are feeding on the glucose from the bloodstream. If the patient is hypoglycemic, you may need to consider a dextrose bolus (0.5 ml/kg diluted 1:2 with saline) (Budde 2023).
- Continue to monitor the patient's vitals and check the lactate in this patient.
- If the patient can tolerate it, take three-view abdomen and thorax radiographs. This can help indicate if there is an insidious process (cancer) or if there is some type of foreign body causing a septic process.
- This patient will likely be so hemodynamically unstable that it will need a combination of therapies, including vasopressors for blood pressure support.
- This patient is a good candidate for a central line or a sampling line (PICC) to help facilitate frequent blood draws.
- Continued patient monitoring (every 15–30 minutes) is needed to continue diagnostics and treatments. All efforts should be made to get the patient as stable as possible to pursue the next steps, surgery versus transfer (Norkus 2019).

Diabetic Crisis

Diabetic patients (newly diagnosed and with a history of diabetes) can be quite sick. Diabetes presents many challenges to the patient but also to the family, and it is quite easy for things to become unregulated. Most frequently, we see diabetic patients who are not well regulated on insulin, resulting in diabetic ketoacidosis, and sometimes we will see incorrect insulin administration resulting in an insulin overdose. More information on this subject can be found in Chapter 9.

- First, one team member can place an IVC and obtain full blood, if possible, while another team member obtains vitals.
- Run a blood glucose test immediately to gauge the level of derangement. Full bloodwork or a blood gas can also be considered to determine if there is an acid–base disturbance (metabolic acidosis).
- If the blood glucose is high, as I expect it will be, then fluids are an important first step. Starting the patient on IVF can help to lower the blood glucose as the patient becomes rehydrated. This can also help to correct electrolyte derangements.
- Blood pressure should be obtained, and an abdominal POCUS should be done to look at the internal organs and determine if there is another underlying cause for the clinical signs.
- A diabetic crisis can be caused by human error in administering insulin, unregulated new diabetics, but it can also be caused by underlying disease. Diabetics tend to get pancreatitis and can often have one or more concurrent underlying diseases, such as hyperadrenocorticism (Norkus 2019).

"Ain't Doin' Right" (ADR)

This is a common acronym that we use in the ER. We can apply this to a broad number of patients. Often, they are just not themselves, and the owner cannot describe in detail what has been going on with the pet. They can come in bright, dull, or completely lateral.

- Depending on the patient, obtaining vitals alone is sufficient before the doctor sees the patient. If the patient is not stable (has abnormal vital signs, difficulty breathing, etc.), then place an IVC and obtain blood and blood pressure.

- A lactate value can indicate tissue perfusion.
- Radiographs (three-view chest and abdomen) can be helpful in a case like this to determine any underlying cause for the presenting complaints, such as a cancerous process.
- Abdominal and thoracic POCUS can indicate if there is any free fluid present in either cavity (Mathews 2017).

Seizures

- IVC – to administer anticonvulsant medications (midazolam/diazepam) as needed. If the patient is having an active seizure and IV access cannot be obtained safely, then rectal anticonvulsants can be considered. Intranasal/mucosal atomizers can also be used if you have them stocked in your clinic.
- Minimum database – CBC + PCV/TS, Chemistry, and electrolytes.
- Blood pressure – patients who are having prolonged seizure activity can be hypertensive.
- There can also be many causes for “lookalike” seizure activity, such as medication administration (ketamine), pyrethrin toxicity in felines, and postpartum hypocalcemia. Obtaining a thorough patient history from the owner can help identify these “lookalikes” (Mathews 2017).

Works Cited

Balli, S. Shumway, K. (2023) “Physiology, Fever”. Available at: https://www.ncbi.nlm.nih.gov/books/NBK562334/ (accessed 22 April 2025)

Budde, J.A. (2023). *Plumb's Veterinary Drug Handbook*. Hoboken: Wiley-Blackwell.

Colorado State University James L. Voss Veterinary Teaching Hospital. (2025). Animal Pain Scores. Retrieved from vetmedbiosci.colostate.edu: vetmedbiosci.colostate.edu/vth/services/anesthesia/animal-pain-scales

Cornell University College of Veterinary Medicine. (2025a). Chemistry. Retrieved from Eclinpath: eclinpath.com/chemistry

Cornell University College of Veterinary Medicine. (2025b). Hemogram Baics. Retrieved from eclinpath.com: https://eclinpath.com/hematology/hemogram-basics/

Mathews, K. (2017). *Veterinary Emergency and Critical Care Manual*. Guelph: LifeLearn Inc.

Norkus, C. (2019). *Veterinary Technician's Manual for Small Animal Emergency and Critical Care*. Hoboken: John Wiley & Sons, Inc.

Royal Canin. (2025). Pain Assessment in the Dog: The Glasgow Pain Scale. Retrieved from: https://academy.royalcanin.com/en/veterinary/pain-assessment-in-the-dog-the-glasgow-pain-scale

Salik, I. and John V. Ashurst. (2023). Closed-loop communication training in medical simulation. StatPearls. Retrieved from https://www.ncbi.nlm.nih.gov/books/NBK549899/

6

Better Living Through Pharmaceuticals

Puja Wright

BluePearl Pet Hospital, 1 Taft Ct., Rockville, MD, USA

When a pet presents in distress or pain for an urgent situation, it is important to address the cause of distress and pain, but it's equally important to address the pet's stress, fear, nausea, and pain from the cause. These symptoms are often discerned from continued or repeated observations, which fall into the realm of the veterinary technician. While vets may sometimes pick up on these symptoms on their exam, they will then often need to move on to the next patient, making what they see more of a snapshot in time. The vet tech will often be the one who is doing continuous treatments on these patients and will be the one to notice the small signs that would lead the clinician to believe that a pet is painful, nauseous, or has an elevated fear, anxiety, or stress (FAS) level.

Pain has become an important part of the physical exam for all veterinary professionals, often touted as the "fifth vital sign" (Tabor 2016). Stress and pain often play into each other, magnifying the effects of each other and making each other worse. Pain is a source of stress for the patient, and stress can lead to bodily dysfunction. Furthermore, stress can enhance pain in strange ways, sometimes leading to an experience of lessened pain, but it can also lead to an experience of heightened pain (Gaynor 2014) (Image 6.1).

Pain can alter behavior in pets and affect respirations, movement, and eliminations if the associated movements cause elevated pain. Pets can be more likely to bother areas that are painful, causing wounds. Pain leads to catecholamine release in the body, increasing heart rate and blood pressure, which can lead to increased oxygen demand by the heart; this can have severe effects on the heart muscle that is already compromised (Tabor 2016). Increased cortisol levels released by the adrenal glands during stress can disrupt insulin and glucose levels in the body. Pain and associated stress can lead to increased clotting activity and coagulopathies. Prolonged effects from pain-induced stress can also lead to immune system suppression, delaying and preventing healing (Tabor 2016).

In the clinic, there are many drugs that can be used in combination to treat both pain and FAS in a synergistic way to benefit the patient and make the experience better for the patient, client, and veterinary professionals involved (Image 6.2).

Pain Control

Opioids

Often, when a pet comes in on an urgent or emergent patient basis, they are experiencing a higher level of pain. Opioids often cause respiratory depression and increase intracranial pressure, so they should be used with caution in patients who may be prone to these issues, with the availability of ventilatory support if needed (Budde 2023). They can cause gastrointestinal side effects, like nausea, vomiting, and slowed GI motility. Opioids can also cause increased external urethral tone and decreased voiding reflex, sometimes leading to urine retention (Gaynor 2014). However, opioids tend to have minimal cardiovascular effects; they can cause increased vagal tone, leading to

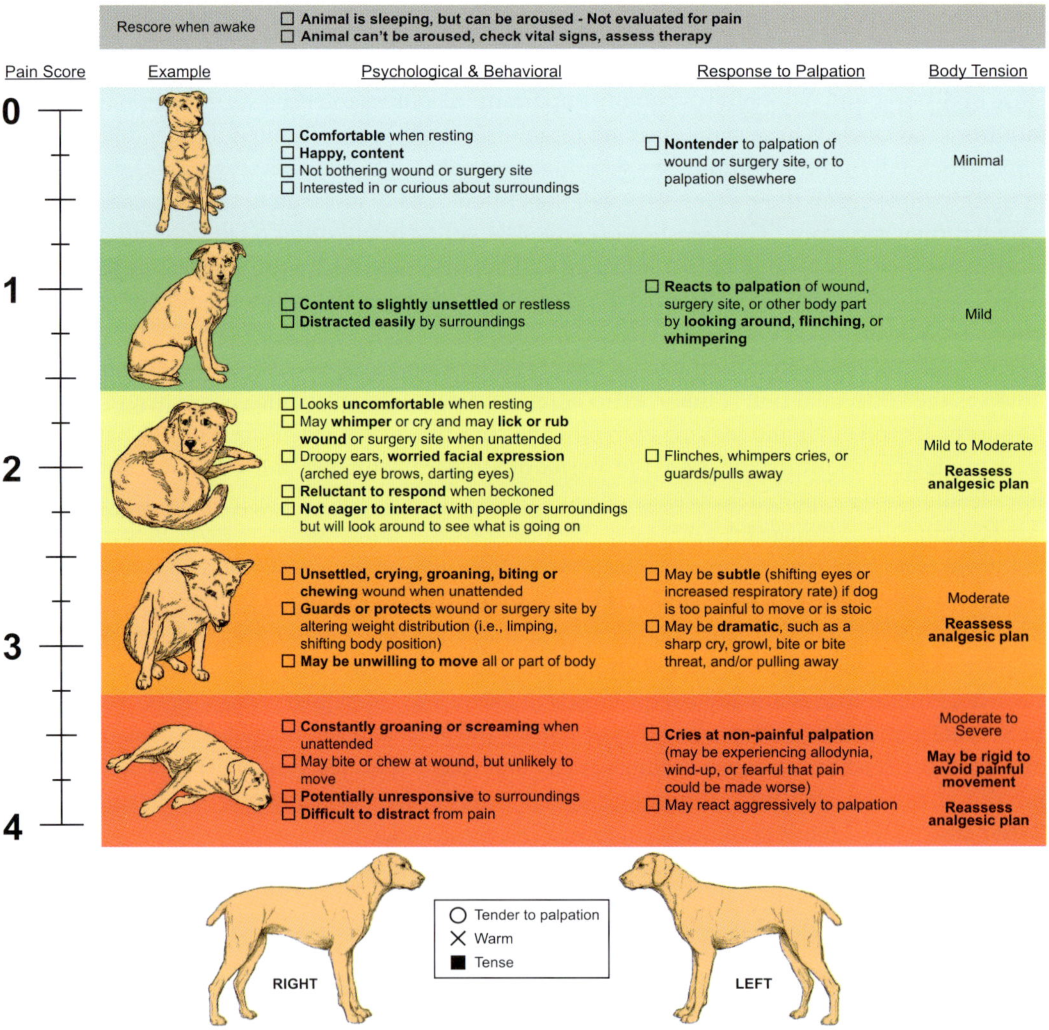

Image 6.1 Examples of the canine and feline Colorado State Pain Scale Worksheet. *Source:* Illustration by PW Hellyer, SR Uhrig, NG Robinson.

Pain Score	Example	Psychological & Behavioral	Response to Palpation	Body Tension
	Rescore when awake	☐ **Animal is sleeping, but can be aroused - Not evaluated for pain** ☐ **Animal can't be aroused, check vital signs, assess therapy**		
0	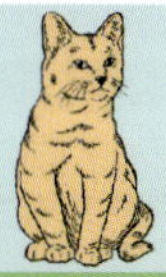	☐ **Content and quiet** when unattended ☐ **Comfortable** when resting ☐ Interested in or **curious** about surroundings	☐ **Not bothered** by palpation of wound or surgery site, or to palpation elsewhere	Minimal
1	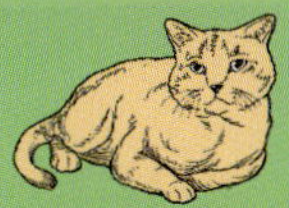	☐ **Signs are often subtle and not easily detected in the hospital setting**; more likely to be detected by the owner(s) at home ☐ Earliest signs at home may be **withdrawal from surroundings or change in normal routine** ☐ In the hospital, may be content or slightly unsettled ☐ **Less interested** in surroundings but will look around to see what is going on	☐ May or may not react to palpation of wound or surgery site	Mild
2	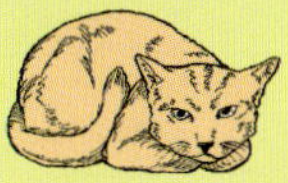	☐ Decreased responsiveness, **seeks solitude** ☐ **Quiet**, loss of brightness in eyes ☐ **Lays curled up or sits tucked up** (all four feet under body, shoulders hunched, head held slightly lower than shoulders, tail curled tightly around body) with eyes partially or mostly closed ☐ **Hair coat appears rough** or fluffed up ☐ May intensively groom an area that is painful or irritating ☐ Decreased appetite, **not interested in food**	☐ **Responds aggressively or tries to escape** if painful area is palpated or approached ☐ Tolerates attention, may even perk up when petted as long as painful area is avoided	Mild to Moderate **Reassess analgesic plan**
3	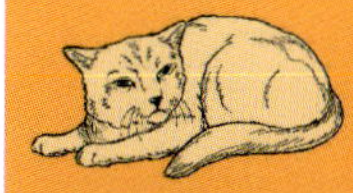	☐ Constantly **yowling, growling, or hissing** when unattended ☐ May bite or chew at wound, but **unlikely to move** if left alone	☐ **Growls or hisses at non-painful palpation** (may be experiencing allodynia, wind-up, or fearful that pain could be made worse) ☐ **Reacts aggressively** to palpation, **adamantly pulls away** to avoid any contact	Moderate **Reassess analgesic plan**
4	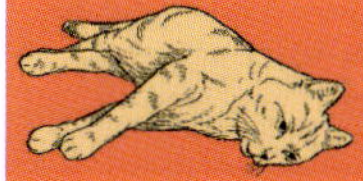	☐ Prostrate ☐ Potentially **unresponsive** to or unaware of surroundings, difficult to distract from pain ☐ Receptive to care (even aggressive or feral cats will be more tolerant of contact)	☐ **May not respond** to palpation ☐ **May be rigid to avoid painful movement**	Moderate to Severe **May be rigid to avoid painful movement** **Reassess analgesic plan**

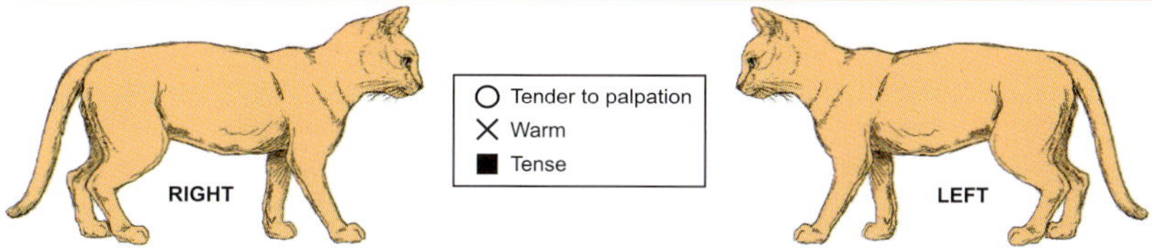

Image 6.1 (Continued)

bradycardia, but there is no vasoconstrictive effect and minimal vasodilatory effects. While the bradycardia can lead to some hypotension, this means there is minimal effect on systemic blood pressure as well (Budde 2023).

For mild–moderate to severe pain, the veterinary world will often lean on opioids. The most prominent type of opioids used for moderate to severe pain is full-mu agonists. All these drugs are for injectable use, mostly just for use within the clinic. Full-mu agonists bind to the mu opioid receptor found in multiple areas of the brain and in the spinal cord, which leads to analgesia (Tabor 2016). Commonly used full mu agonists in veterinary medicine include morphine, hydromorphone, methadone, and fentanyl. Lower doses than recommended should be used for neonates, critically ill patients, and elderly patients, as well as those with hepatic and renal disease (Budde 2023).

Morphine can cause histamine release, and it is contraindicated in cases of ileus and GI obstruction (Budde 2023). If it is given too quickly intravenously, it can cause severe vasodilation; this

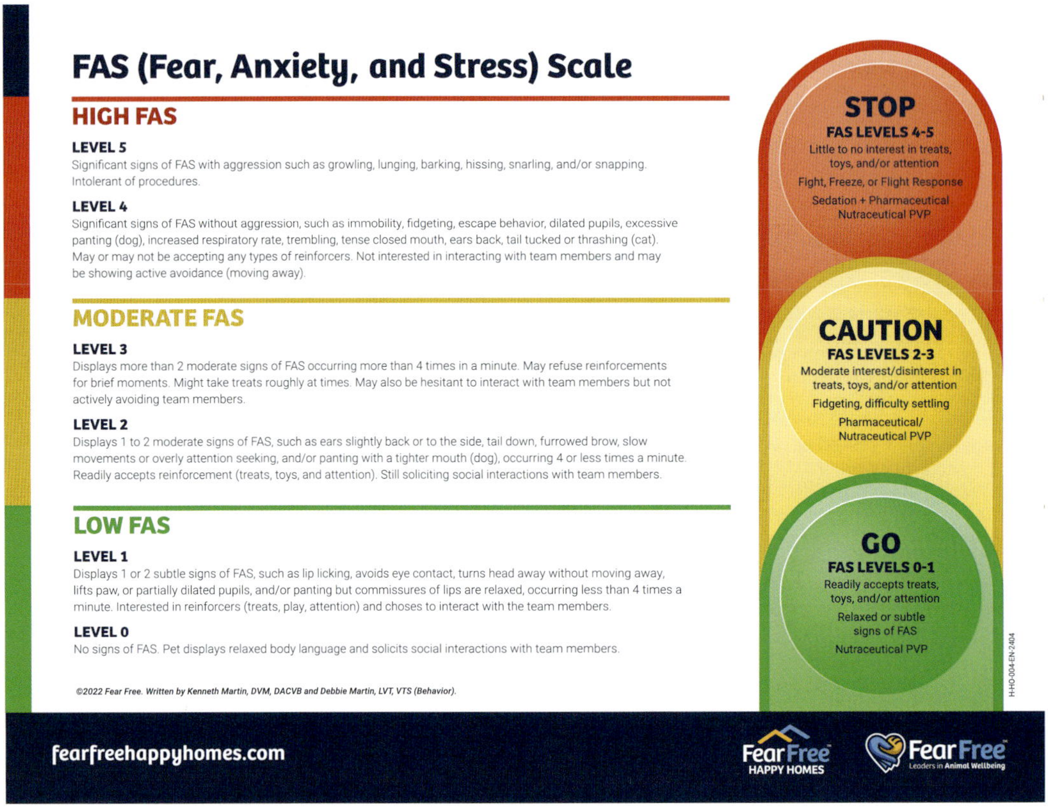

Image 6.2 Fear, anxiety, and stress scale from Fear Free.

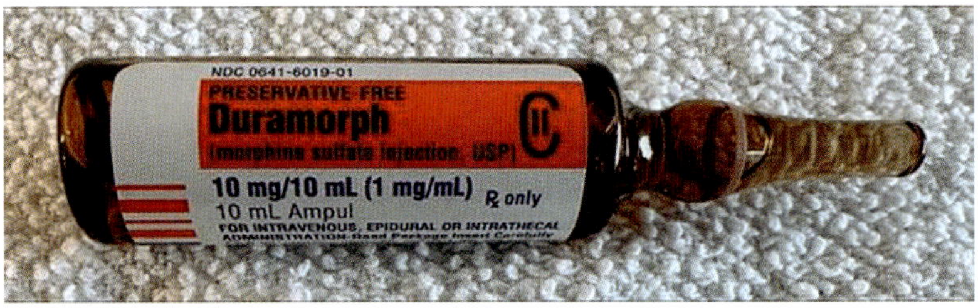

Image 6.3 Example of preservative-free morphine used for epidurals. *Source:* Photo courtesy of Puja Wright, RVT.

effect can be avoided by giving the drug intramuscularly, subcutaneously, or very slowly intravenously. There are preservative-free formulations (like Duramorph) that can be used for epidural applications. Used in lumbosacral epidurals, the effects of morphine can migrate cranially and last up to 18 hours in dogs and 12 hours in cats (Budde 2023) (Image 6.3).

Hydromorphone can cause intense nausea and vomiting in patients, although giving it intravenously may make the impact lesser than other routes (Budde 2023). It can have a similar histamine release like morphine, but at a much lower level (Gaynor 2014). If other options are available, hydromorphone should still be avoided in situations like mast cell tumors to skirt the slight possibility of histamine release. Hydromorphone can also cause hyperthermia in cats that tends to be self-limiting and resolves with cessation of the opioid (Budde 2023) (Image 6.4).

Methadone, while a pure-mu agonist, also has some N-methyl-D-aspartate (NMDA) receptor antagonist activity that can be helpful for neuropathic pain (Gaynor 2014). It can cause more significant bradycardia than morphine. Greyhounds may also need higher doses than listed (Budde 2023) (Image 6.5).

Fentanyl is only available in injection for intravenous usage. This is because its duration of action is up to 15–30 minutes (Gaynor 2014). As modalities like intramuscular and subcutaneous injection can take nearly that long to take effect, giving fentanyl in those ways is not effective. Fentanyl also requires a constant rate infusion (CRI) to provide effective analgesia due to its quick duration. However, when run at higher CRI rates, it can have a significant minimum alveolar concentration (MAC) sparing effect as well. There is a preservative-free version available that can be used in epidurals (Budde 2023) (Image 6.6).

There are also opioids that only partially activate opioid receptors. One such drug is buprenorphine, a partial mu agonist and kappa antagonist. Buprenorphine is better for mild to moderate pain, but not appropriate for severe pain. It has a very high affinity for mu receptors, making it hard to reverse with an antagonist, as well as making it harder to replace on the mu receptors with other mu opioids (Budde 2023). This means that if buprenorphine is given and the patient is not adequately pain controlled, giving a pure-mu agonist after buprenorphine can make the pure-mu less effective. However, buprenorphine can be absorbed transmucosally via the gums, making it an attractive option for pain control in cats. It can cause some mild hyperthermia in cats (Budde 2023).

Another opioid that falls into the partial activation category is butorphanol. Butorphanol is a kappa agonist and a partial mu antagonist. In some places, it can be used to partially reverse full mu agonists to aid anesthetic recoveries without completely reversing pain control as well (Budde 2023). Butorphanol should be primarily used as a sedative in cats and dogs. While it technically has some analgesic effects, it does not touch somatic (superficial) pain or severe pain (Gaynor 2014). There are some studies suggesting that it can be effective for visceral (deep organ) pain and mild pain, but it needs to be redosed frequently for analgesic effects (Gaynor 2014). Analgesic effects last less than an hour, while sedation lasts up to 2–4 hours (Budde 2023) (Image 6.7).

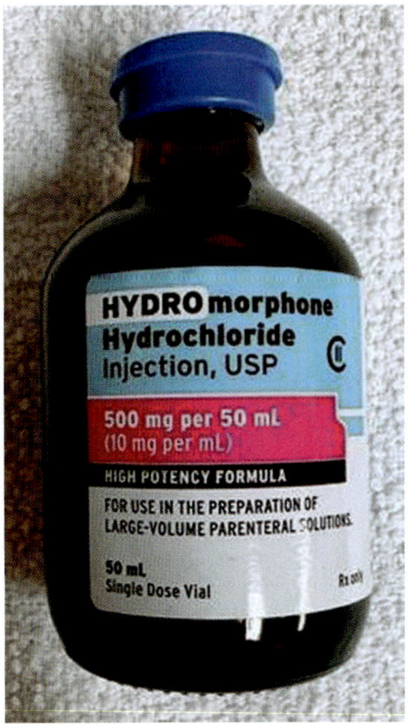

Image 6.4 Hydromorphone bottle. *Source:* Photo courtesy of Puja Wright, RVT.

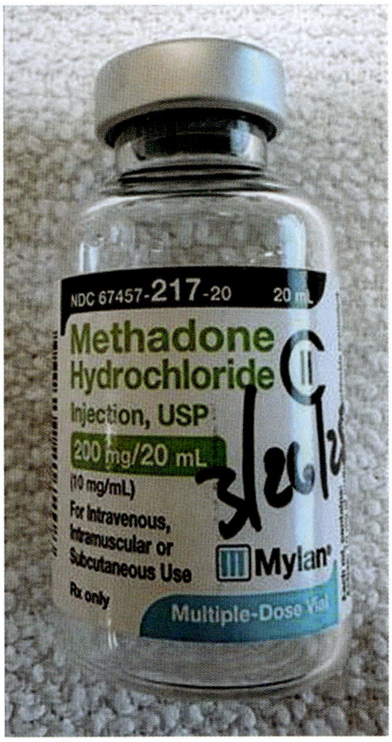

Image 6.5 Methadone bottle. *Source:* Photo courtesy of Puja Wright, RVT.

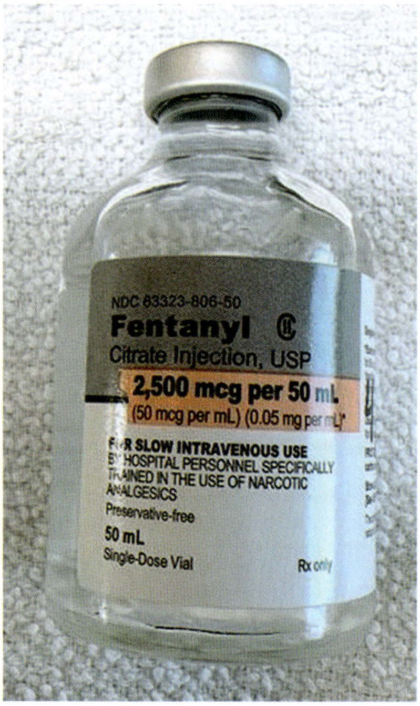

Image 6.6 Fentanyl bottle. *Source:* Photo courtesy of Puja Wright, RVT.

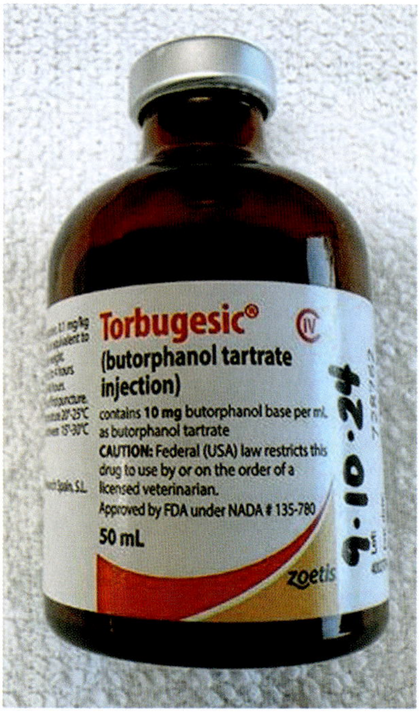

Image 6.7 Bottle of butorphanol. *Source:* Photo courtesy of Puja Wright, RVT.

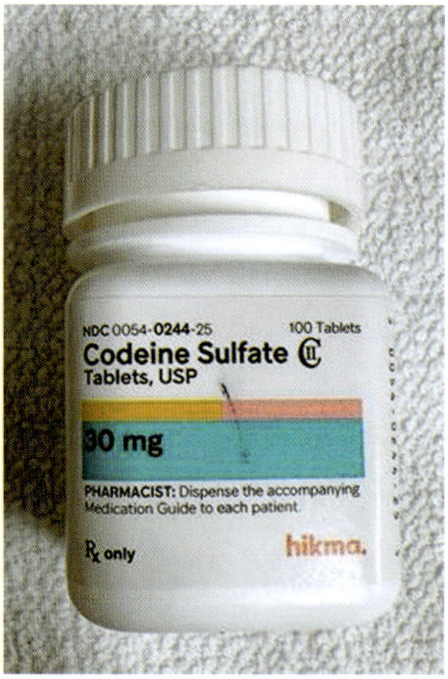

Image 6.8 Bottle of codeine. *Source:* Photo courtesy of Puja Wright, RVT.

Tramadol is an oral opioid mu receptor agonist. Oral opioids have questionable efficacy in small animals since liver metabolism of oral opioids converts a relatively small amount to a usable mu receptor agonist. There is a high "first pass effect" in dogs, where they metabolize too much of the opioid before it can be used for pain control in the body. However, cats make more of the active M1 metabolite, making oral tramadol a possible good option in cats. Naloxone, however, can only partially reverse tramadol. Doses are recommended to be adjusted for patients with renal and hepatic issues (Budde 2023).

Codeine is another oral opioid that is used in small animals. It has a similar high first-pass effect with hepatic metabolism in dogs, making for very low bioavailability. There are no studies done in cats, but since they have a lower first-pass effect with other oral opioids, it is potentially more effective in cats than dogs, like tramadol. Codeine can cause side effects similar to injectable opioids, with sedation, constipation, and respiratory depression (Budde 2023) (Image 6.8).

Opioid	Receptor it works on	Suggested dosing	Routes	Uses
Morphine	Mu-agonist	**Canine:** 0.5–1 mg/kg q 2–4 h CRI: 0.1–1 mg/kg/hr IV **Epidural:** PF 0.1 mg/kg diluted to a volume of 0.3 ml/kg (max volume 6 ml) for up to 18 hr **Feline:** 0.1–0.25 mg/kg a 2–4 hr **CRI:** 0.05–0.1 mg/kg/hr IV **Epidural:** PF 0.1 mg/kg diluted to 0.22 ml/kg volume for 12 hr	IV, IM, SC epidurally	Moderate to severe pain
Hydromorphone	Mu-agonist	**Canine:** 0.1–0.2 mg/kg q 3–5 hr **Feline:** 0.05–0.1 mg/kg q 2–6 hr **Epidurally:** 0.05 mg/kg for 3 hr	IV, IM, SC	Moderate to severe pain
Methadone	Mu-agonist, NMDA antagonist	**Canine:** 0.1–1 mg/kg CRI: 0.1 mg/kg/hr IV **Epidural:** 0.1–0.3 mg/kg, 0.5 mg/kg at LS **Feline:** 0.2–0.5 mg/kg q 4–6 hr CRI: 0.12 mg/kg/hr IV **Epidurally:** 0.2–0.3 mg/kg for 18+ hr	IV, IM, SC	Moderate to severe pain
Fentanyl	Mu-agonist	**Canine:** 2–10 mcg/kg IV, followed by 2–10 mcg/kg/hr CRI (can go up to 20–40 mcg/kg/hr for PIVA or TIVA) **Feline:** 5 mcg/kg IV, followed by 5 mcg/kg/hr CRI (can go up to 20 mcg/kg/hr for PIVA or TIVA)	IV, continuous infusion	Moderate to severe pain
Buprenorphine	Partial Mu-agonist, kappa-antagonist	**Canine:** 0.01–0.04 mg/kg IM or IV q 4–6 hr 0.12 mg/kg OTM **CRI:** 0.0025 mg/kg/hr IV for 6 hr **Feline:** 0.01–0.03 mg/kg IM, IV, OTM q 4–8 hr **Simbadol:** 0.24 mg/kg SC q 3 d **Zorbium:** 2.7–6.7 mg/kg transdermally q 4 d **CRI:** 0.0025 mg/kg/hr IV for 6 hr	IV, IM, SC, OTM	Mild to moderate pain
Butorphanol	Kappa-agonist, partial mu-antagonist	**Canine:** 0.1–0.5 mg/kg SC, IM, IV q 2–4 hr for sedation **Feline:** 0.1–0.5 mg/kg SC, IM, IV q 2–4 hr for sedation. Q 1–2 hr for pain.	IV, IM, SC	Sedation
Tramadol	Mu-agonist	**Canine:** 4–10 mg/kg PO q 6–8 hr, questionable efficacy as a single agent **Feline:** 1–2 mg/kg PO q 12 hr, 4 mg/kg PO q 6 hr	PO	Mild to moderate pain
Codeine	Mu-agonist	**Canine:** 0.5–1 mg/kg PO q 4–6 hr, up to 4 mg/kg suggested due to high first pass **Feline:** 0.5–2 mg/kg PO q 6–8 hr	PO	Mild to moderate pain

Dosages from Plumbs (Budde 2023).

NMDA Antagonists

Ketamine is an N-methyl-D-aspartame (NMDA) antagonist. While it has pain control, it is not sufficient for most types of pain on its own, and it works best as an adjunct pain therapy, especially with opioids (Budde 2023). Ketamine stimulates catecholamine release by the adrenal glands – this, in turn, raises the heart rate and cardiovascular output, as well as causes an increase in blood pressure from vasoconstriction. However, since ketamine stimulates the adrenal glands to release endogenous catecholamines, like norepinephrine, which are already things that the body releases in stressful situations, the drug can have negative inotropic effects (Budde 2023). This can be seen in very sick animals, where ketamine administration can decrease the force of cardiac output, causing a decrease in circulating blood volume and blood pressure. Ketamine can also cause muscle rigidity, making it necessary to lubricate the patient's eyes frequently as they won't blink or close them (Budde 2023). This can also affect their breathing, causing it to become erratic, with varying depths of breaths and pauses between breaths. It makes it contraindicated for procedures involving the throat, as it can affect the normal functions of the trachea, larynx, and pharynx. It is less than ideal for assessing laryngeal function (Budde 2023).

However, many of these side effects are dose-dependent and more significant at higher anesthetic doses. The analgesic effects from ketamine are palpable at much lower doses, which also works to lower the rate of the less desirable side effects (Budde 2023). NMDA antagonists also play an important role in adjunct pain control through modulating central nervous system sensitization to the perception of pain. When a patient has an increased sensitivity to a painful stimulus that appears to be hard to affect with other pain modalities, it can be what is called "wind-up" pain. Ketamine reduces the effects of wind-up pain on the central nervous system, so other modalities can then effectively do their job to control the synthesis of pain. Ketamine can be an effective adjunct therapy in acute and chronic pain situations (Gaynor 2014). This phenomenon has been taken advantage of in patients with chronic pain by using subcutaneous doses to deliver longer-lasting, subanesthetic amounts of NMDA antagonist to affect wind-up pain (Carmack 2023) (Image 6.9).

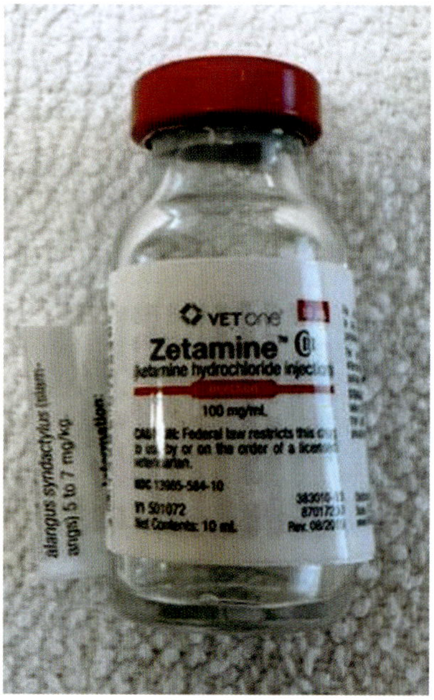

Image 6.9 Ketamine bottle. *Source:* Photo courtesy of Puja Wright, RVT.

Amantadine is an oral NMDA antagonist medication. It can work well for neuropathic pain and to alleviate wind-up pain and allodynia. It can also help with opioid tolerance and let pets need lesser opioid doses for pain control. With excessive doses or delayed clearance in renal patients, behavioral side effects can be seen (Gaynor 2014).

Alpha-2 Agonists

Dexmedetomidine is an alpha-2 receptor agonist (Budde 2023). It belongs in the same category as other drugs such as xylazine, medetomidine, detomidine, and clonidine. Alpha-2 agonists are often used for their sedative properties. Dexmedetomidine is often used in small animal settings for sedation, as it can be given intramuscularly, making it easier to sedate patients that may be fractious (Budde 2023). It does have some mild analgesic properties that are amplified by using it in conjunction with an opioid (Gaynor 2014). Most alpha-2 agonists, such as dexmedetomidine, are easily reversible with agents like atipamezole, making them ideal for sedation (Image 6.10).

Depending on the opioid it is paired with, sedative effects can be more profound as well. Alpha-2 agonists can have a profound effect on the cardiovascular system, though. They cause significant vasoconstriction, leading to increased blood pressure readings (Budde 2023). The patient's heart rate can become profoundly bradycardic as a protective measure to keep it from having to work too hard to pump blood against the vasoconstricted vessels. This leads to bradyarrhythmia, such as sinus arrhythmia and first- and second-degree atrioventricular (AV) blocks (Budde 2023). The vasoconstriction can also lead to challenges in accurate noninvasive blood pressure readings and pulse oximetry readings due to the degree of constriction in the peripheral vessels that these monitoring devices normally use. Dexmedetomidine can also lead to increased urine production through affecting the renal and endocrine systems, so caution should be used in patients with renal disease and any kind of urinary outflow obstruction (Gaynor 2014).

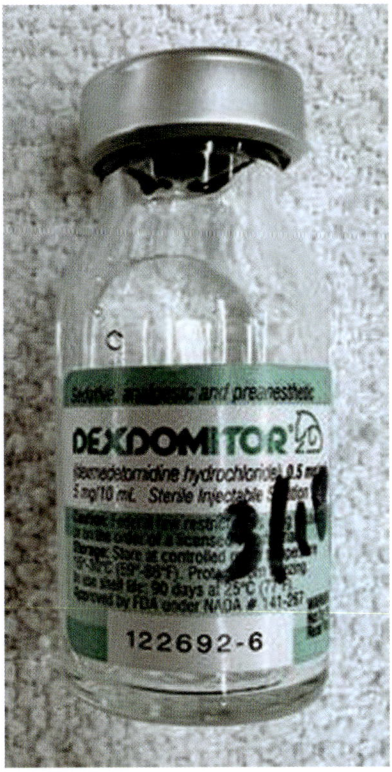

Image 6.10 Bottle of dexmedetomidine. *Source:* Photo courtesy of Puja Wright, RVT.

Drug	Receptor it works on	Suggested dosing	Routes	Uses
Ketamine	NMDA antagonist	**Canine:** 0.5 mg/kg IV, then 0.1–0.6 mg/kg/hr IV CRI **Feline:** 0.5–1 mg/kg IV, then 0.1–0.6 mg/kg/hr IV CRI	IV, IM, SC	Adjunct for moderate to severe pain
Amantadine	NMDA antagonist	**Canine/Feline:** 3–5 mg/kg PO q 12–24 hr	PO	Adjunct for moderate to severe pain, oncological pain
Dexmedetomidine	Alpha-1 agonist	**Canine:** 125–375 mcg/m^2 1–2 mcg/kg IV, then 0.72–1 mcg/kg/hr IV CRI 25 mcg/m^2, then 25 mcg/m^2/hr IV CRI Addition to nerve blocks: 0.5 mcg/kg added to bupivacaine or lidocaine **Feline:** 5–15 mcg/kg SC, IM, IV, up to 40 mcg/kg 0.5 mcg/kg IV, then 0.5 mcg/kg/hr IV CRI	IV, IM, SC	Adjunct for mild to moderate pain

Local Anesthetics

Local anesthetics are sometimes overlooked and overshadowed by "fancier" drugs. However, local anesthetics are the only drugs that block the initiation of pain when looking at the pain conduction pathways. They also block the conduction of pain (Gaynor 2014). While the usage of local anesthetics often requires more knowledge of techniques, practically, they can be some of the most easily accessible of pain control drugs. Many techniques don't need special equipment and use inexpensive, widely available instrumentation and drugs (sterile syringes, small gauge needles, and cheap, common drugs like lidocaine). Often, they do require some investment in the training of the staff administering to make sure they are proficient in the techniques used for particular blocks, but this increases technician utilization overall and contributes to better engagement. Higher engagement from employees leads to increased revenue and better employee retention (see Chapter 19 for further information about employee engagement) (Images 6.11 and 6.12).

Common local anesthetics used in small animal medicine include lidocaine, bupivacaine, ropivacaine, and proparacaine. Proparacaine often comes as eye drops that can be used for patient comfort during procedures involving the eye. They can also be used to apply to the nares to numb the area for things such as nasogastric tubes and nasal oxygen lines. Lidocaine, bupivacaine, and ropivacaine are found mostly in injectable formats; however, there are topical formulations of lidocaine that can be used in surprising ways. The efficacy of local anesthetics is largely determined by the condition of the tissue to which it is applied; local blood flow, local pH, and local temperature can all affect how well a local agent works (Gaynor 2014). For example, acidosis can reduce the effectiveness of a local block. The use of local anesthetics to block the beginnings of the pain conduction pathways greatly reduces MAC for general anesthesia. Used in local blocks for peripheral nerve blocks and in topical fashions, local anesthetics tend to have minimal side effects (Budde 2023). They can be used topically, locally, regionally, systemically (for lidocaine), and epidurally. Lidocaine is often used as a CRI for its antiarrhythmic properties, but it also is thought to provide visceral pain relief for patients requiring abdominal surgery (Budde 2023). Caution needs to be used when using lidocaine systemically, especially in cats, as they have a lower toxic dose, and it can cause cardiac issues (Budde 2023). If a larger volume is used epidurally, caution needs to be taken as large volumes can migrate cranially and affect the muscles used for respiration. Smaller doses of local anesthetics can reduce the side effects of motor dysfunction (Budde 2023).

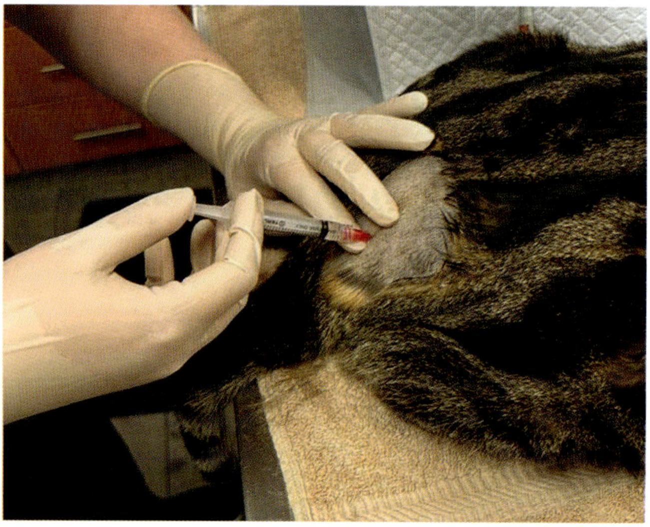

Image 6.11 Example of a sacrococcygeal epidural: the only equipment needed is a standard 25 g needle, local anesthetic, and sterile prep. *Source:* Photo courtesy of Simone Conwell, RVT.

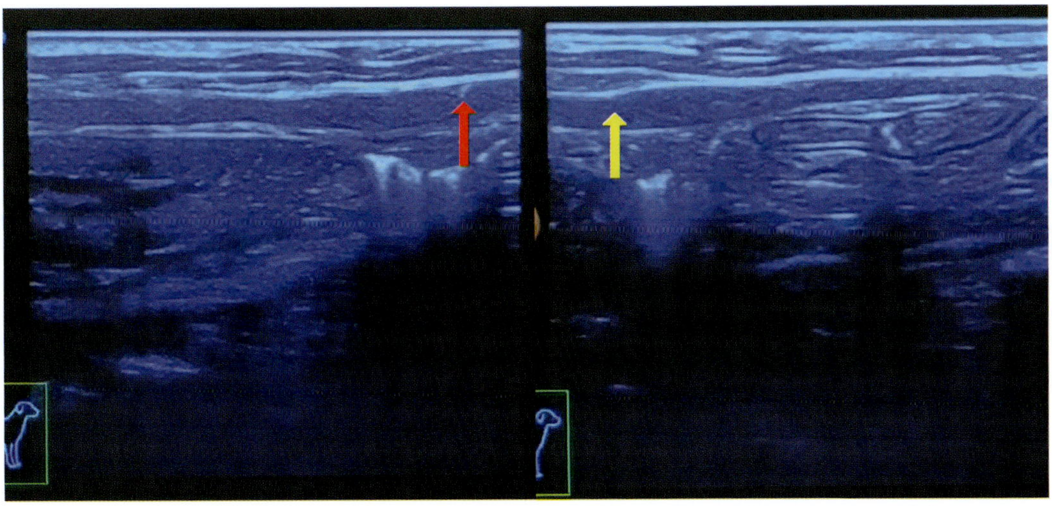

Image 6.12 Still of an ultrasound image of the internal oblique and transversus abdominus muscles (red arrow) from a cadaver during a training wetlab. Successful TAP (transversus abdominus plane) block from the same wet lab (yellow). *Source:* Photos courtesy of Simone Conwell, RVT, VTS (ECC).

Nonsteroidal Anti-Inflammatories

Nonsteroidal anti-inflammatories (NSAIDs) are a class of pain control that can be very helpful, but often can be limited in their usage due to their side effects. NSAIDs are potent anti-inflammatories, antipyretics, and analgesics (Budde 2023). Most NSAIDs work along the inflammation pathway to inhibit the production of prostaglandins, specifically on cyclooxygenase (COX) receptors (Budde 2023; Gaynor 2014). Prostaglandins are responsible for inflammation, and inflammation in turn leads to hyperalgesia of pain pathways (Gaynor 2014). NSAIDs appear to work both peripherally, at the site of injury, and centrally, mostly at the spinal cord (Budde, Gaynor 2014). Peripherally, they work to decrease inflammation at the injury site, while centrally, they can help with central sensitization, where the nervous system becomes extra sensitive to pain signals. NSAIDs can be a good choice for both acute and chronic pain. They are reported to be just as effective as opioids in many cases of musculoskeletal and visceral pain (Gaynor 2014).

However, there is a list of contraindications with NSAIDs. They cannot be used in conjunction with steroids or other NSAIDs, as both drugs would also inhibit parts of the inflammation cascade, which can significantly raise the rate of undesirable side effects (Budde 2023). As some COX inhibitors can affect coagulation as well, caution should be used in patients with coagulopathies (Gaynor 2014). COX inhibition can also cause gastrointestinal issues, so this class of drugs can be counterintuitive in pets with gastrointestinal disease. Newer NSAIDs that are targeted toward COX-2 over COX-1 tend to have less gastrointestinal side effects (Budde 2023). NSAIDs can also affect the renal system and the liver, so caution must be used in patients where renal or hepatic compromise exists. This includes patients where adequate perfusion may be a concern, such as those with hypotension (Budde 2023; Gaynor 2014). Routine bloodwork is recommended to check for any side effects on the liver and renal values. Giving oral NSAIDs with food reduces the chances of gastrointestinal upset as well (Budde 2023).

Carprofen is available as an injectable and oral medication. It is an NSAID that is more selective for COX-2 receptors than COX-1 in canines, making it less likely to have gastrointestinal side effects than some other NSAIDs. In felines, it is suspected to have more COX-1 activity (Budde 2023). Carprofen has had relatively little interference with platelet function and hemostasis in studies with healthy animals (Gaynor 2014). In the United States, this NSAID is registered for usage in dogs only; however, in some countries, a single injectable dose of carprofen is allowed in cats, but repeated use is not recommended (Budde 2023; Gaynor 2014). It has been used long-term in dogs for chronic pain control with success and periodic bloodwork to check for hepatic dysfunction (Budde 2023; Gaynor 2014). It is also frequently used in dogs for postoperative pain management.

Meloxicam is another NSAID available in both oral and injectable formats, as well as transdermal. This NSAID is COX-2 receptor preferential; however, with higher dosages, it shows less preference for COX-2 over COX-1 receptors (Budde 2023). This NSAID can be used in dogs and cats, but there are some reports of acute kidney injury with the labeled dosage in cats (Budde 2023). Still, meloxicam tends to be one of the preferred NSAIDs in cats, particularly for long-term oral usage. Repeat doses of the injection are not recommended in cats (Budde 2023). Long-term dosages in cats have been shown to be safe in cats with renal dysfunction as well. Studies have also shown insignificant alteration to platelet function with usage in both dogs and cats (Gaynor 2014).

Deracoxib is an NSAID available in oral form. It is COX-2 selective and COX-1 sparing. It is labeled for canines only. It performs well for acute and chronic orthopedic pain and has been used for soft tissue surgeries as well. However, there has been a study that implicates deracoxib with serious gastrointestinal complications. It has not been studied in cats, and usage in cats is not recommended (Gaynor 2014).

Firocoxib is another oral-only NSAID for dogs. It is also COX-2 selective like deracoxib. Its use for acute and chronic orthopedic pain is well documented. It also provides effective postoperative analgesia. Clinical data for firocoxib shows a low rate of side effects, mostly related to the GI tract (Gaynor 2014).

Robenacoxib is a COX-2 selective NSAID available in both injectable and oral formats for both cats and dogs (Budde 2023). In dogs, it has about a 130 times higher affinity for COX-2, while in cats that number is closer to 500 times the affinity (Budde 2023). Robenacoxib has been shown to be good for acute surgical pain, as well as chronic orthopedic pain in some places (Gaynor 2014). It is labeled for 3 days of usage in cats in the United States, but up to 11 days in other countries. It has been shown to have a good safety profile in healthy cats up to 42 days (Gaynor 2014).

Grapiprant is a newer oral NSAID for dogs that is not a COX inhibitor. It is a prostaglandin EP4-receptor antagonist, so it works further downstream in the inflammatory pathway (Budde 2023). This makes it less likely to have hepatic and gastrointestinal side effects. However, caution should still be used with hepatic and renal dysfunction in patients. Doses for MDR1-positive patients should be decreased (Budde 2023).

Drug	Species	Suggested dosing	Routes
Carprofen	Canine, single dose in felines	**Canine:** 4.4 mg/kg PO, SC q 24 hr 2.2 mg/kg PO, SC q 12 hr **Feline:** 4 mg/kg SC, IV once 2.2 mg/kg PO prior to surgery	IV, SC, PO
Meloxicam	Canine, feline	**Canine:** 0.2 mg/kg PO, SC, IV first day, then 0.1 mg/kg PO q 24 hr For dogs <4.5 kg put on food, do not give PO directly **Feline:** One dose 0.3 mg/kg SC OR 0.1–0.2 mg/kg PO first day, then 0.05 mg/kg PO q 24 hr. Further titrate down to the lowest effective dose. 0.01–0.035 mg/kg PO q 24	IV, SC, PO

Other Medications

Acetaminophen

Acetaminophen often gets grouped with nonsteroidal anti-inflammatories, but it is not an NSAID. Acetaminophen is also known as paracetamol. It has analgesic and antipyretic properties, but does not work on the inflammatory pathways the same way other NSAIDs (Budde 2023) do. There is little known about the actual pathways that acetaminophen works on. It is highly toxic to cats and should not be used on them, as it causes oxidative damage to red blood cells. This damage can be seen in the form of Heinz body anemia (Budde 2023). Dogs can acquire similar toxicity, but toxicity generally occurs at higher doses (75–100 mg/kg) than dosages used for analgesia (10–20 mg/kg). While it has been traditionally avoided in the United States, acetaminophen has been used successfully for years in the United Kingdom (Budde 2023). While generally found in oral form, there is an injectable form that can be used as rescue medication for postoperative patients.

Gabapentin and Pregabalin

Gabapentin has become frequently used in small animal medicine for pain. It works well for chronic pain, especially hyperalgesia and allodynia, and neuropathic pain (Budde 2023; Gaynor 2014). Despite its name, the drug does not actually function on the gamma-aminobutyric acid receptor, but instead by reducing the release of stimulating neurotransmitters, like substance P (Gaynor 2014). It does not work well for acute pain alone, but can help in a multimodal protocol.

Gabapentin works well as an anxiolytic as well, so it can be well used as a preoperative medication to help prevent hyperalgesia, as well as to reduce FAS preoperatively to help reduce anesthetic needs. Sedation and ataxia can be common side effects. Using gabapentin can be safe in most patients, but it should be used with caution in patients with renal compromise (Budde 2023). Anxiolytics work best before patient arousal, so pre-visit pharmaceuticals are more effective than giving medication when the pet is already in the hospital (Rodan 2022). However, just because it might be less effective does not mean that anxiolytics should be avoided. It reaches peak effect 2–3 hours after administration. Gabapentin has been shown to be a very effective anxiolytic in cats, over other drugs and supplements (Rodan 2022).

Pregabalin works very similarly to gabapentin in terms of action (Gaynor 2014). It is five times more potent than gabapentin. It should also be used with caution in renal patients, like gabapentin, and caution should be taken in pets with cardiac disease and respiratory impairment (Budde 2023). Pregabalin is approved by the Federal Drug Administration (FDA) in the United States for use for fear and anxiety associated with veterinary visits (Budde 2023).

Maropitant

Maropitant is an antiemetic that works as a neurokinin-1 (NK-1) receptor antagonist. It works by binding substance P so it cannot work on the NK-1 receptors, both centrally and peripherally. While being a powerful antinausea and antiemetic, it does not affect gastrointestinal (GI) transit times or gastric emptying. There is some research that shows it has MAC-sparing effects through the mediation of visceral pain. The injection can have some pain on the subcutaneous route, but it can be mitigated by refrigeration (Budde 2023). Nausea, while observable in cats and dogs, can be hard to associate with emotional distress in pets because that can be so subjective. However, there have been multiple reports in humans of antinausea medications reducing the need for postoperative pain control. In fact, there are studies suggesting a correlation between pain and nausea in humans (Johnson 2017). One of the biggest classes of pain medications used in small animal medicine is opioids, which are notorious for causing vomiting and nausea. Usage of an antinausea and antiemetic with these drugs can allow postoperative patients eat sooner and appear to return to normal sooner at home with their owners (Johnson 2017).

Ondansetron

Ondansetron is another commonly used antinausea medication that is commonly used as it is more cost-effective than maropitant. It is a 5-HT3 receptor antagonist. These receptors are found peripherally on the ends of the vagus nerve and centrally in the chemoreceptor trigger zone, one of the centers in the brain that regulates nausea and vomiting (Budde 2023). In humans, it is approved as an antiemetic and antinausea for both postoperative and post-chemotherapy vomiting and nausea. However, in a study comparing maropitant and ondansetron specifically for the treatment of opioid-induced nausea, ondansetron was effective at reducing nausea but not vomiting (Burke 2022). Maropitant was more effective than ondansetron at relieving nausea and vomiting associated with anesthetic opioid usage (Burke 2022). While ondansetron is not as effective in that study, it is an effective antinausea and antiemetic in other situations (particularly with post-chemotherapy-induced nausea) and can be an effective option if maropitant is unavailable or cost-prohibitive (Budde 2023).

Trazodone

Trazodone is a serotonin antagonist (or reuptake inhibitor) – it antagonizes alpha-1 receptors. It can cause decreased blood pressure (Budde 2023). Trazodone is often used as a pre-visit pharmaceutical, as it is an anxiolytic. Pets taking trazodone are at a higher risk for serotonin syndrome. It is often given together with gabapentin. It should be used with caution in dogs with systemic diseases such as cardiac disease, hepatic disease, and renal disease (Budde 2023). It has not been studied as extensively in cats as in dogs, but it appears to have minimal cardiovascular effects in cats (Rodan 2022). It is often used as part of or as an adjunct to the "Chill Protocol" (Budde 2023).

Benzodiazepines

Benzodiazepines do have their place in anesthetic protocols as excellent anxiolytics (Budde 2023). They also provide good muscle relaxation. However, there is not enough research on them as pre-visit pharmaceuticals for reduced FAS associated with veterinary visits. Often, benzodiazepines, such as midazolam, can cause a refractory excitatory phase, especially in cats, which makes them less than ideal for sedation (Rodan 2022). They can cause disinhibition and repulsion behaviors in cats, often increasing FAS scores in cats (Rodan 2022).

Acepromazine

Acepromazine is a phenothiazine that is available in oral and injectable formats. While it is excellent purely as a sedative, it has no anxiolytic effects (Budde 2023). In cats, it can also cause disinhibition and repulsion behaviors in cats, making the situation worse rather than helping (Rodan 2022). Acepromazine can be helpful in conjunction with other anxiolytics for the purpose of sedation, but otherwise, it is not going to help much with FAS management (Rodan 2022).

Drug	Suggested dosing	Routes	Uses
Acetaminophen	10–15 mg/kg PO, IV q 8 hr, possibly up to 10–20 mg/kg q 6 hr	IV, PO	Pain, antipyretic
Gabapentin	**Canine:** **Pain:** 10–20 mg/kg PO q 8 hr **Anxiolytic:** 25–30 mg/kg, 50 mg/kg PO 90–120 min prior to stress. In addition to other drugs, it can range from 10 to 25 mg/kg PO night before and 2 hr prior to stress. **Feline:** **Pain:** 5–10 mg/kg PO q 8–12 hr. **Anxiolytic:** 10 mg/kg PO q 12 hr, 20–35 mg/kg PO 2 hr prior to 10 mg/kg PO	PO	Neuropathic pain, hyperesthesia, allodynia, anxiolytic
Pregabalin	**Canine:** **Pain:** 2–5 mg/kg PO q 8–12 hr **Feline:** **Pain:** 1–3 mg/kg PO q 8–12 hr **Anxiolytic:** 5 mg/kg PO 90 min prior to stress, can be given 2 d in a row	PO	Neuropathic pain, hyperesthesia, allodynia, anxiolytic
Maropitant	**Canine:** 1 mg/kg PO, IV, SC q 24 hr 2 mg/kg PO q 24 hr for nausea from chemo **Feline:** 1 mg/kg PO, IV, SC q 24 hr	IV, SC, PO	Antinausea, antiemetic
Ondansetron	**Canine:** 0.3–1 mg/kg IV, PO q 8–12 hr **Feline:** 0.5–1 mg/kg PO, SC, IM, IV q 8 hr	IV, PO	Antiemetic, antinausea when associated with chemotherapy
Trazodone	**Canine:** doses from 5 to 10 mg/kg PO 90–120 min prior to stress Can be given 3–7 mg/kg PO q 8–12 hr for sedation/anxiety in hospital or postop **Feline:** 5 mg/kg PO added to gabapentin dosage 120 min prior to stress Has to be dosed 50–100 mg/CAT PO 60–90 min prior to stress as a single agent.	PO	Sedative, anxiolytic
Midazolam	**Canine:** 0.1–0.5 mg/kg IV, 0.2–0.5 mg/kg IM **Feline:** 0.1–0.5 mg/kg IV, 0.2 mg/kg–0.5 mg/kg IM **Antiseizure:** 0.2 mg/kg IV, PO, rectal, intranasal	IV, IM	Anxiolytic for anesthesia, antiseizure

(*Continued*)

Drug	Suggested dosing	Routes	Uses
Diazepam	**Canine:** 0.1–0.5 mg/kg IV, recommended to use with multimodal to reduce dosages. **Anxiolytic:** 0.5–2 mg/kg PO 30–60 min prior to stress **Feline:** 0.1–0.3 mg/kg IV Oral diazepam not recommended in cats.	IV, PO	Anxiolytic for anesthesia, antiseizure
Acepromazine	**Canine:** 0.01–1 mg/kg IV, IM, SC generally as a single dose **Max dose:** 2–3 mg/dog **Oral:** 0.55–2.2 mg/kg PO q 6–8 hr 0.025–0.05 mg/kg of injectable solution OTM 30 min prior to stress as part of "chill protocol" **Feline:** 0.01–1 mg/kg IV, IM, SC generally as a single dose **Max dose:** 1 mg/cat 0.05–0.1 mg/kg of injectable solution OTM 30–60 min prior to stress as part of "chill protocol"	IV, IM, SC, PO	Sedative, NOT anxiolytic

Your local emergency room (ER) will thank you for giving appropriate medications to your patients before you transfer. Control the nausea. Control pain. If the only options for pain control at your clinic are not sufficient for the level of pain experienced by the patient, please reach out to the hospital the patient will be transferring to and ask them directly what they recommend, given your available options.

Works Cited

Budde, J.A. (2023). *Plumb's Veterinary Drug Handbook*. St. Louis, Missouri: Wiley-Blackwell.

Burke, J.H. (2022). Effectiveness of orally administered maropitant and ondansetron in preventing preoperative emesis and nausea in healthy dogs premedicated with a combination of hydromorphone, acepromazine, and glycopyrrolate. *Journal of the American Veterinary Medical Association* 260 (S1): S40–S45. https://doi.org/10.2460/javma.21.02.0082.

Carmack, T. (2023). Advanced pain management protocols in veterinary hospice and palliative care. *dvm360*. Retrieved from www.dvm360.com/view/advanced-pain-management-protocols-in-veterinary-hospice-and-palliative-care

Gaynor, J.A. (2014). *Handbook of Veterinary Pain Management*. St. Louis, Missouri: Mosby.

Johnson, C. (2017). Fear, stress, and pain - what about nausea? *dvm360*. Retrieved from www.dvm360.com/view/fear-stress-and-pain-what-about-nausea

Rodan, I.D. (2022). 2022 AAFP/ISFM cat friendly veterinary interaction guidelines: approach and handling techniques. *Journal of Feline Medicine and Surgery* 24 (11): 1093–1132. https://doi.org/10.1177/1098612x221128760.

Tabor, B. (2016). Pain recognition and management in critical care patients. *Today's Veterinary Nurse*. Retrieved from todaysveterinarynurse.com/emergency-medicine-critical-care/pain-recognition-and-management-in-critical-care-patients

7

I Can't Pee! – The Blocked Cat

Puja Wright

BluePearl Pet Hospital, 1 Taft Ct., Rockville, MD, USA

What do you do when a cat presents to your clinic for a possible urinary tract obstruction? What would it look like? Is this something that can be handled by your clinic, or does it immediately need to make its way to an emergency clinic?

As most veterinary professionals who have been in the field for any length of time can tell anyone, the urinary obstruction cat tends to skew largely male. The feline male anatomy lends itself to easy obstruction, as they have a long narrow urethra in comparison to female cats (Cléroux 2023). The urethra in males also tends to narrow further along its length as it gets to the distal end of the penis. This is where most obstructions tend to get stuck. Obstructions in cats can consist of urinary stones or crystals, urethral plugs, neoplasia, and stricture (the last two are less common). Muscle spasms, as well as edema in the urethra, have been suggested as secondary factors to urinary obstruction (Pratt 2020). Critical patients often present with severe azotemia, hypotension with decreased tissue perfusion due to hypovolemia, metabolic disturbances, and associated venous dilation from backup of urine filtration from the kidneys and the associated decreased cardiac output (Cléroux 2023).

Presentation

When examined, the classic sign is a palpable, firm bladder that could be enlarged. A urinary obstruction cannot be ruled out just because there is no palpable urinary bladder, as these patients can occasionally present with a ruptured bladder. Additionally, their body temperature can range from hypothermia to hyperthermia, while their heart rate ranges from bradycardic to tachycardic. They can also be tachypneic, depressed, or comatose; dehydrated with tacky, pale mucous membranes; skin tenting; prolonged capillary refill times; and halitosis (O'Brien 2014; Plunkett 2000). Some cats will have been overgrooming the preputial area, which can make the area and the penis look edematous, hyperemic, cyanotic, or necrotic, depending on how long it has been (Plunkett 2000).

A certain number of diagnostics need to be run to evaluate the state that the patient is in. Bloodwork includes a packed cell volume/total solids (PCV/TS), a blood urea nitrogen (BUN) from an Azostick or serum BUN/creatinine, electrolyte levels, a serum glucose, and venous blood gas (Plunkett 2000). Urinary obstruction is the most common cause of acute kidney injury in cats. This can lead to azotemia, which only shows up on bloodwork once less than 25% of the renal tubules

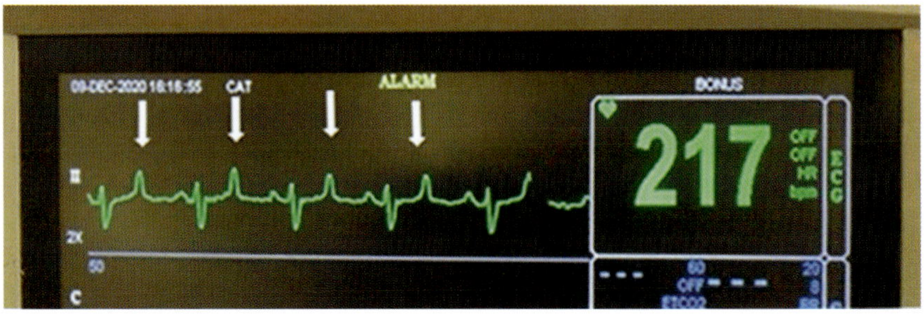

Image 7.1 Photo of an ECG showing increased T wave amplitude (white arrows). *Source:* Photo courtesy of Simone Conwell, RVT, VTS (ECC).

have normal perfusion (Cléroux 2023). BUN will show increased urea nitrogen levels that would indicate azotemia. A PCV and TS help pinpoint how dehydrated the obstructed patient may be. If the patient is unable to urinate for extended periods of time, the body loses its thirst response in an attempt at compensation. Commonly, metabolic acidosis will be found on venous blood gas. The inability of the body to remove the accumulated hydrogen ions in the body via the kidneys due to renal injury causes the pH of the blood to rise and cause an acidosis (Randels-Thorp 2017). Other bloodwork, such as a full blood chemistry and complete blood count, can also help determine the severity of the patient's disease. A urinalysis can also help determine if crystalluria is present as well as infection (O'Brien 2014). However, bacterial infections are rarely involved with urinary obstructions (UO) in cats (Cléroux 2023).

The dysfunction of the renal tubules can lead to electrolyte abnormalities, like a buildup of potassium in the system, or hyperkalemia (Plunkett 2000). This is dangerous, as it can lead to cardiac arrhythmias along with poor perfusion (Plunkett 2000). Hyperkalemia needs to be corrected before cardiac arrhythmias can become fatal. An electrocardiogram (ECG) is necessary in these patients to determine if there is an arrhythmia present. Mild elevations in serum potassium can cause the T-wave in the ECG tracing to have an increased amplitude and be narrower. The QT interval can be shortened as well (Cléroux 2023) (Image 7.1). With more moderate hyperkalemia, the ECG can have a prolonged PR interval with a decreased amplitude in the P waves and a widened QRS complex. With patients with severe hyperkalemia, the P wave can be completely absent (atrial standstill) and bradycardia. This can worsen to the QRS complex merging with the T-wave, a sine wave ECG, as well as ventricular fibrillation and ventricular asystole (Cléroux 2023).

Further diagnostics can include urine culture and sensitivity, abdominal radiographs, and abdominal ultrasound (O'Brien 2014). Abdominal radiographs can confirm the presence of radiopaque uroliths, as well as display if the urinary bladder is still intact. Abdominal ultrasound can also help visualize uroliths, especially radiolucent ones. Contrast cystogram and/or urethrogram studies with radiography can also show if the urinary bladder and urethra are intact. These can be negative, done with air, or positive, performed with contrast. Contrast radiographs are generally only done after urinary obstruction is relieved, as a urethral catheter needs to be in place to do a study (O'Brien 2014).

Stabilization

Treatment to relieve the obstruction is the most definitive way to prevent further damage to the patient. The prognosis for a cat with a urethral obstruction can be good to grave, dependent on the presence or absence of hematuria, vomiting, hypothermia, depression, azotemia, and arrhythmias

(Plunkett 2000). Conversations with the clients deciding what type of treatment to pursue should include not just prognosis, current diagnostics and treatments needed, and associated costs, but also the fact that most of these felines need additional lifelong care of varying degrees – whether that looks like just a prescription diet or additional episodes of urinary obstruction and future surgeries.

Furthermore, electrolyte, fluid, and acid/base abnormalities need to be fixed as a first step (Cléroux 2023). The order of treatment is determined by the patient's clinical signs, presence of arrhythmias, and bladder distention. One of the first items needed for these patients is at least one intravenous (IV) catheter, as this will need to be used for treatment of the patient's fluid and metabolic abnormalities, as well as administration of sedation or anesthesia used to unblock the patient.

Fluid imbalances should be treated based on an assessment of dehydration status. If there is no heart murmur or gallop rhythm present on auscultation and examination, then a 10 ml/kg fluid bolus of isotonic fluids is recommended if poor perfusion is found, with continuation of IV fluids afterward until urinary de-obstruction (Cléroux 2023). However, care needs to be taken to regularly reevaluate the patient to make sure there is not a development of a new heart murmur or gallop rhythm to aid in the prevention of fluid overload, especially if there is a delay in returning the patient to normal urine flow (Cosford 2020).

Metabolic imbalances need to be corrected as soon as possible. Hyperkalemia can be treated with regular insulin given IV. Insulin given IV can help shift potassium ions from the bloodstream to the intracellular space, to relieve the load of extra potassium in the bloodstream that can lead to cardiac arrhythmias. Too little or too much potassium can disturb the normal electrical activity of the heart. It is recommended to add IV dextrose to patients' fluids in addition to the insulin administration to keep the patient from developing hypoglycemia from the insulin dose.

Administering a dose of IV insulin will last about 4–6 hours to treat hyperkalemia (Cléroux 2023). Dextrose administration alone in a nondiabetic animal will also help potassium ions move intracellularly. Another treatment to move excess potassium to the intracellular compartment is the administration of sodium bicarbonate IV. The effects of this drug can last up to 2 hours (Cléroux 2023).

If a patient is having severe cardiac arrhythmias due to hyperkalemia, a 10% calcium gluconate IV bolus given slowly over 10 minutes can be used to quickly undo the electrical changes to the heart (Budde 2023). A common misconception is that calcium gluconate is affecting the hyperkalemia; it is reinforcing the myocytes and is a cardiovascular protectant (Plunkett 2000). The effect can last 10–15 minutes, and it is imperative to have ECG monitoring on the patient while administering the calcium gluconate to ensure the medication is not working too quickly (Plunkett 2000). On ECG tracing, this could look like a prolonged PR interval, widening of the QRS complex, shortening of the QT interval, shortening or absence of the ST segment, as well as a widening T wave. These can progress to bradycardia and complete heart block, asystole, or, conversely, to ventricular fibrillation; either way, cardiac arrest occurs quickly (Cléroux 2023).

With any treatment to correct metabolic imbalances, repeated blood gases are indicated to monitor the effects of the treatments and metabolic status, as treatment of electrolyte and acid/base derangements can easily tip in the opposite direction.

Further Treatment

Once any life-threatening metabolic and fluid abnormalities are corrected, the patient needs to be heavily sedated or fully anesthetized to pass a urinary catheter to "unblock" the urinary obstruction. Recommended protocols are often lacking adequate pain control for these patients based on the assumption that it may not be necessary since the patient is presenting laterally or comatose to begin with. However, without adequate pain control, there is the likelihood that the urethra and patient will not have adequate muscle relaxation to make urethral catheterization as smooth, successful, and nontraumatic as possible (Plunkett 2000). In addition to pain medications, there are other drugs that may be more helpful than others with the muscle relaxation they offer, as well as local anesthetic techniques that can minimize the effects of the drugs on the whole patient.

This can be helpful, especially in critical patients where systemic drugs may be limited due to the status of the patient.

Care needs to be taken with any drugs given to the cat with a urinary obstruction; these patients are often azotemic, which can cause changes in the blood–brain barrier permeability, which would cause drug dosages to affect patients more than normal (Steagall 2018). As such, dosages should be reduced to avoid unwanted effects from overdoses.

Benzodiazepines, such as midazolam, diazepam, and zolazepam, are often used in urethral obstruction cats as a sedative or anesthetic agent. It is important to note that benzodiazepines have no analgesic effects. Many emergency technicians have a visceral reaction to giving a cat midazolam because it can cause excitatory behaviors, increasing aggression in cats that are already stressed. However, benzodiazepines do have an anxiolytic effect on the nervous system, as well as having minimal effects on the cardiovascular system. In addition, this class of drugs produces skeletal muscle relaxation (which is a type of muscle present in the distal feline male urethra) by working in the central nervous system (Steagall 2018; Wiese 2018). Benzodiazepines are also well tolerated by patients with renal compromise, such as acute kidney injury (Schroeder 2015). Diazepam is hydrophobic, making it not very effective with intramuscular injection (Budde 2023). Diazepam, while hepatically metabolized, is renally excreted, which can make the effects of diazepam longer lasting in cats with lessened renal function (Budde 2023). Midazolam can be given intravenously as well as intramuscularly, with less hepatic side effects in cats with repeat doses, making it the benzodiazepine of choice for cats (Steagall 2018). Zolazepam is available in some countries as part of a combination drug with tiletamine; however, since tiletamine is renally

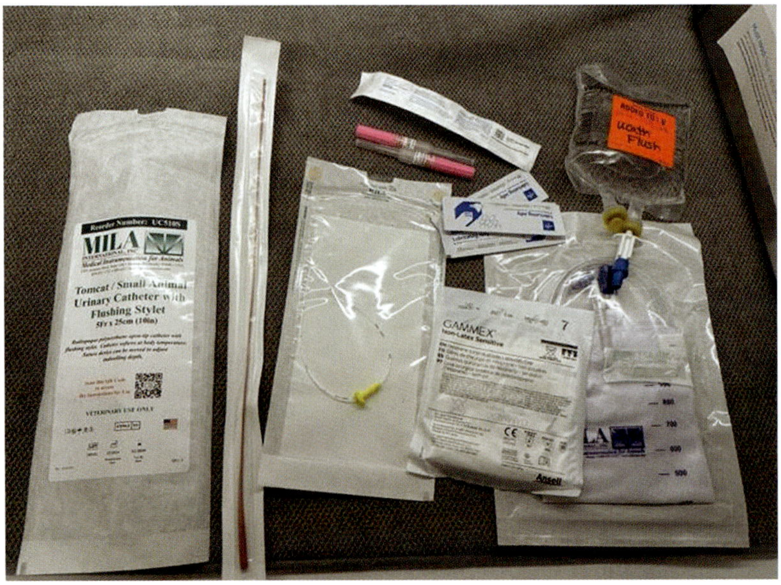

Image 7.2 Set up for a urethral catheterization with sterile flush, sterile gloves, sterile lube, sterile catheters, and a sterile urinary collection bag. *Source:* Photo courtesy of Simone Conwell, RVT, VTS (ECC).

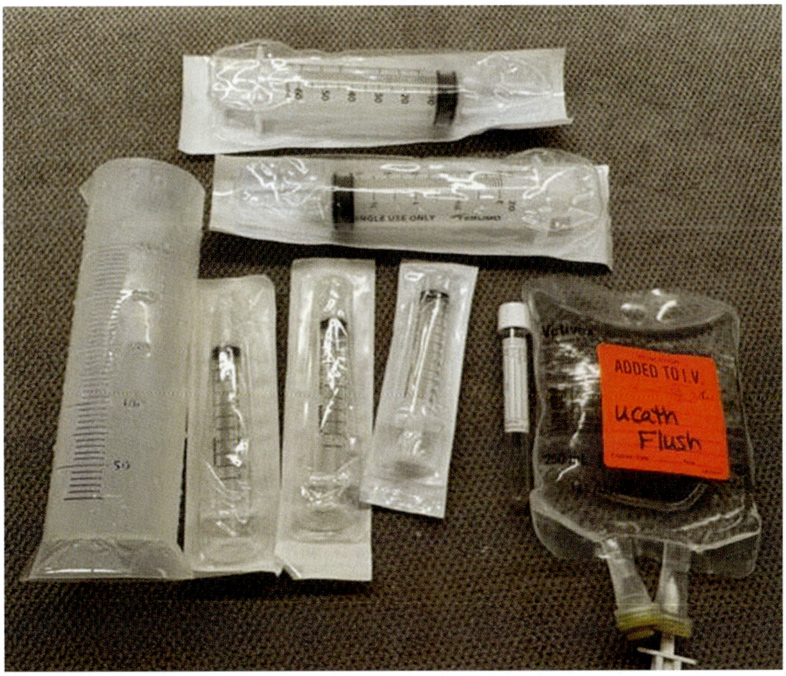

Image 7.3 A white top tube for sample collection, a variety of catheters, and a graduated cylinder to quantify urine removed during unblocking. *Source:* Photo courtesy of Simone Conwell, RVT, VTS (ECC).

excreted, telazol is not recommended in felines with renal compromise or felines with cardiac dysfunction, such as the UO patient (Zoetis 2022).

Sedatives such as alpha-2 agonists, like dexmedetomidine, should be avoided in patients with current urinary obstruction as well. Alpha-1 agonists can inhibit insulin release, causing an elevated blood glucose level, and can inhibit antidiuretic hormone, both of which can cause increased urine production (Schroeder 2015; Steagall 2018). In a currently blocked cat, adding more urine to the already stressed bladder could lead to bladder rupture. In addition, UO cats are often cardiovascularly unstable, so a drug that causes increased cardiovascular load would not be ideal.

Phenothiazines, such as acepromazine, can work well for sedation. Acepromazine can cause smooth muscle relaxation; however, this would likely be unhelpful in unblocking a male cat, as the distal urethra (post-prostate) is comprised of striated muscle (Steagall 2018). Acepromazine is also a poor anxiolytic drug, having purely sedative effects instead. It also has a high potential for causing vasodilation and hypotension. These effects make it a poor choice in patients where cardiovascular status is questionable, as well as in cases where preserving adequate blood pressure to preserve ideal renal blood flow is imperative.

Opioids are the pain medication of choice for urinary obstruction cases. Specifically pure-mu agonists should be used to provide adequate analgesia for the visceral and somatic components of pain for UO patients. Pure-mu or full-mu agonists should be considered first for the level of pain seen in UO patients, especially since these patients may need surgery for a cystotomy or perineal urethrostomy (PU) soon after hospitalization. Oftentimes, a pure-mu agonist given to a sick patient can cause a level of sedation as well (Steagall 2018). Full-mu opioids to consider include morphine, hydromorphone, methadone, and fentanyl. Full-mu agonists tend to be relatively hemodynamically stable; while they can cause some increase in vagal tone and subsequent bradycardia, there is very little change in vascular resistance. This makes the side effects easier to treat, like an anticholinergic to treat increased vagal tone (Steagall 2018). Other opioids, such as buprenorphine, which is a partial mu agonist, should only be used if a full-mu agonist is unavailable, as the analgesia provided is weaker. Kappa agonists like butorphanol should not be used as pain control in UO patients, as they primarily only provide sedation, with some possible level of visceral pain control (Steagall 2018).

Local anesthesia for the UO cat is the sacrococcygeal epidural, also called a caudal epidural or coccygeal block. This technique is relatively available to most clinics as it does not require any specific instrumentation, simply the knowledge on how one is performed, unlike regular epidurals. The caudal epidural can be performed with a local anesthetic, such as lidocaine or bupivacaine. An opioid like morphine can be added as well to the mix. The sacrococcygeal block covers the nerves of the tail, perineum, rectum, penis, and urethra, making it ideal to help relax and provide analgesic coverage for unblocking a cat (Pratt 2020). In a study comparing the effectiveness of bupivacaine or bupivacaine and morphine caudal epidural usage to no epidural in relieving urethral obstruction in cats, the groups that received caudal epidurals needed roughly half the propofol required for the non-epidural group when unblocking the cats (Pratt 2020) (Images 7.4–7.7).

Generally, nonsteroidal anti-inflammatories should be avoided in UO felines, as they often present with concurrent renal injury (Budde 2023).

If anesthesia is to be induced, there are several options available. Propofol is a widely available and used single-drug induction agent. It can be combined with benzodiazepine for a co-induction to decrease the volume of propofol used and try to limit the cardiovascular depression and vasodilation seen with propofol boluses. If vasodilation and resultant hypotension are limited and managed appropriately, propofol is well tolerated in patients with renal compromise, which makes it a good choice for UO patients (Budde 2023). Cardiovascular depression can be more pronounced in hypovolemic patients, which some UO patients are (Steagall 2018). Propofol can cause significant respiratory depression as well, which makes preoxygenation and being ready to intubate very important when using this drug (Budde 2023).

Alfaxalone is another single-agent induction agent that is gaining more popularity. It can also cause dose-dependent cardiovascular depression, which can be mitigated with a co-induction such as a benzodiazepine (Budde 2023). There is some dose-dependent respiratory depression noted as well, though it is generally less severe than what is seen with propofol (Budde 2023). If repeat doses

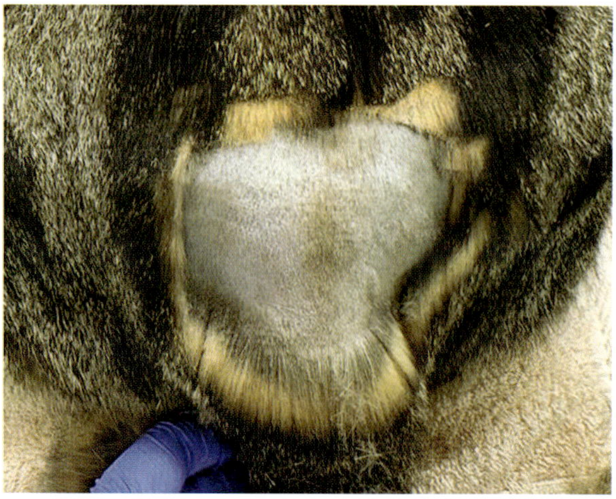

Image 7.4 The sacrococcygeal space can be found by pumping the tail up and down while palpating for the intervertebral space in between the cranial vertebra that is still and the caudal vertebra that is moving. *Source:* Photo courtesy of Simone Conwell, RVT, VTS (ECC).

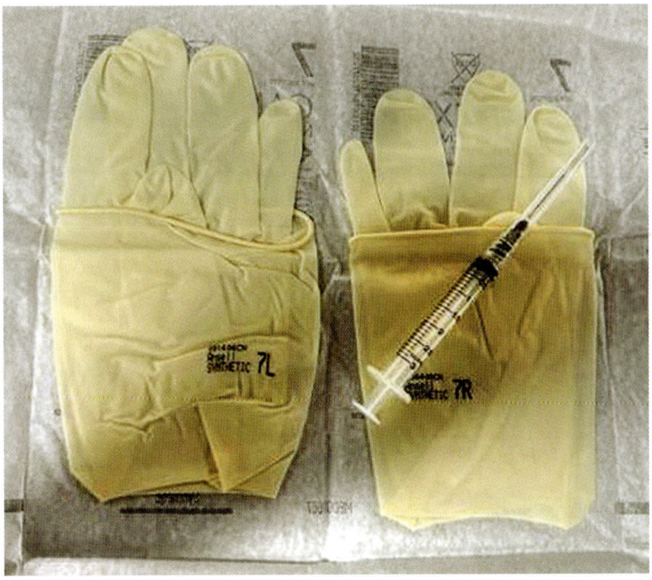

Image 7.5 Sterile gloves and a sterile syringe with a 25 g (or 22 g, depending on patient size) needle are the only tools that are needed. *Source:* Photo courtesy of Simone Conwell, RVT, VTS (ECC).

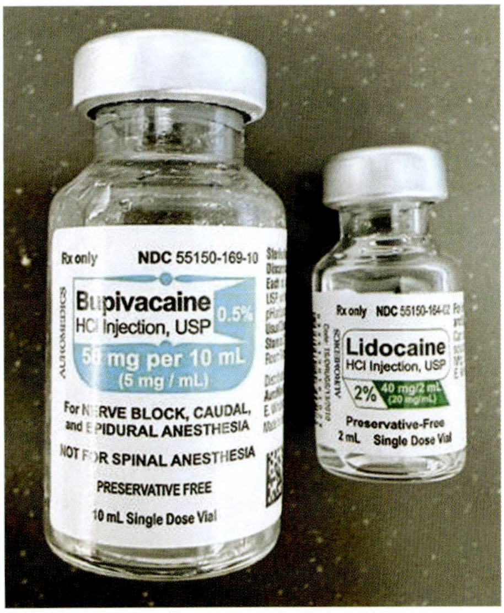

Image 7.6 Example of preservative-free local anesthetics that can be used for sacrococcygeal epidurals. *Source:* Image courtesy of Puja Wright, RVT.

or total intravenous anesthesia is required, alfaxalone is preferable over propofol in cats to avoid dose-dependent Heinz body formation in red blood cells (Steagall 2018).

Dissociative anesthetics, like ketamine and tiletamine, are not ideal induction agents in UO felines. While N-methyl-D-aspartate (NMDA) antagonists can have some analgesic effects, especially when used in conjunction with opioids, they do not cause muscle relaxation (can cause muscle rigidity in some cases), can increase cardiovascular load, are excreted by the kidneys, and work by causing catecholamine release in the body (Steagall 2018). In healthy animals, catecholamine release can be beneficial by boosting heart rate and blood pressure, but in sick animals,

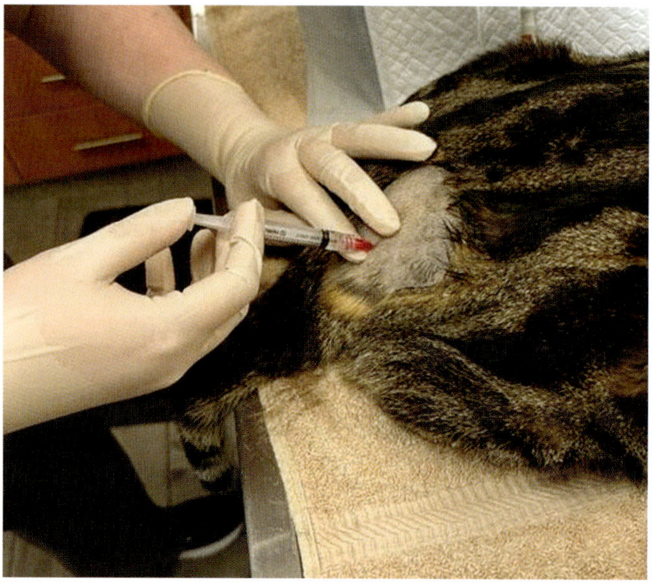

Image 7.7 Example of a sacrococcygeal epidural being performed with a 25 g needle. *Source:* Photo courtesy of Simone Conwell, RVT, VTS (ECC).

endogenous catecholamines will already be low. By causing this release in an already stressed system, instead of the positive inotropic effect that is helpful, it can have a negative inotropic effect (Budde 2023).

Etomidate can be considered as an induction agent that is friendlier to the cardiovascular system, as it causes less cardiovascular and respiratory depression (Budde 2023). However, it is primarily excreted by the renal system and should be avoided in felines with renal disease (Steagall 2018).

Once a cat is adequately pain-controlled and sedated or anesthetized, a rigid urethral catheter needs to be passed through the penis and urethra, into the urinary bladder to break up any obstruction to urine flow (Images 7.2 and 7.3). Aseptic technique needs to be used to prevent any iatrogenic introduction of infection into the compromised urinary tract (Cléroux 2023). The penis is extracted and massaged to relieve any possible mucus plug at the tip. A lubricated rigid Tom Cat catheter can be used. If that is not rigid enough to pass, an ophthalmic lacrimal duct cannula or olive tip catheter can be used to reestablish urine flow (Plunkett 2000). If obstruction is relieved, a softer, sterile, indwelling urinary catheter needs to be placed, such as a red rubber urinary catheter or a Foley catheter (Cléroux 2023). A rigid polypropylene Tom cat catheter left in place can lead to compromise of the bladder wall via trauma to already fragile tissues (Cléroux 2023). However, MILA has a Tom Cat catheter that can be left in place for up to 3 days, as it is rigid at room temperature and becomes pliable at body temperature (MILA n.d.). This should be secured in place with sutures around the sheath of the penis and then attached to a sterile urine collection system. The line of the urine collection system should be secured at the tail of the patient as well to prevent further trauma to the penis if excessive tension is applied to the line. An Elizabethan collar (e-collar) needs to be used in conjunction with an indwelling urinary catheter to prevent self-traumatization (Cléroux 2023) (Images 7.8 and 7.9).

There is some evidence that points to a smaller urinary catheter size, leading to less chances of re-obstruction when the pet's urinary catheter is pulled. The theory is that the smaller urinary catheter size causes less traumatization to the urethral walls, leading to less inflammation and lesser narrowing of the urethra from inflammation (Cosford 2020). The indwelling MILA Tom Cat

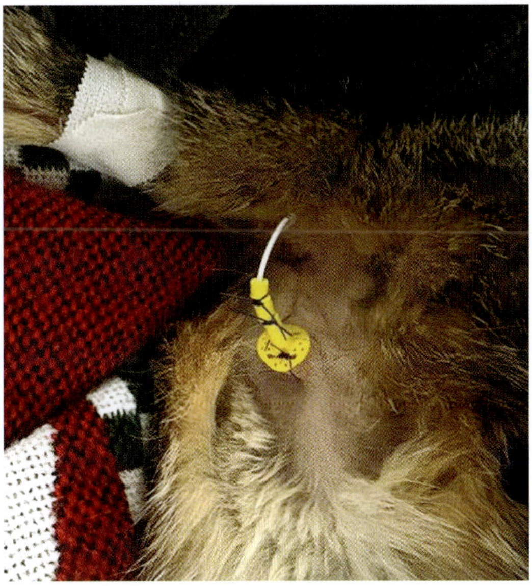

Image 7.8 Urinary catheter anchored to the prepuce, and the anchor is cinched down to prevent slippage from the penis. *Source:* Photo courtesy of Simone Conwell, RVT, VTS (ECC).

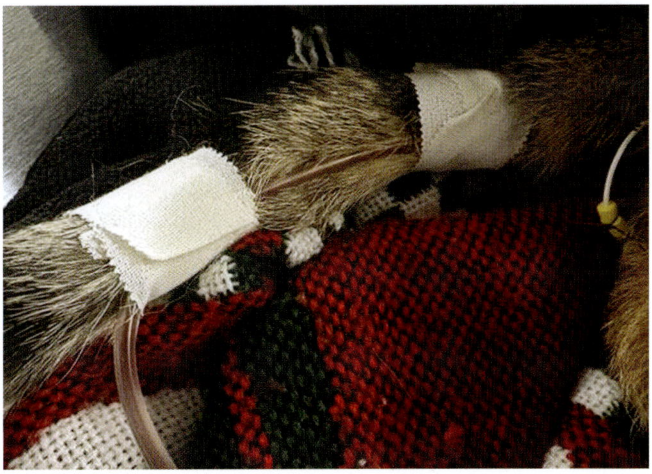

Image 7.9 Tension loops of the line connecting the urinary catheter to the urine collection bag are placed on the cats tail to avoid causing trauma to the penis. *Source:* Photo courtesy of Simone Conwell, RVT, VTS (ECC).

catheter works on a similar theory that by using one urinary catheter to unblock and stay in the cat, there is less trauma to the urethra from re-catheterization (MILA n.d.).

In the case that a urinary catheter cannot be passed and urethral obstruction cannot be relieved to reestablish urine flow, a decompressive cystocentesis should be performed to relieve pressure on the bladder wall (Plunkett 2000). Repeated cystocentesis is not recommended due to the increased risk of bladder rupture and uroabdomen. If a patent urethral catheter cannot be achieved, a cystotomy tube of some sort needs to be inserted to have a way of repeated bladder evacuation until a urethral catheter can be placed, while lowering the risks of multiple cystocentesis (Cléroux 2023).

If there is concern for urethral rupture with traumatic urinary catheterization, a contrast study with positive contrast can be done to check for urethral latency. While usually done with fluoroscopy, it can be done with serial radiography as well to make it more accessible to facilities without access to fluoroscopy. Iodine contrast, diluted with saline, can be given via the urethral catheter in small aliquots between radiographs to see if it is in the bladder and as the catheter is pulled out normograde in small amounts. The radiographs should highlight if the contrast goes outside the urethra, which would indicate a urethral tear. If a urethral tear is present, treatment is determined by the severity of the tear and the ability to pass a catheter into the bladder. If a urethral catheter can be placed into the bladder despite the tear, the catheter can be kept in place to drain the bladder and give the urethra time to heal (Cléroux 2023). If a urinary catheter cannot be passed into the bladder, then a cystotomy catheter can be placed to try to relieve the bladder. However, surgical correction may be required in cases of complete or extensive tearing of the urethra with little to no resolution with indwelling urinary catheterization (Cléroux 2023).

Once a urinary catheter is in place and urine flow is reestablished, urine output needs to be monitored on an hourly basis, as well as monitoring the fluids going into the patient; this is generally referred to as checking "ins and outs" on the intensive care unit (ICU) floor. This is generally why hospitalization is recommended even in the most stable of urinary obstruction patients (Cléroux 2023). These patients need to be sent home with appropriate recommendations for dietary and environmental changes to prevent further episodes of urinary obstruction in the future.

Recurrence rates in cats with urinary obstruction range from 15% to 40% (Cléroux 2023). Perineal urethrostomy is often recommended in male cats that have repeated urinary obstructions despite medical management (Cléroux 2023).

In patients where hospitalization may not be a viable financial option, sedation with a one-time urethral catheterization to relieve the obstruction with outpatient care may work in some patients (Cléroux 2023). However, there are studies that suggest higher rates of recurrence of urinary obstruction in cats with outpatient therapy, which implies that these treatment options should be considered only when hospitalization is not possible (Cosford 2020). When considering this route of therapy, there should be a very frank conversation with the client about the possibility of re-obstruction, so they are prepared to take the cat in for further, more extensive care if necessary.

If diagnostics show the presence of uroliths, the cat will generally need to be hospitalized with a urinary catheter in place to prevent re-obstruction until a cystotomy can be performed to remove the uroliths. In repeat offenders, a perineal urethrostomy should be considered along with cystotomy. This surgery removes the penis and creates a new urethral opening in the perineum. Ideally, this new opening is larger, removing the narrowing of the urethra in the penis that tends to be where male cats get blocked. There is a risk of urethral stricture causing an obstruction postoperatively; however, the risk is minimized when done by an experienced surgeon, avoiding postoperative catheterization, and keeping the patient from self-traumatizing (Milgram 2016). There is a higher reported risk of urinary tract infections after PU surgery as well (Milgram 2016).

Works Cited

Budde, J.A. (2023). *Plumb's Veterinary Drug Handbook*. Wiley-Blackwell.

Cléroux, A. (2023). Urologic emergencies: ureters, bladder, urethra, GN, and CKD. In: *Feline Emergency and Critical Care Medicine* (ed. K. Drobatz), 223–242. Hoboken, NJ: John Wiley & Sons Inc.

Cosford, K.A. (2020). In-hospital medical management of feline urethral obstruction: a review of recent clinical research. *The Canadian Veterinary Journal* 61 (6): 595. Retrieved from http://pmc.ncbi.nlm.nih.gov/articles/PMC7236633.

MILA. (n.d.). MILA Urinary Catheters for Cats [Format - Pdf Instructions]. Retrieved from www.milainternational.com: www.milainternational.com/pub/media.wysiwyg/pdf/urinary_catheters_for_cats.pdf

Milgram, J. (2016). Feline perineal urethrostomy. In: *Complications in Small Animal Surgery* (ed. D.A. Griffon), 500–503. Ames: John Wiley & Sons, Inc.

O'Brien, M. (2014). Renal and urinary emergencies. In: *Handbook of Canine and Feline Emergency Protocols* (ed. M. McMichael), 189–195. Ames, Iowa: Wiley.

Plunkett, S. (2000). Urogenital and reproductive emergencies. In: *Emergency Procedures for the Small Animal Veterinarian* (ed. S. Plunkett), 211–248. St. Louis, Missouri: Elsevier.

Pratt, C.E. (2020). A prospective randomized, double-blinded clinical study evaluating the efficacy and safety of bupivacaine versus morphine-bupivacaine in caudal epidurals in cats with urethral obstruction. *Journal of Veterinary Emergency and Critical Care* 30: 170–178. https://doi.org/10.1111/vec.12944.

Randels-Thorp, A.A. (2017). *Acid-Base and Electrolyte Handbook for Veterinary Technicians*. Ames, Iowa: John Wiley & Sons, Inc.

Schroeder, C. (2015). Renal disease. In: *Canine and Feline Anesthesia and Co-Existing Disease* (ed. L.A. Snyder), 116–128. Hoboken, NJ: Wiley-Blackwell.

Steagall, P.R. (2018). *Feline Anesthesia and Pain Management*. Hoboken, NJ: John Wiley & Sons, Inc.

Wiese, A. (2018). Sedation for cats with cardiovascular disease. *Today's Veterinary Practice*. Retrieved from https://todaysveterinarypractice.com/anesthesiology/sedation-for-cats-with-cardiovascular-disease

Zoetis. (2022). Telazol (Tiletamine and Zolazepam for Injection) [PDF of Package Insert]. Retrieved from www.zoetisus.com: www.zoetisus.com/content/_assets/docs/telazol_pi.pdf

8

Communicating and Supporting Clients While Supporting Yourself

Valerie Bogie[1,2,3,4,5]

[1] *Insight Animal Behavior Services, USA*
[2] *Valerie Bogie, LLC, USA*
[3] *National Empowerment Center, USA*
[4] *International Association of Veterinary Social Work, USA*
[5] *MSSW, Veterinary Social Worker, USA*

Communication with Clients During High Stress Times

Veterinary technicians in an emergency and critical care setting often meet pet parents for the first time on one of the worst days of that client's life. Their beloved animal is sick, so sick in fact, that they have opted for emergency services. Take a moment to think about the experience from the client's point of view. Maybe they have been observing the pet at home and recognize that the pet is struggling or in distress. Or they watched their animal get into a fight or get hit by a car. There is panic. The quick online searches to see where they can take their pet. There is fear. Driving to get to the emergency veterinary clinic, hoping the experts there can make everything okay. It is an overwhelming situation for any pet parent. One of the key components to supporting clients in emergency situations is to first understand the brain's response to stress.

Understanding the Human Stress Response

Humans, after all, are just large mammals. As a veterinary technician, there is an understanding of the stress response of the smaller patients. Too many triggers or stressful events in a short amount of time take the prefrontal cortex offline and send the animal into flight, fight, or freeze. Humans are wired in a similar way. "Functionally, it has been suggested that the emotional responses are of relevance for coping reactions to short-term aversive events and for the initiation of fight-flight-freezing reactions, which serve the subject to deal effectively with a source of danger and to return into a state of safety" (Steckler et al. 2005). Understanding that both the human client and pet patient are under large amounts of stress, which reduces the ability to problem-solve and regulate emotions, is key to being supportive as a staff member. It can be a helpful reminder that while the acute stress of their pet being ill contributes to the pet owner's stress response, individual differences such as genetic factors, physiological, developmental, and lifetime experience also contribute to how they are reacting (Steckler et al. 2005). There is no way to know these details when a client walks in with their pet, so it is imperative that every client is met with unconditional positive regard and kindness. A helpful model of the human brain states is Conscious Discipline's Brain State Model (2025), which clearly defines the key parts of the brain and how they respond to stress (Image 8.1). Typically, a pet owner bringing their ill

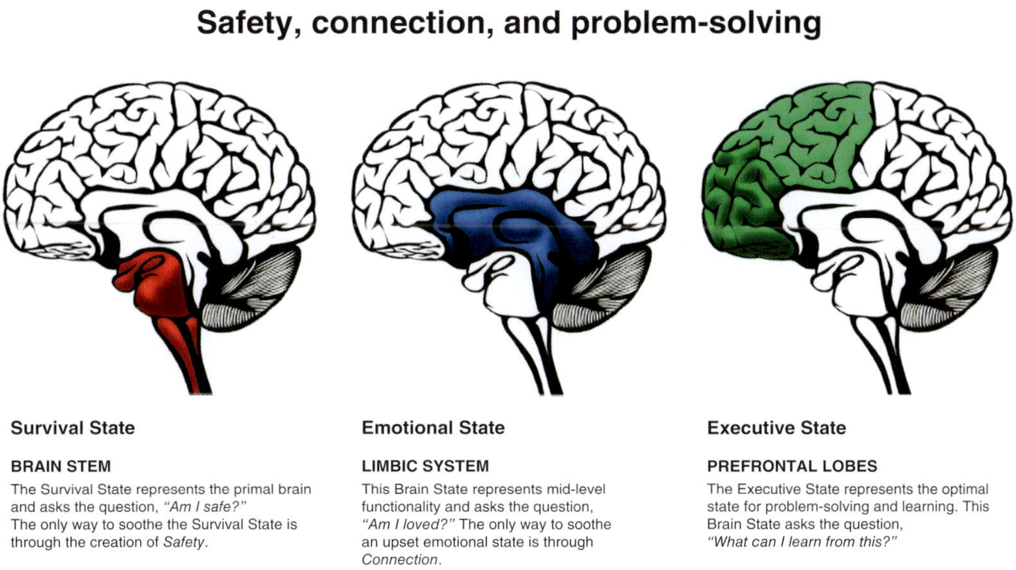

Image 8.1 Visualization of brain states and which parts of the brain are active in response to different types of stress – Conscious Discipline (2025).

pet to the emergency room is in the survival state. Note that with the prefrontal cortex offline, it is very difficult for them to problem solve, learn, and regulate their emotions.

Another advantage to an emergency room veterinary technician is to remember that brain states are contagious. If there is a very stressed-out client and the vet tech and staff are able to stay calm, that can actually help the client start to regulate their emotions more effectively. There are times that it can also go the opposite way, though. This can occur when the highly stressed brain of the client brings others around them up to a higher stressed state, so it is important to practice grounding and breathing techniques to reduce that possibility. There is a lot of research about unconscious emotional processing, meaning that as humans, we can view a facial expression and have our own emotional reaction from viewing it (Boggio et al. 2023). This also ties into co-regulation. Scientifically, the term coregulation is used "to capture the adaptation of partners in adjusting to each other's biology and behavior. Coregulation is defined as the continuously unfolding individual attributes and actions that are susceptible to being modified by the changing attributes and actions of a partner" (Bornstein and Esposito 2023).

Moral of the story? The pet parent is under a large amount of stress because their pet is sick, and therefore, their brain is unable to function as normal. There are actions that veterinary technicians and staff can take to support the human while caring for the patient.

Six ways to communicate effectively in high-stress situations

1) Provide visual aids or printouts to help explain common situations more effectively to a stressed-out client, such as what CPR entails.
2) If CPR is performed, it is ideal to have a staff member with the client to explain what is happening.
3) Pare down or disseminate the information being shared in smaller, more digestible pieces.
4) Be clear and concise when explaining diagnosis, prognosis, and potential outcomes of treatment.

5) It may be helpful to repeat the information in different ways and ask the client if they understand what is being shared.
6) This emergency has thrown time into hyperdrive, so try to slow things down for them. Take a big deep breath to subconsciously encourage them to take one as well.

Active Listening and Emotional CPR

Another way to help a stressed pet parent is to practice active listening. This can help them share their story and what has happened with their pet without being interrupted. Active listening is a skill that is typically only learned if the adults in our lives modeled it. The good news is that we can continue to build this skill no matter where we might be with it. Active listening might seem counterintuitive when working with a client who is coming to the emergency clinic in search of help and answers. The key is to incorporate active listening to build connection and trust with the client while you are caring for their pet.

Emotional CPR is a helpful evidence-based framework that teaches humans how to support another human going through an emotional crisis. The purpose of eCPR is "to assist another person through emotional distress by connecting through feelings first, respecting each other as equally human, enabling us to be together without fixing, judging, or imposing our beliefs, allowing us to explore the unknown together, in the present moment, releasing our power to create a new voice, new purpose, and new hope" (National Empowerment Center 2022, p. 3). The training focuses on three main points – Connection, emPowerment, and Revitalization (Image 8.2). By flowing in and out of these three areas, the resonator (person supporting the person in crisis) guides the person in crisis toward a more emotionally regulated state. The full certification is a 12-hour training course that can be completed online or in person. Check https://emotional-cpr.org/training/ for upcoming public trainings. The National Empowerment Center and the International Association of Veterinary Social Work sponsored the creation and RACE certification of a prerecorded 1-hour "Intro to Emotional CPR" workshop. At the time of publishing, the workshop was hosted by the National Empowerment Center on the Teachable platform: https://nationalempowermentcenter.teachable.com/p/emotional-cpr-connection-empowerment-revitalization-to-support-others (National Empowerment Center 2025).

What might this look like in real time? While the order of operations may differ depending on the severity of the patient's issue and patient's stability, here are two examples. Scenario #1: Mona, a 15 year old, female spayed, 9 pound chihuahua, got into a fight with another dog in the household. Mona's owner is visibly upset, speaking quickly and breathing heavily. Mona appears bright, alert, and responsive with broken skin around her left eye. Mona is content in her owner's arms. In this instance, you are able to allow Mona's owner to explain what happened and utilize Emotional CPR right away.

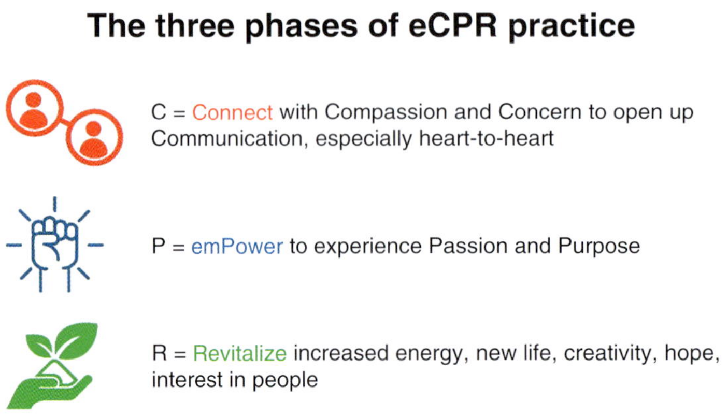

Image 8.2 Courtesy of National Empowerment Center (2022). Emotional CPR: Assisting People Through Emotional Crisis Participant Workbook.

You may ask a few clarifying questions for the patient record, but for most of the initial part of the conversation, Mona's owner is able to speak freely which builds connection. You then ask if she is ready to go over next steps with Mona's treatment plan. You can share potential outcomes to increase the owner's feelings of safety by reducing the fear of the unknown. As you speak clearly and breath deeply, you notice that Mona's owner also takes a deep breath and seems more calm. You can continue to utilize active listening throughout the visit to help empower Mona's owner to make decisions for Mona's care. This can help Mona's owner recover in the moment, moving towards revitalization. Note that the issue causing the emotional distress (Mona's bite wounds) does not need to be completely solved to transition to the other phases of eCPR. Scenario #2: Boopie, a 4 year old, male neutered, 12 pound cat, is brought in by a concerned owner. Boopie is lethargic, dehydrated, and the owner shared he has not eaten in 24 hours. The owner is not sure what could be causing Boopie's illness. The owner is visibly nervous- wringing his hands and pacing. You do a brief check and Boopie's gums are pale- time is of the essence. You ask a few more crucial questions then take Boopie for the team to start triaging. If there is another staff member available, they could sit with Boopie's owner and utilize Emotional CPR. Alternatively, you could return to the owner with an update, utilize eCPR, and gain additional details for the medical record. Because Boopie's condition was critical, patient care took precedence. Notice that in either scenario, even just 5 minutes of Emotional CPR can make a world of difference for a scared and stressed out pet parent.

Quality of Life and Euthanasia

The reality of a visit to an emergency veterinary clinic is that it may result in euthanasia. Asking the pet parents if they want life-saving measures performed on their pet can be the first of many difficult decisions they will have to make. In the stressed, survival brain state they are in, it can be challenging to make decisions due to the changes in brain function. "Although there are times when the decision may need to be made immediately, you usually will have some time to review the facts and discuss the situation with your family and friends, before deciding how to proceed" (American Veterinary Medicine Association (AVMA) 2025). This is another opportunity for veterinary technicians and staff to slow down and provide expertise to the client so they can make a fully informed decision.

Quality of Life Discussions

There are several Quality-of-Life scales that can be used to help collect objective data about the pet. These can provide a more concrete representation of the pet and help the owner navigate a discussion about their pet's quality of life and potential for euthanasia.

Quality of Life Scales

Focused on Physical Health

- Lap of Love (2025) https://www.lapoflove.com/how-will-i-know-it-is-time/lap-of-love-quality-of-life-scale.pdf
- Ohio State University Veterinary Medical Center (2024) https://vmc.vet.osu.edu/sites/default/files/documents/how-will-i-know_rev_mar2024ms_0.pdf
- HHHHHMM Scale (2024) https://awionline.org/awi-quarterly/summer-2019/quality-of-life-scale-for-aging-and-ailing-pets/

Focused on Behavioral Health

- Ohio State University Veterinary Medical Center (2024) https://vmc.vet.osu.edu/sites/default/files/documents/behavior-qol-scale-2024.pdf

It is also important to take the client's quality of life into consideration. If the pet could potentially go home but only with a very intense treatment plan that will be difficult to maintain, that needs to be taken into consideration. If the client has already been caring for the pet with a high level of physical and time-consuming care, that matters. Resources are not infinite, even for the most compassionate pet owner. Resources such as time, emotional bandwidth, physical ability, and finances can run out. Because of its significance, the topic of financial discussions has its own chapter (Chapter 20).

Caregiver Burden

ZBI

To help assess a client's stress levels and quality of life, a caregiver burden survey called the Zarit Burden Interview (ZBI) can be utilized. Spitznagel et al. first validated an 18-question version of the ZBI (originally created to measure burden when a human is caring for another human) for pet owners in 2017. While more thorough, this might not be as easy to administer in settings when time is of the essence with decision-making. In 2019, Spitznagel et al. validated an abbreviated seven-question ZBI to be used in assessing veterinary client caregiver burden.

> This brief, 7-item scale can easily be completed during an office visit, lending itself to use as a quick secondary outcome measure for clinical trials. It might also be of use in standard practice as a tool to facilitate client communications, as greater understanding of the client's experience while caring for a seriously ill companion animal could help the veterinarian better appreciate the client's perspective (Spitznagel et al. 2017).

The higher the score, the more burdened the client is. This can be used in conjunction with a quality-of-life scale for the pet to give the veterinary team a clearer picture of the well-being of the entire household.

When discussing the diagnosis and prognosis of the patient, it is imperative to be clear about the amount of time and physical effort the treatment plan will take. Brené Brown (2012) shared "Clear is kind," which applies to these situations perfectly. We already know that stress levels are high for the client, and they cannot problem-solve or absorb information as effectively as usual. Share details in layman's terms, and when possible, utilize visual aids and repeat the most important facts.

Euthanasia Decisions

Think again of the client's experience. Their emotions are swirling, their stress levels are high, and they have made the impossible decision to euthanize their pet. As long as the pet is stable, this can be another opportunity to give the client time and space to ask questions and process what is coming next. As the veterinary technician, be present and stay in the moment. While euthanasia is a daily occurrence in an emergency clinic, it is important to remember the gravity of the situation for the clients. It is helpful to gauge the needs of the client at that moment. It may be helpful for some to walk step by step through a handout together; others may need time to themselves before moving forward with the procedure. There are many resources to support these conversations.

Euthanasia Handout for Clients

- Animal Welfare Foundation (2013) https://www.animalwelfarefoundation.org.uk/wp-content/uploads/2017/06/Saying-Goodbye.pdf

Euthanasia Handout for Staff

- Lap of Love (Gardner & McVety 2016) https://todaysveterinarypractice.com/wp-content/uploads/sites/4/2016/05/TVP_2016-0102_PB_Euthanasia.pdf

In a study conducted to explore veterinarians' role for pet owners facing pet loss, Fernandez-Mehler et al. (2013) shared "The veterinarian has to fulfil in sequence the very different roles of first attempting to save the ill animal, to then convincing the client of euthanasia when a severely ill animal cannot be cured, and thereafter, to provide support to the client." This changing of roles can also occur for veterinary technicians. It is helpful to build awareness around this because this constant switching of roles can increase confusion and stress for the client.

Euthanasia Procedure

Pet parents hope for a peaceful passing, usually at their home or with their primary care vet-- not at the emergency clinic. This can be an additional layer to an already difficult situation- the owner is now grieving the pet they are about to lose as well as the loss of the option to euthanize their pet in the manner they hoped to. The 2013 Fernandez-Mehler et al. study found that "Of 1272 (owners) who had lost an animal by euthanasia, 1173 (92%) were completely satisfied with the procedure of the euthanasia." There were several reasons for dissatisfaction with the euthanasia procedure, including "inability to be present during euthanasia ($n = 28$), too cold and quick treatment ($n = 22$), insufficient information about the procedure ($n = 21$), inappropriate treatment by staff ($n = 8$), too detailed explanations ($n = 3$)" (Fernandez-Mehler et al. 2013). It is important to take stock in how the treatment of the client and how much information is shared can affect their perception of the entire procedure. There may be factors out of the staff's control related to the client's inability to be present during the euthanasia, which might be due to severe suffering of the pet requiring an immediate euthanasia, clients being out of town, and more.

In a time when a client may feel like the entire situation is out of their control, it is imperative to offer as many choices as are reasonable and available. This starts with asking the client if they want to be present for the procedure. Based on the 2019 study by Adrian and Stitt (2019), "results indicate that physically attending a companion animal's euthanasia is not correlated with CG (Complicated Grief) or PTSD (Post-Traumatic Stress Disorder). As the experience of pet loss itself may be more indicative of psychological distress than whether or not the owner was present at the moment of euthanasia, veterinary staff need not dissuade pet owners from sharing their pet's final moments." While dissuading a client from attending the euthanasia of their pet may be coming from a compassionate place, it is important to leave that decision up to the client. We are each the expert in our own lives, and we must trust the client will make the best decision for them as an individual. Additional choices that are important to offer pet owners may include:

> 659 persons (33%) wished that their companion animal could die at home, 663 owners (33%) wanted to personally choose the time of euthanasia, 1403 persons (70%) wanted to be together with their pet during euthanasia, 563 persons (28%) did not want to wait in the waiting room before euthanasia, 309 persons (15%) did not want to pay the bill immediately, 94 persons (5%) wanted to have the possibility to talk to the veterinarian sometime after euthanasia (Fernandez-Mehler et al. 2013).

Even if the decisions made by the client seem small, they can still have a big impact. "Making the client feel included and supported during the decision-making process can help reduce their feelings of distress" (Uccheddu 2021). Speak clearly about each step of the euthanasia process and allow the client to give consent to move onto the next step. Once the pet has passed, allow them to spend time with their pet. Depending on the urgency of euthanasia, body care options can be discussed before or after the euthanasia procedure. Laws regarding pet burial on personal property vary greatly by location, so it is helpful to know what the laws are for the most common areas the clinic clientele lives in. Options for memorial items such as nose prints, paw prints, and fur clippings should be offered when possible, even if the pet is going to a third-party crematorium. The memorial items from the emergency clinic are something tangible the owner can take with them on a difficult day when their pet is not going home with them.

Grief

Grief is a natural reaction to loss. The Kubler-Ross five stages of grief model, while being one of the most well-known models for grief and loss, is not often used by mental health professionals. "Critics have focused on the fact that her research and use of 'stages' have not been empirically validated" (Tyrrell et al. 2025). The Kubler-Ross model can also give a false sense of progression for the griever, as if once they reach the final step of acceptance, they should be done grieving. The reality is that the grief journey of every individual is as unique as their fingerprint – no two journeys are alike. There are two grief models that are used more frequently with the pet loss. They can be applied to anyone grieving the animal, such as the owner, veterinarians, veterinary technicians, support staff, and more.

Dual Process Model

The guilt commonly associated with grief makes many people feel as though they do not deserve to experience happiness or hope. Many feel that if they experience joy, that means they have forgotten about or no longer miss their animal. But to stay forever in the dark depths of loss is not sustainable. The Dual Process Model (DPM) "identifies two types of stressors, loss- and restoration-oriented, and a dynamic, regulatory coping process of oscillation, whereby the grieving individual at times confronts, at other times avoids, the different tasks of grieving" (Stroebe and Schut 1999). There will be the heavy, not leaving the house days with lots of tears- which are the loss-oriented stressors. Over time, there will be days that feel lighter. These are days the griever might think of fond memories of the pet and smile, or feel hope or joy about an upcoming event. These are examples of restoration-oriented stressors. This can make the intense waves of grief more manageable by allowing for moments with an absence or less intense grief. The goal of this model is to increase the ability to cope with grief. "Coping refers to processes, strategies, or styles of managing (reducing, mastering, tolerating) the situation in which bereavement places the individual" (Stroebe and Schut 2010). The DPM can help an individual with their acute grief as well as help build resilience for future grief. This can be a helpful way to honor an animal and just an additional way the animal improved the human lives around them.

Continuing Bonds

When we lose an animal, there is a significant disruption in the routines and rhythms of our day that involved them. The Continuing Bonds (CB) theory helps remind the bereaved that while the animal is no longer physically present, there can be ways to keep their memory alive. "CB examples may include looking at photos, reminiscing, engaging in memorials and rituals such as altars or yearly birthday dinners, talking to the deceased, dreams, and holding onto special possessions" (Habarth et al. 2017). It is important to recall the uniqueness of the individual's grief journey and understand that the CB options that are most comforting are also unique to each person. "In the current study, CB strategies were almost universally experienced as more comforting than distressing, a finding that is consistent with our earlier pilot study on pet loss" (Habarth et al. 2017). It is still beneficial to provide pet owners with options to let them choose what they feel will be most supportive – paw prints, nose prints, fur clippings, collars, etc. This helps to give the family options as they navigate life without their furry family member. Maybe they want to carry the collar when they walk the same route they used to with their dog. Maybe they want to create a memorial area with photos, paw prints, and fur in their home and visit that at the same times of day they would normally feed their cat. Keeping parts of our routine consistent as we grieve can help remind us of our special bond with our loved one.

Veterinary Team Well-Being

Veterinary emergency clinics can be a high-stress environment for many reasons. Challenging conversations, burden transfer, euthanasia, and grief are just a few of the contributing factors to staff well-being. There have been multiple studies conducted regarding the mental health of veterinarians, but those results cannot be assumed to be true for veterinary technicians. The 2024 Merck Animal Health Veterinary Team study by Volk et al. focused on non-veterinarian employees, including vet techs, vet assistants, hospital/practice managers, and reception/client service representatives (CSRs). "Serious psychological distress was twice as prevalent among team members as among veterinarians and well-being was lower than that of veterinarians" (Volk et al. 2024). Thankfully, the study also found several factors (listed below) that "are associated with higher well-being, lower burnout, and less serious psychological distress" (Volk et al. 2024).

Supportive factors

- Positive practice culture that fosters teamwork, trust, open communication, and sufficient time for high-quality care
- Openly discuss mental health in team meetings
- Increase opportunities for staff advancement
- Develop reliable methods for coping with stress
- Manage work-life balance
- Utilize mental health professionals

It is important to recognize that unless you are taking care of your own mental and physical well-being, you are unable to provide the best patient care possible. You cannot pour from an empty cup. The number of resources for veterinary professional well-being and mental health continues to grow. You are not alone, and you deserve the same high level of care you provide to your patients.

Resources

Veterinary Social Work

The term veterinary social work was coined by Dr. Elizabeth Strand, PhD, LCSW, founding director of the University of Tennessee, Knoxville, Veterinary Social Work program in 2002 (Loue and Linden 2022). Veterinary social work focuses on the human side of human–animal interactions. There are four main areas of focus, including intentional well-being, animal-assisted interventions, the link between human and animal violence, and animal-related grief and bereavement (Loue and Linden 2022). Veterinary social work can be found in veterinary hospitals, colleges of veterinary medicine, animal shelters, and more. As the field grows and gains popularity, there has been an increase in veterinary social work positions. The titles vary, including Veterinary Social Worker, Wellness Counselor, Human–Animal Interaction Specialist, and more. The roles and job descriptions also vary within veterinary social work. Some focus solely on the pet owners, some focus solely on providing support and therapy to the staff, and some do a gentle blend of both. If a client receives emotional support from a veterinary social worker, that can help reduce the stress of the staff. If the staff receive support, it could be in individual sessions, team debriefs, or psychoeducation about work-life balance, compassion satisfaction, and communication skills.

If your clinic does not have a veterinary social worker, there is now a directory of veterinary social work and human–animal interaction professionals (https://bit.ly/VSW-HAI-directory). I created this free, public access directory to help connect veterinary staff and clients to professionals trained to support them. It is also important to note that there are other certificates, such as Pet Grief Counselor, Pet Death Doula, Human–Animal Interactions, Veterinary Human Support Certificate, and more. While they are different than veterinary social workers, those holding other qualifications may be able to support your team or clients.

Veterinary team

- Not One More Vet https://www.nomv.org/
  - Peer support, private online forum, resource lists
- Veterinary Hope Foundation https://veterinaryhope.org/
  - Support groups
- Measures
  - Burden Transfer Inventory-abbreviated (Spitznagel et al. 2022)
  - Professional Quality of Life (https://proqol.org/)

Clients

- Lap of Love (2025) https://www.lapoflove.com
  - Support groups, individual sessions with grief counselors
- Love, Baxter (2025) https://lovebaxter.com
  - Senior pet end-of-life and pet loss grief resource center
- Measures
  - Caregiver Burden Survey (ZBI) (Spitznagel et al. 2019).

There are most likely additional options in your city, state, or country. It can be supportive to have handouts for clients with local and international resources for them.

Works Cited

Adrian, J.A.L. and Stitt, A. (2019). There for you: attending Pet Euthanasia and whether this relates to complicated grief and post-traumatic stress disorder. *Anthrozoös* 32 (5): 701–713. https://doi.org/10.1080/08927936.2019.1645515.

American Veterinary Medical Association (AVMA). (2025) Euthanasia. Retrieved from https://www.avma.org/resources-tools/pet-owners/petcare/euthanasia

Animal Welfare Foundation. (2013) Saying Goodbye - The Ultimate Kindness. Retrieved from https://www.animalwelfarefoundation.org.uk/wp-content/uploads/2017/06/Saying-Goodbye.pdf

Boggio, P.S., Wingenbach, T.S., da Silveira Coêlho, M.L. et al. (2023). *Social and Affective Neuroscience of Everyday Human Interaction: From Theory to Methodology*, 1e. Cham: Springer Nature.

Bornstein, M.H. and Esposito, G. (2023). Coregulation: a multilevel approach via biology and behavior. *Children* 10 (8): 1323. https://doi.org/10.3390/children10081323.

Brown, B. (2012). *Daring Greatly: How the Courage to Be Vulnerable Transforms the Way We Live, Love, Parent, and Lead*. New York, NY: Gotham Books.

Conscious Discipline. (2025). Brain State Model. Retrieved from https://consciousdiscipline.com/methodology/brain-state-model/#brainstatemodel

Fernandez-Mehler, P., Gloor, P., Sager, E. et al. (2013). Veterinarians' role for pet owners facing pet loss. *Veterinary Record* 172 (21): 555–555.

Gardner, M. and McVety, D. (2016). Handing euthanasia in your practice. *Today's Veterinary Practice*. https://todaysveterinarypractice.com/wp-content/uploads/sites/4/2016/05/TVP_2016-0102_PB_Euthanasia.pdf

Habarth, J., Bussolari, C., Gomez, R. et al. (2017). Continuing bonds and psychosocial functioning in a recently bereaved pet loss sample. *Anthrozoös* 30 (4): 651–670.

Lap of Love. (2025). Lap of Love Quality of Life Scale. Retrieved from https://www.lapoflove.com/how-will-i-know-it-is-time/lap-of-love-quality-of-life-scale.pdf

Loue, S. and Linden, P. (2022). *The Comprehensive Guide to Interdisciplinary Veterinary Social Work*, 1e. Cham: Springer International Publishing AG.

National Empowerment Center. (2025). Emotional CPR. Retrieved from https://emotional-cpr.org/

National Empowerment Center. (2022). Emotional CPR: Assisting People through Emotional Crisis Participant Workbook.

Ohio State University Veterinary Medical Center. (2024). How Will I Know? Retrieved from https://vmc.vet.osu.edu/sites/default/files/documents/how-will-i-know_rev_mar2024ms_0.pdf

Spitznagel, M.B., Martin, J.T., Carlson, M.D., and Fulkerson, C.M. (2022). Validation of the Burden Transfer Inventory-abbreviated and examination across veterinary medicine positions and settings in the United States. *Veterinary Record Open* 9 (1): e46. -n/a.

Spitznagel, M.B., Jacobson, D.M., Cox, M.D., and Carlson, M.D. (2017). Caregiver burden in owners of a sick companion animal: a cross-sectional observational study. *Veterinary Record* 181: 321–321. https://doi.org/10.1136/vr.104295.

Spitznagel, M.B., Mueller, M.K., Fraychak, T. et al. (2019). Validation of an abbreviated instrument to assess veterinary client caregiver burden. *Journal of Veterinary Internal Medicine* 33: 1251–1259. https://doi.org/10.1111/jvim.15508.

Steckler, T., Kalin, N.H., and Reul, J.H.M. (2005). *Handbook of Stress and the Brain Part 1: The Neurobiology of Stress*. Amsterdam: Elsevier Science & Technology.

Stroebe, M. and Schut, H. (1999). The dual process model of coping with bereavement: rationale and description. *Death Studies* 23 (3): 197–224. https://doi.org/10.1080/074811899201046. PMID: 10848151.

Stroebe, M. and Schut, H. (2010). The dual process model of coping with bereavement: a decade on. *Omega: Journal of Death and Dying* 61 (4): 273–289.

Tyrrell, P., Harberger, S., Schoo, C., and Siddiqui, W. (2025). Kubler-Ross stages of dying and subsequent models of grief. In: *StatPearls*. Treasure Island (FL): StatPearls Publishing Retrieved from https://www.ncbi.nlm.nih.gov/books/NBK507885/.

Uccheddu, S. (2021). Improving vet-client communication through understanding the client perspective. *Veterinary Record* 188 (9): 349–351.

Volk, J.O., Schimmack, U., Strand, E.B. et al. (2024). Merck animal health veterinary team study reveals factors associated with well-being, burnout, and mental health among nonveterinarian practice team members. *Journal of the American Veterinary Medical Association* 262 (10): 1330–1337.

Part III

Internal Medicine Emergencies

9

Diabetes

Simone Conwell[1,2] *and Julia Conny*[1]

[1] *VeG ER for Pets, 1858 Reisterstown Road, Pikesville, MD, USA*
[2] *Veterinary Emergency and Critical Care Society Member, USA*

What Is Diabetes?

While owners and even less experienced veterinary staff may be familiar with diabetes in people, they do not always understand it well and that it is not identical to human diabetes and that while we use the same terms, they are not entirely accurate (Norkus 2019). There are two types of diabetes mellitus (DM) in cats and dogs: primary insulin-dependent (type 1) that occurs due to destruction of insulin-producing beta cells in the pancreas and non-insulin-dependent (type 2) due to insulin resistance, beta cell dysfunction, and increased gluconeogenesis. Type 1 typically requires insulin for life and may be congenital, immune-mediated, or idiopathic, and typically acutely presents. Type 2 has insulin present, but typically not in sufficient concentration to overcome insulin resistance, and can be managed with diet. Specifically, the diet should be higher in protein and lower in carbohydrates. Type 2 is seen in cats and is the type they can go into remission from, though it can progress to insulin-dependent if not addressed (Norkus 2019). Diets for all diabetics should be modified to help minimize postprandial glucose changes, and maintaining a lean body weight should also be prioritized for these patients. There are several commercial diets available that are designed to have higher fiber content and geared specifically to diabetes. If the patient is insulin dependent, it is important to modify their feeding schedule to coincide with insulin administration (usually twice daily). Consultation with a board-certified internal medicine doctor can be considered, and then the disease can be mostly managed by the primary care veterinarian.

More recently, for newly diagnosed diabetic cats that have never been on insulin and have no other comorbidities, sodium-glucose cotransporter 2 (SGLT2) inhibitors have recently become an option for treatment instead of the traditional insulin injections. These medications lower blood glucose by increasing excretion through the kidneys. Some owners may be particularly interested in this option, particularly if they themselves are diabetic, as this class of medications has been available for over a decade in human medicine, and feeding on a specific schedule is less important. It is a pill, so owners who are shy around needles may also be particularly interested in using SGLT2 inhibitors. Bexacat™, the first of these drugs, was only released in 2022, so we do not have significant data about how many cats go into remission (Elanco n.d.). There are reports of an increased risk of euglycemic diabetic ketoacidosis (DKA) in cats on SGLT2 inhibitors, which will be touched on later in the chapter. SGLT2 inhibitors are not used to treat DKA or hyperosmolar hyperglycemic syndrome (HHS), so we in the emergency room (ER) are not currently as familiar with them as our GP counterparts.

DM has historically been monitored by performing a fructosamine, a test that reflects glucose concentrations over 2–3 weeks, or in-hospital glucose curves. More recently, flash glucose monitor systems (FGMS) have become more popular. While they are off-label in pets, there are some studies exploring their efficacy. Continuous glucose monitors (CGM) tests glucose using interstitial readings, while fructosamine and inhospital curves use venous blood, raising questions about the accuracy. A 2020 study comparing FGMS such as the freestyle libre and portable blood glucose meters (PBGM) for monitoring dogs with diabetes concluded that FGMS allow for "more accurate identification of the glucose nadirs and hypoglycemic episodes compared to the use of a PBGM and assessment of day-to-day variations in glycemic control" (Baldo 2020). This is where owners and less experienced staff may get confused with DM; the trends matter in veterinary patients more than the individual readings. Humans give themselves a glucose reading-dependent dose of insulin, while veterinary patients get the same dose each time, and that dose is adjusted based on the overall trend. It is important to monitor for clinical signs of diabetes in patients still – are they still polyuric and polydipsic? (Images 9.1–9.5)

Diabetic Ketoacidosis

The majority of the diabetic patients we see in the ER present with DKA. The lack of insulin results in blood glucose not being metabolized into components that cells can use, and eventually the body will start breaking down fat, which converts to ketones. Because the body is not meant to use ketones in place of glucose, pH and electrolyte derangements occur. While there are multiple types of ketones, including acetone and acetoacetate that cause reactions on ketostix, beta-hydroxybutyrate is found in blood (Drobtaz 2012). Blood ketones should be prioritized over ketostix for a more accurate diagnosis of ketosis. Newly diagnosed diabetes are commonly diagnosed in the ER as being diabetic when they present in DKA, with the owners noting that they have been experiencing polyuria/polydipsia, lethargy, anorexia, weight loss, and sometimes vomiting. They may be laterally recumbent or have altered mentation. They will be dehydrated, sometimes severely, and in a state of shock. Some people can smell a "fruity" odor associated with ketones.

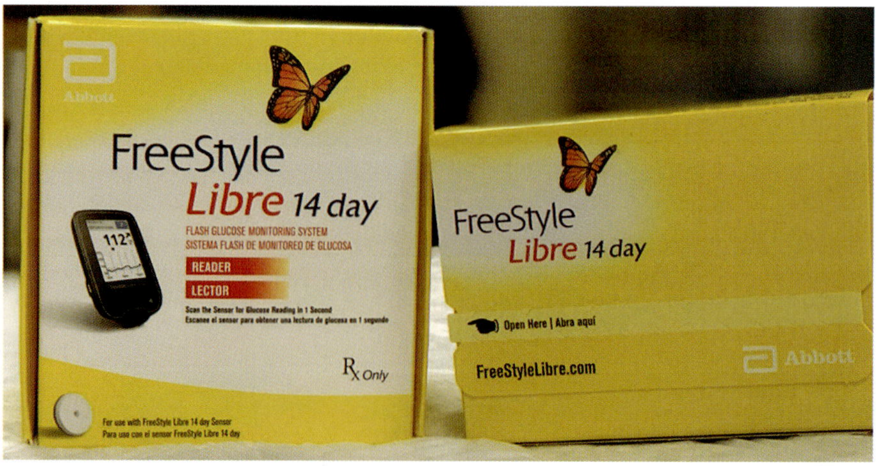

Image 9.1 Freestyle Libre sensor and reader. *Source:* Photo courtesy of Julia Conny, RVT.

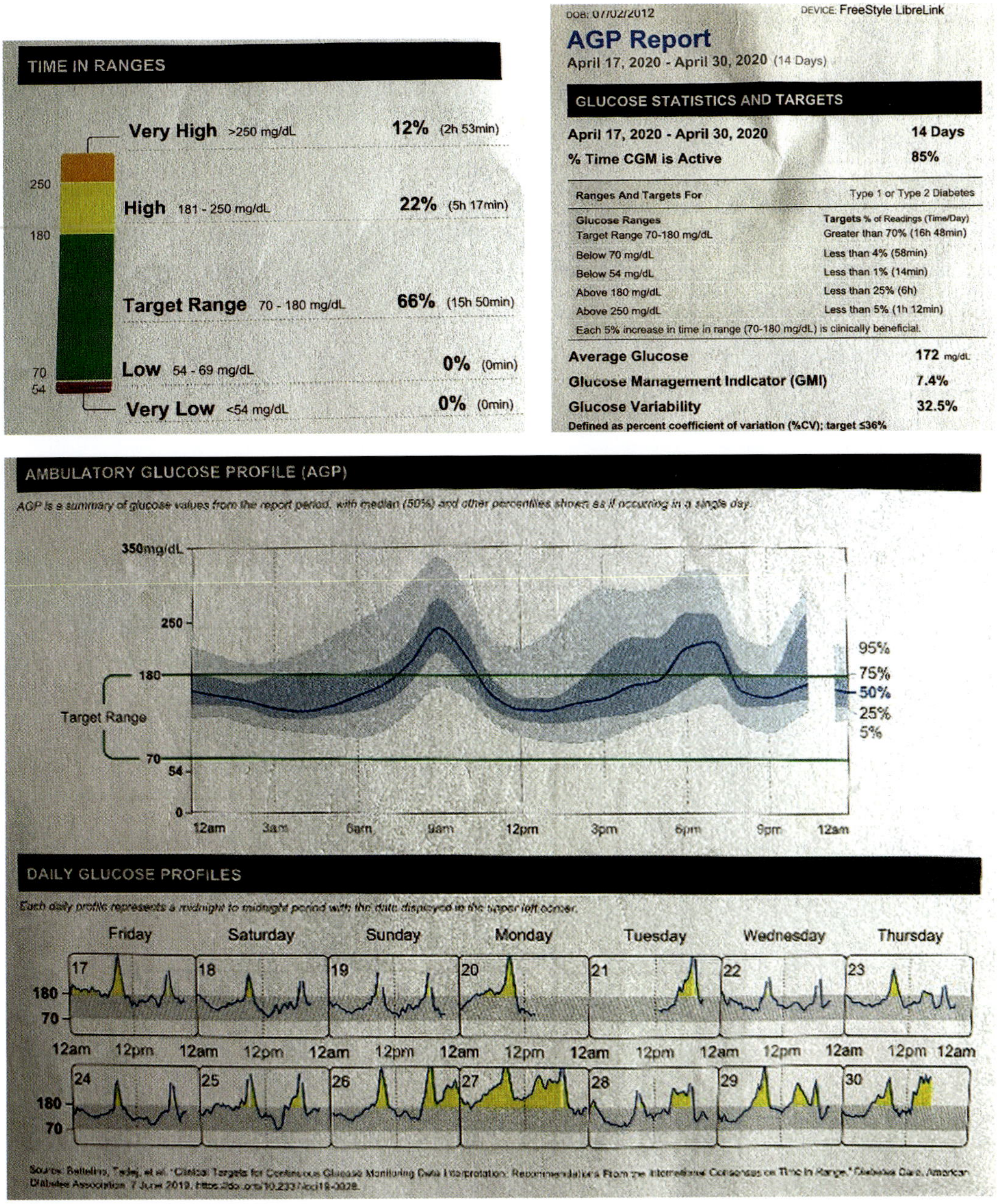

Image 9.2 Image of the reports generated by the Freestyle libre sensor. *Source:* Photos courtesy of Julia Conny, RVT.

A full chemistry, complete blood count, and urinalysis should be run, as should a blood gas to confirm acidosis. Common laboratory findings include hyperglycemia, glucosuria, ketonemia +/− ketonuria, metabolic acidosis, hyperosmolarity, azotemia, electrolyte derangements, and mild anemia (Schermerhorn 2005). For the best outcome, this patient should be hospitalized and rehydrated prior to starting an insulin therapy (Schermerhorn 2005). Dilution of blood glucose and loss through

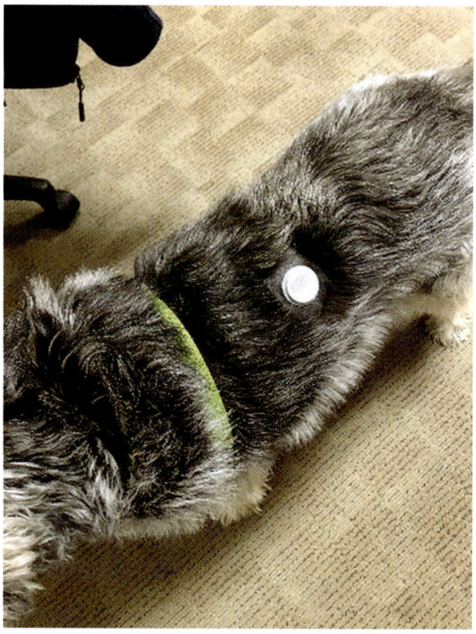

Image 9.3 Photos of dogs with Freestyle Libre attached in various spots. To place: shave a window caudal or the shoulder blade (a), at the tail base/dorsum, or on the lateral neck. Lightly scrub the skin. "Skin-Tac," or tissue glue, in a thin layer, should be applied to the sensor to ensure it sticks better. Tegaderm may be placed on top. *Source:* Photos and instructions courtesy of Julia Conny, RVT.

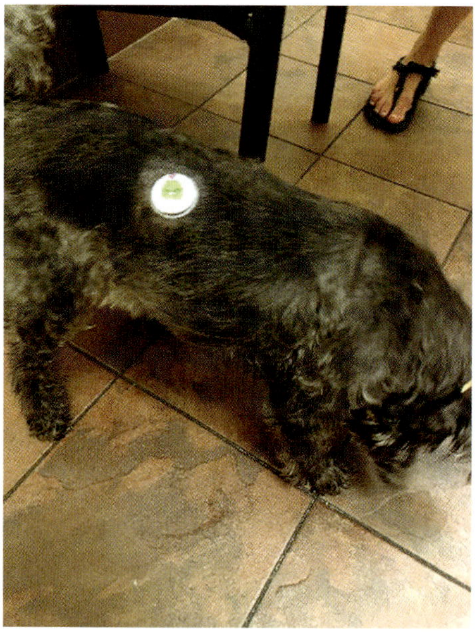

Image 9.4 Photos of dogs with Freestyle Libre attached in various spots. To place: shave a window caudal or the shoulder blade, at the tail base/dorsum (b), or on the lateral neck. Lightly scrub the skin. "Skin-Tac," or tissue glue, in a thin layer, should be applied to the sensor to ensure it sticks better. Tegaderm may be placed on top. *Source:* Photos and instructions courtesy of Julia Conny, RVT.

urinary excretion enhance renal glucose loss, ultimately leading to a decrease in blood glucose. There are multiple ways to introduce insulin to this patient, but a continuous rate infusion (CRI) of insulin is one of the most common. As far as specific protocols go, those are more hospital-dependent and if a specialty is involved. Most ERs will use regular insulin at a dose of 2.2 U/kg in a 250 ml bag of normal saline for dogs and 1.1 U/kg in a 250 ml bag of normal saline for cats. The insulin CRI rate will change based on the patient's blood glucose, but starts at 10 ml/h, and dextrose supplementation may be needed. Internal medicine will sometimes use a novel insulin protocol, which has the

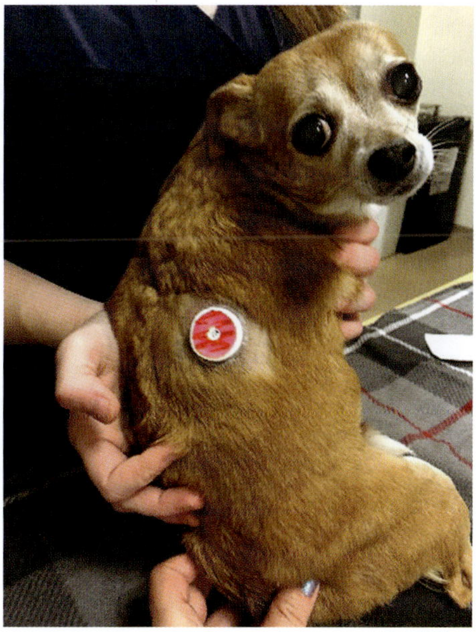

Image 9.5 Photos of dogs with Freestyle Libre attached in various spots. To place: shave a window caudal or the shoulder blade, at the tail base/dorsum, or on the lateral neck (c). Lightly scrub the skin. "Skin-Tac," or tissue glue, in a thin layer, should be applied to the sensor to ensure it sticks better. Tegaderm may be placed on top. *Source:* Photos and instructions courtesy of Julia Conny, RVT.

insulin at a much higher dose, and brings the patient out of ketosis more quickly. This should be done in hospitals with a specialty or with doctors who learned this protocol from specialists. It is important to remember that insulin binds to plastic, and 50 ml of the CRI needs to be run through the fluid line prior to attaching it to the patient. The bag of insulin needs to be remade every 24 hours. It is also important to account for the rates of all CRIs running when calculating a total fluid rate. For example, if the patient's total fluid rate should be 20 ml/h, and the insulin CRI is running at 10 ml/h, the fluids without insulin should be running at 10 ml/h as well. Blood glucose levels should be checked every 1–2 hours, and blood ketones and electrolytes should be monitored as well. A central line of some sort is imperative for these cases to be managed appropriately. The insulin CRI will run until ketosis is resolved, and intermittent insulin dosing can be started.

Glucose (mg/dl)	Dextrose supplementation	Insulin CRI (ml/hr)
>250	0	10
200–250	2.5%	7
150–200	2.5%	5
100–150	5%	5
<100	5%	**STOP**

Hypokalemia is frequently associated with DKA and should be treated aggressively from the start (Drobtaz 2012). Recall from the blocked cat chapter that insulin drives potassium into cells, so even patients who start eukalemic develop hypokalemia. Potassium supplementation must stay lower than K_{max}, which is 0.5 mEq/kg/hr. Potassium chloride (KCl) is the most common supplement for hypokalemia, but DKA patients may also become hypophosphoric and need supplementation when the phosphorus drops below 2.0 mg/dl (Schermerhorn 2005). The supplement for phosphorus comes in potassium phosphate (KP), and when creating a CRI of it, care must be taken to use the correct concentration, as the concentrations of potassium and phosphorus are different; there are generally 3 mmol/ml phosphorus and 4.4 mEq/ml potassium. Because potassium is in this fluid, that too must be accounted for when monitoring K_{max}. DKA patients are typically started on a KP CRI at 0.03 mmol/kg/hr, and it is titrated up as needed based on bloodwork rechecks. KP is a hyperosmolar medication and requires dilution before use; KCl can burn at higher rates, and any dextrose supplementation over 5% needs to be run through a central line. These points must be considered when catheter selection for DKA is being made. A triple-lumen central line will allow for the gold standard of care (Images 9.6 and 9.7).

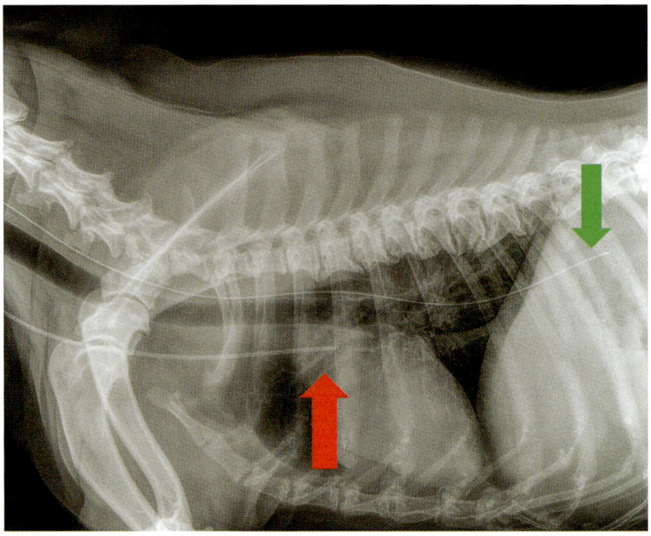

Image 9.6 Radiographic confirmation of a central line (red arrow) and nasogastric tube (green arrow). Notice the central line terminates between the 3rd and 4th ribs. *Source:* Photo courtesy of Alli Opishinski, CVT.

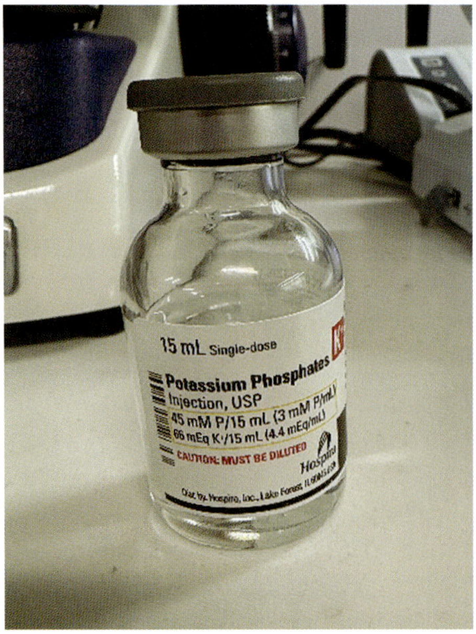

Image 9.7 Potassium phosphate bottle showing that the potassium concentration is 4.4 mEq/ml and the phosphorous concentration is 3 mM/ml. *Source:* Photo courtesy of Simone Conwell, RVT, VTS (ECC).

Potassium level (mmol/l)	mEq/l KCl supplementation to be added
>3.5	20
3–3.5	30
2.5–3	40
2–2.5	50
<2	60

Euglycemic DKA

A euglycemic DKA (eDKA) is what it sounds like: a diabetic crisis with a normal blood glucose. Symptoms include anorexia/hyporexia, lethargy, and vomiting (Mott 2025). Any cat that is on SGLT2 inhibitors and exhibiting these symptoms should have blood ketones checked to rule out eDKA. The treatment is the same as with traditional DKA, though it may need to be more aggressive to resolve ketosis, and feeding tubes may be needed sooner than with a traditional DKA (Mott 2025). Once resolution of eDKA occurs, traditional insulin therapy will need to be instituted for management of diabetes.

Hyperglycemic Hyperosmolar Syndrome

Hyperglycemic hyperosmolar syndrome (HHS) is a rare and dangerous complication of DM. It is characterized by severe hyperglycemia, hyperosmolar blood, a lack of ketones, and a reduction of glomerular filtration rate (Drobtaz 2012). On exam, the patient is dehydrated, has an altered mentation, may be brady- or tachycardic with arrhythmias, and has an increased respiratory rate/effort (Norkus 2019). Because glucose excretion through urine is compromised, profound hyperglycemia occurs, which leads to hyperosmolarity (Drobtaz 2012). Because the blood glucose is so high, it is important to calculate the corrected sodium using the formula

$$\text{Corrected sodium} = \text{measured Na}^+ + \frac{1.6\left(\text{Glucose}_{\text{measured}} - 100\right)}{100}$$

Serum osmolarity should also be calculated. One formula for that is

$$\text{Serum osmolarity:} \left[2\left(\text{Na} + \text{K}\right)\right] + \text{BUN} / 2.8 + \text{glucose} / 18$$

There are multiple formulas available, some of which discount potassium. Which formula to use should be a hospital decision, and that choice should be applied to every patient.

HHS patients will have a serum osmolarity of >350 mOsm/l (Norkus 2019). Sodium needs to be managed as a chronic condition and not reduced at rates greater than 0.5 mEq/l/h to prevent cerebral edema and worsening neurological status (Norkus 2019). Serial blood draws every 2–4 hours are needed to monitor electrolyte and osmolarity changes. Insulin therapy may be started after rehydrating the patient or when they are more stable, and the dose is lower than that for DKA. Electrolyte abnormalities are known to cause ventricular arrhythmias, and HHS causes many electrolyte derangements, making checking an electrocardiogram a reasonable move (Laslett 2020). (Image 9.8).

As technology for monitoring diabetes in humans improves, veterinary staff must strive to keep up by attending continuing education regularly and reading about updates. Many clients come in

TEST	RESULT	REFERENCE VALUE	
Glucose	**641**	**70 – 143 mg/dL**	H
Creatinine	1.1	0.5 – 1.8 mg/dL	
BUN	7	7 – 27 mg/dL	
BUN: Creatinine Ratio	6		
Phosphorus	6.2	2.5 – 6.8 mg/dL	
Calcium	9.4	7.9 – 12.0 mg/dL	
Sodium	156	144 – 160 mmol/L	
Potassium	**3.2**	**3.5 – 5.8 mmol/L**	L
Na: K Ratio	49		
Chloride	112	109 – 122 mmol/L	
Total Protein	**8.5**	**5.2 – 8.2 g/dL**	H
Albumin	3.5	2.2 – 3.9 g/dL	
Globulin	**5.0**	**2.5 – 4.5 g/dL**	H
Albumin: Globulin Ratio	0.7		
ALT	**589**	**10 – 125 U/L**	H
ALP	**315**	**23 – 212 U/L**	H
GGT	0	0 – 11 U/L	
Bilirubin - Total	**1.1**	**0.0 – 0.9 mg/dL**	H
Cholesterol	202	110 – 320 mg/dL	
Amylase	**447**	**500 – 1,500 U/L**	L
Lipase	536	200 – 1,800 U/L	
Osmolality	335	mmol/kg	

Image 9.8 Blood work results of a patient suspected to have HHS. The calculated osmolarity was 354 mOsm, and the corrected sodium was 145 mmol/l. The patient was arrested and CPR was performed. She eventually went into ventricular fibrillation and was shocked three times and given refractory treatment before the owner made the decision to stop CPR. *Source:* Photo courtesy of Simone Conwell, RVT, VTS (ECC).

wearing CGMs themselves; these clients, in particular, should be viewed as partners in their pet's care and educated extensively on the differences in human and animal diabetes.

Works Cited

Baldo, F.C. (2020). Comparison between a flash glucose monitoring system and portable blood glucose meter for monitoring dogs with diabetes mellitus. *Journal of Veterinary Internal Medicine* https://doi.org/10.1111/jvim.15930.

Drobtaz, K.M. (2012). *Manual of Small Animal Emergency and Critical Care Medicine*. Iowa: Wiley-Blackwell.

Elanco. (n.d.). Bexacat. Retrieved from www.elanco.com: https://my.elanco.com/us/bexacat

Laslett, D.C. (2020). Electrolyte abnormalities in patients presenting with ventricular arrythmia (from the LYTE-VT study). *American Journal of Cardiology* https://doi.org/10.1016/j.amj.ard.2020.04.051.

Mott, J. (2025). Recognizing and Managing Euglycemic DKA in Cats on SGLT2 Inhibitors: A Guide for Early Intervention. Retrieved from Florida Veterinary Medical Association: https://fvma.org/recognizing-and-managing-euglycemic-dka-in-cats-on-sglt2-inhibitors-a-guide-for-early-intervention/

Norkus, C. (2019). *Veterinary Technician's Manual for Small Animal Emergency and Critical Care.* Hoboken: John Wiley & Sons, Inc.

Schermerhorn, T. (2005). Understanding diabetic ketoacidosis. *World Small Animal Veterinary Association World Congress Proceedings*. Retrieved from https://www.vin.com/apputil/content/defaultadv1.aspx?meta=Generic&pld=11196&id=3854239

10

Searching for Red Blood Cells – IMHA

Danielle Schuler[1,2]

[1] *VeG ER for Pets, 1858 Reistertown Rd, Pikesville, MD, USA*
[2] *Veterinary Emergency and Critical Care Society Member, USA*

Immune-mediated hemolytic anemia usually shortened to the acronym IMHA. What is it? How and why does it occur? Maybe you've seen it before in your patients; maybe those four words put together are brand new information. I know when I was working in my general practice years ago, I had never encountered it, and when I transitioned to emergency room (ER)/specialty (specifically internal medicine), that is when I was exposed to this disease process. A primary function of erythrocytes (red blood cells), among other important duties, is to carry oxygen to tissues and organs and to carry carbon dioxide back to the lungs to be expelled. IMHA is an autoimmune disease where the body no longer recognizes its own red blood cells and starts destroying them. This causes a plethora of issues, including but not limited to severe anemia due to hemolysis, icterus (also due to hemolysis), and the need for potential transfusions. Depending on severity, signs and symptoms range anywhere from lethargy and pale or icteric mucous membranes (see Images 10.1 and 10.2), to respiratory distress and collapse. It is an incredibly serious disease with a mortality rate of up to 70% within the first 3 weeks of treatment (Piek 2008). Coming to a diagnosis and starting treatment as soon as possible for these patients to have a chance is our number one priority. Typically, when I see these patients present to the ER, it is not an automatic diagnosis of IMHA, unlike when you see the unproductive retching giant breed with a tense, distended abdomen and go, "Oh, I'm immediately worried that is a bloat." These IMHA patients can look anywhere from stable to critical, and a workup is always needed. So, hopefully by the end of this chapter you are thinking about how that patient presents symptomatically, patient history (has it traveled anywhere with known common infections, had vaccines recently, etc.), what diagnostics your doctor would want (always thinking ahead is a great asset to our doctors who are already thinking a mile a minute!), and if you were to transfer this patient to the ER: What would we, as the ER team, appreciate that patient coming with from your practice?

American College of Veterinary Internal Medicine (ACVIM) Consensus Statement

Before we get into that, though, let's talk a little bit about what IMHA is, what can cause it, and how to diagnose and treat these patients. The American College of Veterinary Internal Medicine (ACVIM) has published a consensus statement "to provide clinical guidelines for diagnosis of,

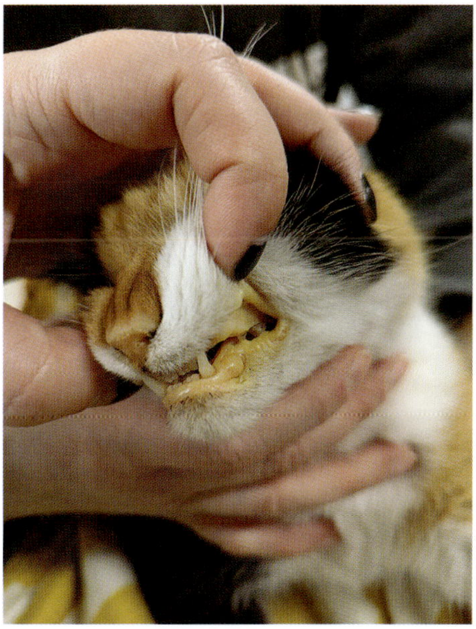

Image 10.1 Icteric mucous membranes in a cat. *Source:* Photos courtesy of Danielle Schuler, RVT.

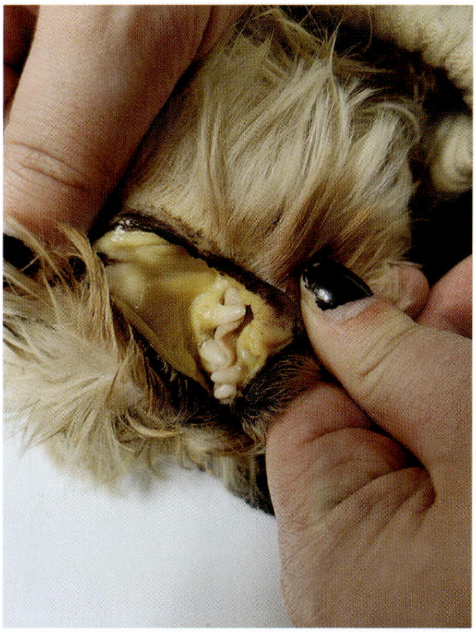

Image 10.2 Icteric mucous membranes in a dog. *Source:* Photos courtesy of Danielle Schuler, RVT.

and underlying disease screening for, IMHA in dogs and cats" (Garden 2019). Because most animals present as anemic, that is not enough to confirm an immune-mediated process. Anemia can be present for different reasons (such as hemorrhage, parasitosis, kidney disease, etc.); that is why it is important to run further diagnostics. Once anemia is established and IMHA is suspected, the next step is to look for markers of immune-mediated destruction and hemolysis. Since our patients can't speak and give us an idea of what diagnostic testing to pursue, allowing

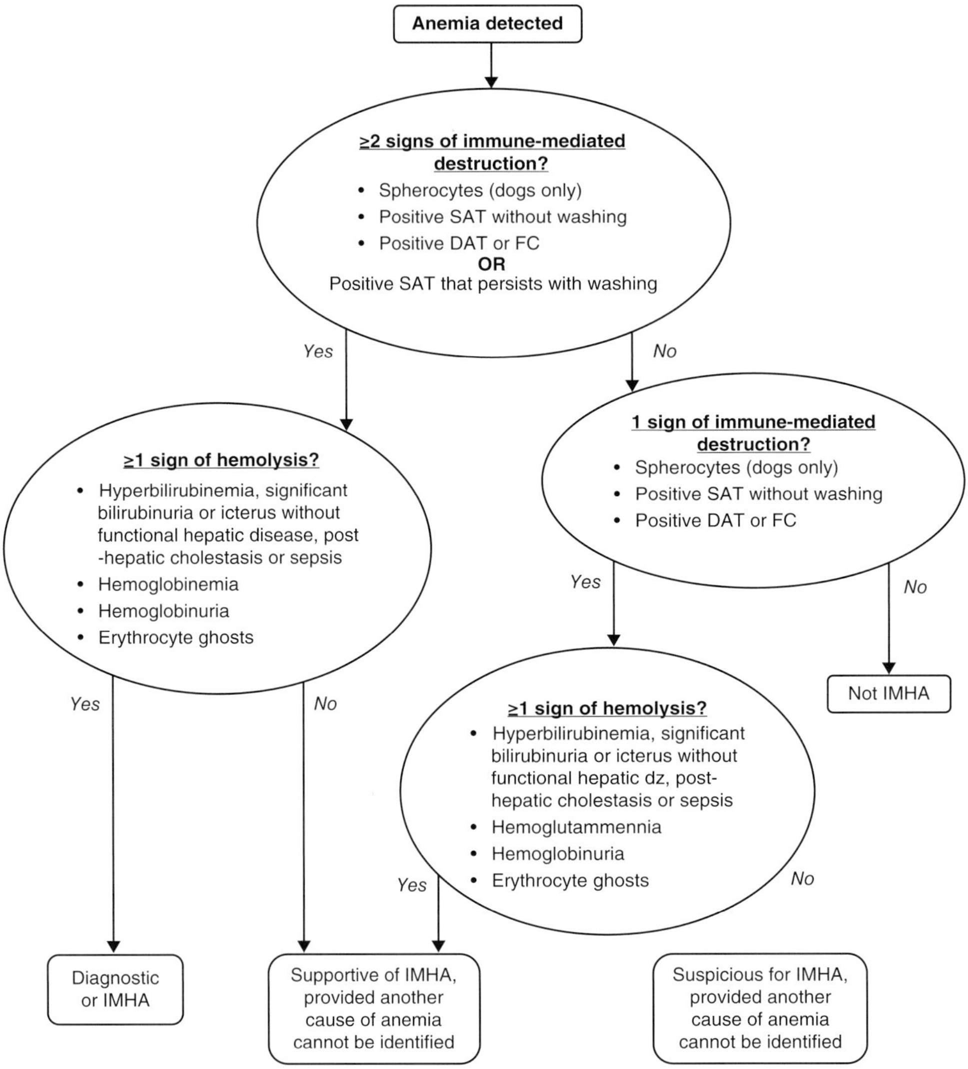

Image 10.3 Flow chart from ACVIM consensus statement on diagnosing IMHA. *Source:* Garden et al. (2019)/with permission of Oxford University Press.

for a diagnostic "gold standard" to give a definitive diagnosis, practitioners rely on interpreting multiple test results to come to the diagnosis of IMHA (see Image 10.3). There must be at least two indicators of immune-mediated destruction and at least one indicator of hemolysis for a definitive diagnosis.

If you have less than the required indicators of each marker, then you have a supportive diagnosis or suspicion of IMHA. Markers of immune-mediated destruction include: spherocytes (in canines only), positive saline agglutination test, positive direct antiglobulin test (DAT) or flow cytometry (FC), or a positive saline agglutination test that persists with washing. Markers of hemolysis include hyperbilirubinemia, significant bilirubinuria or icterus without functional hepatic disease, posthepatic cholestasis or sepsis, hemoglobinuria, and erythrocyte ghosts.

Diagnostics

Pulling blood for a ethylenediaminetetraacetic acid (EDTA) lavender top tube, tiger top/gold top (serum), making a fresh blood smear, and saving the extra to send over with your patient is always ideal. Not only is it helpful for the ER team, but it is imperative for running the abovementioned diagnostics. Making and staining a blood smear to look for spherocytes is something that can be done in-house. Spherocytes are erythrocytes that have lost their central pallor (see Image 10.4). Finding greater than five spherocytes/×100 oil immersion field is supportive of an IMHA diagnosis (Garden 2019). Did you make a beautiful blood smear, stain it, and aren't confident in reading it? Send it with the rest of the blood so your ER team can (1) read it and (2) admire your blood smear technique.

A saline agglutination test is also something that can easily be done in the regular hospital setting to help form a diagnosis. Agglutination is when red blood cells clump angrily together, not to be mistaken with rouleaux formation, which is not considered a positive agglutination. Mix one drop of blood with four drops of saline on a glass slide and rock until the blood is fully mixed with saline. Then observe for agglutination, which can look like cracks forming macroscopically, and confirm clumping microscopically (see Images 10.5 and 10.6). A study done in 2020 has reported that dilutions of up to 49:1 (saline to blood) are beneficial in dispersing rouleaux that can look like agglutination in a crowded field (Sun 2020). This dilution can be difficult to achieve without the proper micropipettes. My coauthor and editor, Simone, will mix one part blood to nine parts saline in a syringe and apply that mixture to a slide to look for agglutination. Another test you can send out to a referring diagnostic laboratory is the direct Coombs test. This test is looking for antibodies coating the surface of red blood cells. However, if your patient is already agglutinating, your test can come back as a false positive, making the diagnosis useless. If the patient receives a blood transfusion, this will also result in false-positive Coombs testing. That's why it's imperative to obtain and save samples prior to starting treatments. Flow cytometry can also be performed via an outside laboratory, but it can oftentimes be cost-prohibitive, and results can take up to 5 days to

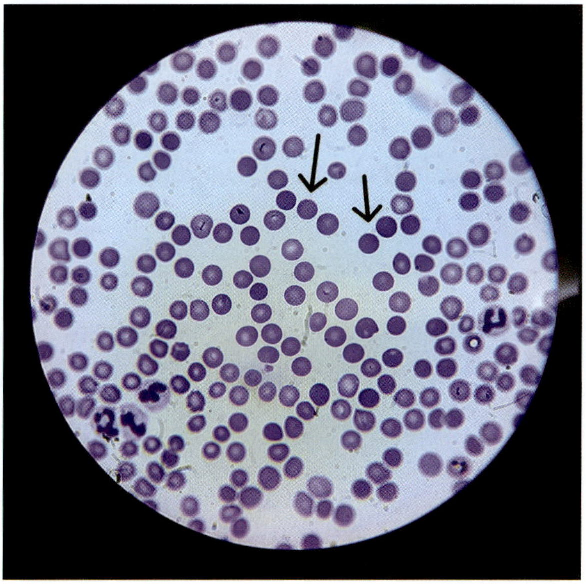

Image 10.4 Wright's solution-stained blood smear on 100× magnification with oil lens showing spherocytes (arrows). *Source:* Photo courtesy of Danielle Schuler, RVT.

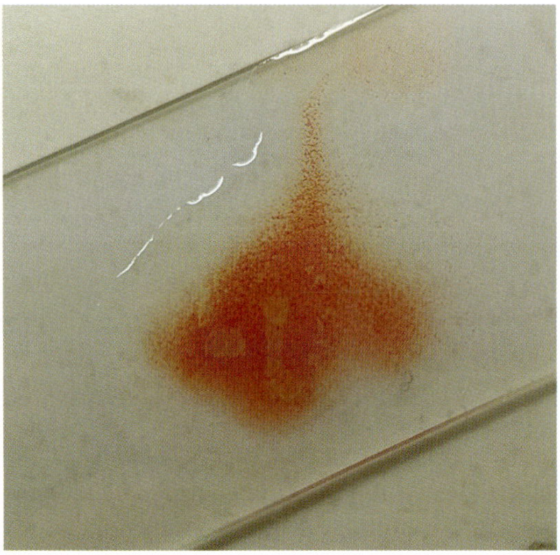

Image 10.5 Macroagglutination provided by Danielle Schuler, RVT.

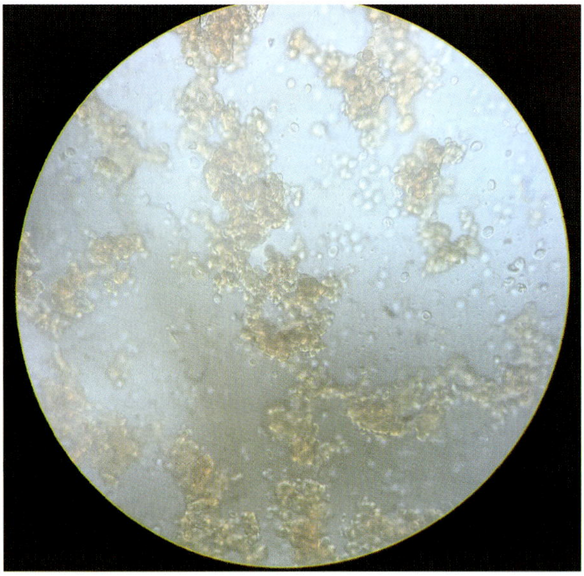

Image 10.6 Microagglutination under 40× magnification (6) provided by Danielle Schuler, RVT.

come back. This should never delay treatment because you need to be fast and aggressive in treating immune-mediated disease. Most often, you can come to a suggestive or firm diagnosis without flow cytometry. Again, this test would need to be run before starting treatments because immunosuppressive medications will impact results.

On top of these specific diagnostics, it's always recommended to run a complete blood count (CBC), biochemistry panel, snap 4DX, and urinalysis. Having a complete blood cell count is helpful for identifying if the anemia is regenerative versus non-regenerative, looking for reticulocytes, and giving insight into what the white blood cells are doing. A biochemical panel will give you key insights into organ function and can tell you if your patient has hyperbilirubinemia. Having a chemistry panel will help rule out other factors that could cause jaundice, including hepatic disease, posthepatic cholestasis, or sepsis (Garden 2019). Looking at the color of your spun serum is also important. Your patient might not look jaundiced, but if you spin down the blood and find the sample is icteric, that is also telling of hemolysis. Finally, running a snap test in-house for anaplasmosis will help determine if IMHA is primary or secondary. If you're able to collect a urine sample, you can spin that down and visually inspect if hemoglobinuria is present. Hemoglobinuria (no red blood cells) can be differentiated from hematuria (red blood cells) by centrifugation; if the supernatant is still red, then hemoglobinuria is present. When hematuria is present, the red blood cells are pulled into the pellet during centrifugation, leaving the supernatant colorless. If you can't run these in-house, send those samples with your patient! That extra blood you pulled saves us time, blood typing, and cross-matching in preparing for a transfusion. And it saves our patients an extra "poke," which is all-around appreciated. ER techs and nurses are vampires, and we want everything we can get because you never know what test your doctor is going to ask for next.

There are two types of IMHA – primary and secondary. Primary IMHA is considered idiopathic and is described as such when all other diagnostics, by process of elimination, rule out other causes. When there is an underlying pathogenesis that is found to be the cause of IMHA, that is considered secondary IMHA. Sixty to seventy-five percent of IMHA cases are considered primary/idiopathic (Piek 2008). It is important to find a potential cause because with treatment of the primary disease process, the immune-mediated process will also be cured. I'll briefly touch on these "trigger factors," but I won't be spending a whole lot of time on them because our immediate problem is that our patient is anemic. We know two things: (1) they are most likely going to need a transfusion (potentially multiple) and (2) they are going to need round-the-clock hospitalization for supportive care and start on immunosuppressive medications.

Causes of secondary IMHA include infection, neoplasia, inflammatory processes, drugs, and vaccines. I won't get into every little thing that could potentially cause an immune-mediated reaction because there are so many things that could potentially trigger a reaction, even if the chances are low. In dogs, a common parasitic infection of *Babesia gibsoni* can cause IMHA. If this is found to be the case, once the infection is controlled, the immune-mediated destruction stops without the need for immunosuppressive medications (Garden 2019). In cats, *Mycoplasma heamofelis* can also cause IMHA. According to the ACVIM consensus statement, organisms may cause IMHA by amplifying normal antibody-mediated removal of aged or damaged erythrocytes. Neoplasia is another factor to consider. While having a low association in both our canine and feline patients, there has not been enough research to rule it out as a trigger factor. Inflammation (i.e., pancreatitis, generalized inflammation) is another trigger factor listed in the consensus statement that ultimately boils down to having anecdotal reports of it happening, but no direct evidence to support it, leading to the need for additional research on the topic to be performed. "The prevalence of drug-induced IMHA in dogs and cats is either rare or underreported" (Garden 2019). Meaning, while possible, it is something that is rarely seen. It's important to include all medications the patient is taking in their history in case they might be associated. The same can be said of vaccines. While adverse reactions are reported to be about 0.002%, less than 5% of those reactions are considered immune-mediated. Meaning less than 0.0001%, or one per one million vaccinated dogs, are having what is considered an immune-mediated response to a vaccine they have received (Duval 1996). While it is important to determine which vaccines and their schedule are best for each immunocompromised patient, the ACVIM considers the current vaccine strategies generally safe. Future vaccines should be considered carefully by each individual patient's doctor because of the risk of relapse. At the end of the day, the ACVIM posits that overall, and more specifically, research that is focused on individual trigger factors needs to be conducted.

Association of Veterinary Hematology and Transfusion Medicine (AVHTM) Position and Transfusion Guidelines

Ultimately, you are considering a transfer for this patient because they are clinically anemic and require a transfusion. Your clinic may have the resources to type, crossmatch, and even have blood products available for administration. Canines have two major blood types, dog erythrocyte antigen (DEA) 1 negative and DEA 1 positive, while felines have type A and type B. Blood types are dependent on specific antigens found on red blood cells. This is incredibly important, and if all you take away from this segment on blood transfusions is this, then I am okay with that: type B cats can absolutely under no circumstances EVER receive type A blood. Reactions are severe and oftentimes fatal (Davidow 2021a, b). We will briefly touch on what to do with a type B cat patient when only type A blood is available later in the chapter. In most scenarios, this is when it is decided to transfer your patient to an emergency hospital and/or specialty clinic. Here is what I want you to think about: Have I done everything I can to help facilitate an easier transition to a specialty facility for my patient to get the care that they need? This may include placing an appropriately sized catheter to receive a blood transfusion, drawing that extra bit of blood to send over to type and crossmatch, and having diagnostics done so that the ER can get right to the need of the patient: getting a transfusion started as soon as possible.

For simplicity's sake, and because this chapter is on IMHA and not transfusion medicine, we'll only talk briefly about it. If you are looking for more information about anything transfusion-related, I cannot recommend Ken Yagi's book on transfusion and blood banking enough (Yagi 2016). The AVHTM is another resource for research and creation of transfusion and blood banking standards. The AVHTM has released comprehensive consensus statements, AVHTM Transfusion Reaction Small Animal Consensus Statement (TRACS) parts 1–3, that go over in detail the clinical signs, prevention and monitoring, and diagnosis and treatment of transfusion reactions (Odunayo 2021). A blood transfusion is a critical life-saving measure and can be a challenge to administer to patients who are nonimmune-mediated. We worry about transfusion reactions as mild as a slight increase in temperature all the way to anaphylaxis (Odunayo 2021). There are even posttransfusion reactions like transfusion-associated circulatory overload (TACO) and transfusion-related acute lung injury (TRALI), but these serious complications are beyond the scope of this book (Odunayo 2021). These complications are expounded on in the Manual of Veterinary Transfusion Medicine and Blood Banking by Ken Yagi and Marie Holowaychuck (Yagi 2016). And even after the transfusion is done, we worry about hemolysis and how much of that unit the patient will actually keep. I've run transfusions where the patient starts hemolyzing the blood product being administered before the transfusion is even completed. Easily visible signs of hemolysis are icterus (of mucous membranes, skin, and serum) and hemoglobin, which is seen as a reddish-orange change in color to urine. It might be difficult to differentiate if the cause of hemolysis is due to a reaction to the transfusion or from the hemolytic nature of the disease process itself. The immune-mediated patient is already destroying its own red blood cells, will likely chew through donor blood given to them, and will require multiple transfusions. In one study, ten out of nineteen cats required a blood transfusion, with half of those cats needing multiple transfusions over a course of 10 days (Kohn 2006). Checking a packed cell volume (PCV) after administering a transfusion is vital in telling you if the transfusion helped or not. Current recommendations tell us that checking a PCV immediately after a transfusion, as opposed to waiting two hours, will give a reliable number and will help clinicians determine if another transfusion is recommended, as well as adjust hospitalization time based on the outcome (Morris 2021).

This is why giving your patient blood that matches their type and cross-matching that product to make sure there is no reaction present. If you cross-match a unit, and it reacts, you should move onto cross matching the next unit until you have a match. There will be scenarios where your patient reacts to every unit you have in the hospital. At that point, it's all about reaching out and seeing who has blood to spare and procuring it. In a pinch, with no other options, you can give a dog that is type DEA 1 negative with no prior transfusion reactions a unit of positive blood, knowing that the risks include reactivity and rejection of that blood (Davidow 2021a, b). Current AVTHM recommendations are to give DEA 1 negative compatible negative blood and DEA 1 positive compatible positive or negative blood. However, for the sake of product availability, you should be reaching for a compatible positive unit of blood for a DEA 1 positive patient before moving on to a negative unit.

Xenotransfusion is also an option and has been successful in interspecies cases, such as giving canine blood to feline patients (Bell 2020). This is used almost exclusively as a last resort in emergency situations where there is no compatible feline blood on hand, and the patient would expire before a suitable match can be found. Remember that scary bit about never giving type A blood to a type B cat? This is a scenario where I would try using canine blood to transfuse until a suitable unit of type B blood can be found. This can only be done once for our feline friends. Cats with no prior cross-species transfusions do not have naturally occurring antibodies to canine red blood cell antigens. However, antibodies are formed rapidly within 4–7 days posttransfusion. The average lifespan of feline red blood cells transfused to the same species is 30 days, while the lifespan of canine red blood cells transfused to a feline patient is less than 4 days (Bovens 2013). Cats requiring multiple transfusions can still be transfused with canine blood within 4–6 days, but after that, they will experience life-threatening anaphylaxis reactions (Davidow 2021a, b). It is incredibly important to note in a patient's record if they have had a previous transfusion, what type of blood they received, if it was from a different species, and any transfusion reactions noted to help prevent reactivity in future transfusion treatments.

Your doctor will give you an estimated amount to transfuse. The equation of volume of packed red blood cells (pRBCs) (ml) = 1.5 × desired increase in PCV × body weight (kg) is an easy and accurate formula to assess how much blood your patient will need (Short 2012). There are other equations as well, which one your hospital uses depends on your doctor. Units of pRBC come in single and double units, commonly in dogs. Once spiked, if you're not using that whole unit, it can be stored in the fridge for 24 hours to use for future transfusion. It is incredibly important that your unit of blood is not past its expiration date. While not immediately dangerous, the cells will start to deteriorate, will not be beneficial to your patient, and can cause incredibly detrimental side effects. A 2013 study by Solomon (2013) showed that 42-day-old expired blood causes "pulmonary hypertension and vascular damage at sites of injury and gas exchange abnormalities, each contributing to the increased risk of death." There are a couple of important things to remember before a blood product even touches your patient. First and most important is typing your patient and cross-matching whatever blood product, whether it be whole blood or packed red blood cells. Crossmatching your unit of blood will help prevent potential transfusion reactions. I am personally familiar with the RapidVet-H Major crossmatching kit because it comes with all the necessary items (minus a centrifuge, but it has a handy paper with how fast/long to spin blood for a plethora of centrifuges) and easy-to-follow instructions. It also comes with a reference picture of what a negative and positive result look like. Once you find a compatible match, you can either spike the whole bag with a filter set and run using a fluid pump calibrated to infuse blood, or you can pull out the required amount into a syringe and give via syringe pump with a hemonate filter. Using a pump not calibrated for blood products will run the risk of damaging the erythrocytes, making the transfusion ineffective while wasting good blood and money. If using a syringe and a hemonate filter, that filter should be replaced every 60 ml of blood administered.

Before you start your transfusion, you should be taking a set of vitals, including heart rate, respiratory rate and effort, mucous membrane color, capillary refill time, and temperature. These will be your baseline vitals and your reference for any changes that you might see while your transfusion progresses. It is common not to premedicate with diphenhydramine or dexamethasone (Davidow 2021a, b). The thinking behind this is that it could potentially mask a reaction during the transfusion, and if a reaction does occur, you can always administer it during the transfusion. That being said, your patient should already have a steroid on board, as that is the primary treatment for IMHA and should not be delayed. There are a handful of monitoring sheets out there, as well as one that the AVHTM has included in their recent consensus statement. I personally use one that is proprietary to Veterinary Emergency Group (VEG). Below is the transfusion monitoring sheet proposed by the AVHTM (Image 10.7).

I start my transfusion at 0.5 ml/kg/h, then after 15 minutes will recheck my patient's vitals. If there is no significant change, then I will increase the rate to 1 ml/kg/h for the next 15 minutes. If there continue to be no major changes to the patient's vitals, you can increase to the full rate for the remaining amount of blood. This can be determined by taking the total amount to be infused and dividing by three and a half hours. I continue to monitor every 15 minutes for the first hour, then every half hour until the transfusion is complete. Once your transfusion is done, you can check a PCV to verify the efficacy of the transfusion (Morris 2021).

Medications

There is no one definitive way to treat IMHA, just like there is no one way to definitively diagnose it. The ACVIM has put out a broad guideline based on research studies and clinician experience to help guide treatment of IMHA. According to the ACVIM's consensus statement, the first line of treatment is to start on an immunosuppressive dose of steroids. This can be done as soon as you have a diagnosis of IMHA and any samples you need have been collected. This does not need to wait for transfer, as most hospitals have injectable dex SP or oral prednisone on hand. While not all patients will need a secondary immunosuppressive medication, it is oftentimes automatically added in because the benefit of a patient potentially needing it outweighs the potential symptoms of the medication. Studies within the past two decades have noted the use of azathioprine, cyclosporine, mycophenolate mofetil, and leflunomide. In my personal experience back in my internal medicine days, we would try to transition our patients off of glucocorticoids to modified cyclosporine, while other contributors to this book worked with doctors who preferred azathioprine or mycophenolate. I've found that the side effects of using the modified cyclosporine were minimal and were lowered by keeping the drug frozen before use. Typical side effects are mostly gastrointestinal-related and can be ameliorated with the use of maropitant, ondansetron, and probiotics.

Steroid use has its own side effects in short- and long-term use. Short-term usage can cause polyuria/polydipsia (pu/pd), increased appetite, and lethargy. In some instances, it can cause behavioral changes such as aggression. An internist I worked with a while ago had his cat on prednisolone as part of his treatment for lymphoma, and he got so aggressive that he attacked his owner, who loved him very much. Fortunately, these side effects should resolve with time after discontinuation of steroids. Long-term usage can cause dermatological problems, insidious urinary tract infections, obesity, muscle weakness, and the potential to develop Cushing's. Continued steroid use can tip a patient into a diabetic crisis, and patients with underlying heart disease can be

TRANSFUSION MONITORING SHEET

RECIPIENT DETAILS
Name: ____________
Signaiment: ____________
Case no: ____________
Blood type: ____________
PCV/TS: ________ Serum/plasma colour: ________
Body weight: ____________

PRODUCT DETAILS
Blood product ID: ____________
Date of collection: ____________
Expiry date: ____________
Blood type: ____________
PCV/TS: ________ Serum/plasma colour: ________
Unit volume: ____________

Previous transfusions: ____________
Reason for transfusion: ____________
Clinician: ____________ Signature: ____________

(Please circle)	PRBC Canine Feline	FFP Canine Feline	FWB Canine Feline	Other (specify): ________ Canine Feline

Administration plan (volume & rate): ____________
Name: Signature:

Cross-matched? Compatible Incompatible Not evaluated	Method of admin: Gravity Syringe driver Fluid pump

Correct patient (initialled by 2): ________ Correct unit (initialled by 2): ________ IV catheter checked: ________
Start time: ________ Date: ________ Person starting transfusion: ________

	Time	Infusion rate ml/hr	Resp. rate	Pulse rate	MM Colour & CRT	Temp °C	Mentation	S/D/M blood pressure	Serum/ plasma/ urine colour	Angiodema /Erythema/ Pruritis (Y/N)	Vomit or diarrhea (Y/N)	Other concerns
Pre-transfusion												
5 mins												
15 mins.												
30 mins.												
60 mins.												
2 hours												
3 hours												
4 hours												
15 mins post transfusion												
1 hour post transfusion												
24 hour post transfusion												

Finish time: ________ Volume infused: ________ Post-transfusion PCV & time: ________

Comments: ____________

FOLLOW TRANSFUSION REACTION GUIDELINES IF YOU SUSPECT A REACTION

Image 10.7 Transfusion sheet proposed by AVHTM. *Source:* Elizabeth et al. (2021)/with permission of John Wiley & Sons.

pushed into congestive heart failure (Dutch 2023). As you can imagine, these are both very serious conditions that will need treatment after the discontinuation of steroids.

As far as the length of their hospital stay goes, it is dependent on each individual's recovery of red blood cells and need for transfusion. I've had patients who only need to stay for 24 hours and some that I spend my whole week's worth of shifts with (for reference, I work three consecutive 12-hour shifts). Starting at the beginning of their stay, we will triage them upon arrival. We will get new vitals, including heart rate, respiratory rate and effort, mucous membrane color and capillary refill time (CRT), and a temperature. We will also make a note of their mentation. From there, we will assess their catheter if transferred with one and draw necessary blood work if not completed at the primary veterinarian. We'll always want a green top or tiger top for plasma or serum in order to crossmatch against packed red cells for transfusion. We may run a new PCV/total solids (TS) if collecting more blood to see if it has dropped further during transfer. Steroids, if not administered by the general practice, will be given via a patent catheter. Antibiotics will also be considered if the underlying problem is pointing toward infection. After we admit the patient to the hospital, we'll get them set up for their blood transfusion. Once the transfusion is administered, we'll recheck the PCV/TS to make sure that the number increases. Due to altered clotting factors, there is a concern for thromboembolism, and decreased platelet counts (unrelated to immune-mediated thrombocytopenia (IMTP) – see next chapter) may be seen. In previous hospitals I have worked at, doctors have utilized enoxaparin, a low molecular weight heparin, as an antithrombotic to decrease the chances of thromboembolism by disrupting the clotting cascade. While enoxaparin is not usually kept in the hospital, it can be prescribed, and the owner can pick it up from a human pharmacy. Clopidogrel is an antiplatelet medication that can be used instead of enoxaparin and is much more readily available in hospitals. Starting an antiplatelet or antithrombotic medication is an important part of treatment because a pulmonary thromboembolism increases our patients' mortality rates. While hospitalized, we will start them on intravenous (IV) fluids and GI protectants such as maropitant, ondansetron, and sucralfate. PCV/TS will be checked at least daily, or more frequently if indicated, while in our care, and if the number drops or is still too low, another blood transfusion will be considered. A second immunosuppressive may be started while hospitalized as well. I have found working in an ER setting for a combined 7 years that once the patient's PCV has stabilized and they are no longer clinical for anemia, we will send them home!

Follow-Up Care

Just because they left the ER doesn't mean your patient is in the clear. These patients will need to continue medications at home with follow-up visits with either their primary care veterinarian or an internal medicine specialty. At these visits, rechecked blood work, including a CBC and PCV/TS, will be monitored. A gradual decrease in medications can be trialed as long as the PCV/TS remains consistent or continues to increase to a normal range (>30%). This is consistent with previous veterinary literature, where a posttransfusion PCV of 25–30% is the goal in anemic dogs. (Short 2012) For some patients, full remission is possible even with primary IMHA. In Piek's 2008 study on the outcome and prognostic factors for patients with IMHA, a majority of dogs in the study went into remission with a 3-month protocol of azathioprine and prednisolone. Per Kohn's 2006 study, feline patients had a greater survival rate if their anemia could be controlled and corrected without secondary complications.

Let's summarize everything from the beginning. You see a patient who is anemic. You find out that it is immune-mediated by doing a slide agglutination, looking for spherocytes on a blood smear, or sending out a direct Coombs antibody test. In preparation to transfer your patient, you place an IV catheter and draw any labs the ER might need, including a purple, green, and gold top. You've thought about the need for a blood transfusion, so you placed an appropriately sized catheter so the cells have less chance of lysing during transfusion. You drew those extra tubes so we can type and crossmatch that patient to a unit of blood at the ER. That also means we have extra blood before giving any type of treatment in case we need to do more testing. Since you had the foreknowledge to pull extra blood, you went ahead and started your patient on steroids before transfer. Now that they've arrived at the ER, we can type, crossmatch, and transfuse pRBC. We will continue to monitor their PC/TS during their stay and start them on an antiplatelet or antithrombotic medication as well as IV fluids and GI protectants. Multiple transfusions will be considered if the patient's PCV doesn't improve over time. A secondary immunosuppressant can and usually will be prescribed. Once the patient is stable, they will be discharged home with instructions for follow-up care with their primary care physician or an internal medicine specialist. Weaning off medications should be done slowly and with regular CBC and PCV/TS monitoring. While remission is possible, considerations for drugs, vaccines, and exposure to infectious diseases will need to be evaluated based on the patient's risk factor with the veterinarian treating the patient.

Works Cited

Bell, A.G. (2020). Successful xenotransfusion in a domestic ferret with spontaneous hemoperitoneum using feline packed red blood cells. *Journal of Veterinary Emergency and Critical Care* 30: 336–341. https://doi.org/10.1111/vec.12943.

Bovens, C.G.-J. (2013). Xenotransfusion with canine blood in the feline species: view of literature. *Journal of Feline Medicine and Surgery* 15: 62–67. https://doi.org/10.1177/1098612X12460530.

Brooks, W. (2023, March 4). Immune mediated hemolytic anemia (IMHA) in dogs and cats. *Veterinary Partner*. Retrieved from https://veterinarypartner.vin.com/default.aspx?pid=1923&id=4951868

Davidow, E.B.-T. (2021a). Association for Veterinary Hematology and Transfusion Medicine (AVHTM) Transfusion Reaction Small Animal Consensus Statement (TRACS) part 2: prevention and monitoring. *Journal of Veterinary Emergency and Critical Care* 31: 167–188. https://doi.org/10.1111/vec.13045.

Davidow, E.B.-T. (2021b). Association of Veterinary Hematology and Transfusion Medicine (AVHTM) Transfusion Reaction Small Animal Consensus Statement (TRACS). Part one: definitions and clinicial signs. *Journal of Veterinary Emergency and Critical Care* 31: 141–166. https://doi.org/10.1111/vec.13044.

Dutch, W.N. (2023). Incidences of steroid induced diabetes mellitus and congestive heart failure in cats given non-immunosuppressive doses of methylprednisolone acetate: 1042 cats. *Canadian Veterinary Journal* 64: 1051–1057. Retrieved from https://pmc.ncbi.nlm.nih.gov/articles/PMC10581361/.

Duval, D.A. (1996). Vaccine-associated immune-mediated hemolytic anemia in the dog. *Journal of Veterinary Internal Medicine* 10: 195–290. https://doi.org/10.1111/j.1939-1676.1996.tb02064.x.

Garden, O.K. (2019). ACVIM Consensus Statement on the diagnosis of immune-mediated hemolytic anemia in dogs and cats. *Journal of Veterinary Internal Medicine* 33: 313–334. https://doi.org/10.1111/jvim.15441.

Kohn, B.W. (2006). Primary immune-mediated hemolytic anemia in 19 cats: diagnosis, therapy, and outcome (1998–2004). *Journal of Veterinary Internal Medicine* 20: 159–166. https://doi.org/10.1111/j.1939-1676.2006.tb02836.x.

Morris, J.B. (2021). The effect of time on packed cell volume following packed red blood cell transfusion in anemic dogs. *Journal of Veterinary Emergency and Critical Care* 31: 215–220. https://doi.org/10.1111/vec.13027.

Odunayo, A.N. (2021). Association of Veterinary Hematology and Transfusion Medicine (AVHTM) Transfusion Reaction Small Animal Consensus Statement (TRACS) part 3: diagnosis and treatment. *Journal of Veterinary Emergency and Critical Care* 31: 189–203. https://doi.org/10.1111/vec.13043.

Piek, C.J. (2008). Idiopathic immune-mediated hemolytic anemia: treatment, coutcome, and prognostic factors in 149 dogs. *Journal of Veterinary Internal Medicine* 22: 366–373. https://doi.org/10.1111/j.1939-1676.2008.0060.x.

Short, J.D. (2012). Accuracy of formulas used to predict post-transfusion packed cell volume rise in anemic dogs. *Journal of Veterinary Emergency and Critical Care* 428–434. https://doi.org/10.1111/j.1476-4431.2012.00773.x.

Solomon, S.W. (2013). Mortality increases after massive exchange transfusion with older stored blood in canines with experimental pneumonia. *Blood* 1663–1672. https://doi.org/10.1182/blood-2012-10-462945.

Sun, P.J. (2020). Effect of dilution of canine blood samples on the specificity of saline agglutination tests for immun-mediated hemolysis. *Journal of Veterinary Internal Medicine* 32: 2374–2383. https://doi.org/10.1111/jvim.15945.

West, L.A. (2014). Treatment of idiopathic immune-mediated hemolytic anemia with mycophenolate mofetil in five dogs. *Journal of Veterinary Emergency and Critical Care* 24: 26–231. https://doi.org/10.1111/vec.12121.

Yagi, K.A. (2016). *Manual of Veterinary Transfusion Medicine and Blood Banking*. Ames, Iowa: Wiley Blackwell.

11

Searching for Platelets: IMTP

Danielle Schuler[1,2]

[1] *VeG ER for Pets, 1858 Reistertown Rd, Pikesville, MD, USA*
[2] *Veterinary Emergency and Critical Care Society Member, USA*

Introduction

Welcome back for round two of immune-mediated disorders! This time we're going to talk about immune-mediated hemolytic anemia (IMHA)'s close relative, immune-mediated thrombocytopenia (IMTP). Another mouthful of a disease process, and it can be as elusive to diagnose and treat as its sister disease. While IMHA targets erythrocytes, IMTP targets platelets. Unfortunately, little research has been done on how and why this happens in dogs and even less in cats. This is most likely due to IMTP being rare in felines while being more common in our canine patients. That makes this disease process no less deadly, with a morbidity and mortality rate of up to 27% (LeVine 2024a). What personally makes this disease so terrifying is that the severity of a patient's thrombocytopenia and their bleeding signs are not always correlated. Meaning that you could have a patient who has presented otherwise perfectly normal (seen for a routine health visit), and you get their blood work back, and their platelets are in the toilet! Is that due to a poor blood draw? (Ideal scenario: we wish all of our patients' abnormal lab work were due to poor phlebotomy). A viral infection or even leukemia? This is why it's important to examine a complete blood cell count, but we'll get to that later. On the flip side, you will also see a patient who is covered snout to tail in bruises and is at an extreme bleeding risk at that exact moment. While both of these theoretical patients have presented clinically differently, there has been little correlation between the severity of their thrombocytopenia and their risk of hemorrhage (LeVine 2024a). Unexplained bruises, small petechiae to the gums, and easily visible abdominal skin should be an immediate tip-off to check their clotting times and perform a manual platelet estimate. When preparing these cases for transfer, it is super important to keep sticks for blood collection and catheter placement to a minimum. Using a slightly smaller size catheter, like a 20 g instead of an 18 g, and using that catheter placement to collect blood saves that patient from multiple sticks and unnecessary risk of hemorrhage.

So what does IMTP mean, and how does it work? First, let's talk about platelets and what they do. Platelets, or their physiological name, thrombocytes, are the smallest component that makes up blood. Platelets can vary in appearance based on species. A canine's platelets are generally circular to oblong-shaped structures that stain purple. Normal feline platelets, because they cannot follow the textbook to save their lives, can range in size with "frothy" edges. Cats' platelets can go into overdrive during blood draws, so seeing some clumping is normal. To help mitigate this, it is important to employ a "clean" stick, do no fishing around to find a vein, and avoid severe agitation

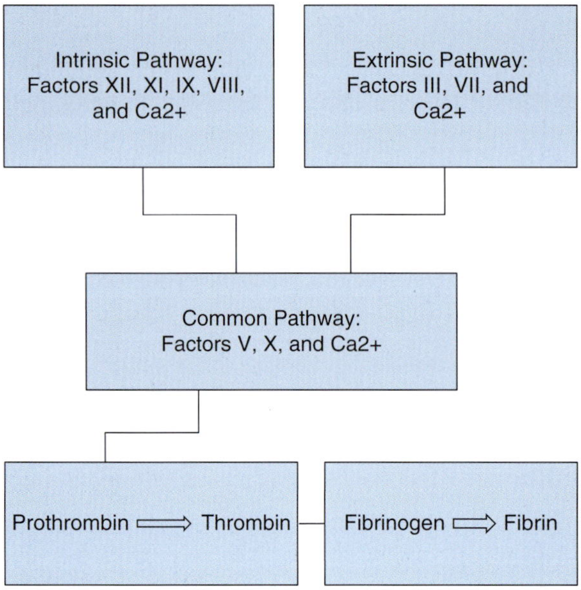

Figure 11.1 Very simplified model of the clotting cascade. The intrinsic pathway (longer, triggered by endothelial collagen exposure) is measured by partial thromboplastin time (PTT) while the extrinsic pathway (activated by endothelial tissue injury) is measured by prothrombin times (PT) on the coagulation machines. They converge in measuring the common pathway, which is the start of clot formation. *Source:* Courtesy of Danielle Schuler, RVT.

of the blood. If you've ever looked at a diagram of the clotting cascade and cried a little bit, don't worry, me too. So, we'll only briefly go over normal hemostasis before jumping into the meat of this chapter. Platelets are the body's first form of action in the clotting cascade called primary hemostasis (Jandrey 2012). In an oversimplified term, they form the "plug" that is the crucial first step in stopping hemorrhage. Secondary hemostasis boiled down to its most basic components, starting with either intrinsic or extrinsic pathways that coalesce into the common pathway, forming a stable clot. The intrinsic pathway starts by surface activation of factors XII, XI, IX, and VIII, and Ca^{2+}, while the extrinsic pathway starts by factor III (tissue factor) interacting with factor VII. Both of these pathways will flow into the common pathway involving factors V and X and Ca^{2+}. From there, prothrombin is converted to thrombin, which then converts fibrinogen into fibrin, thus stabilizing the clot (Cornell 2023) (Figure 11.1).

In this chapter, we're going to discuss what IMTP is, signs and symptoms, potential causes (primary versus secondary), and how to diagnose and treat this disease. IMTP is when the body targets its own thrombocytes with antiplatelet antibodies, destroying them and the body clearing them from its system. New platelet production can also be inhibited by antibodies and T-cells that target megakaryocytes. These are large bone marrow cells that go on to produce platelets. These new immature platelets are called megaplatelets that can be seen as a response that the body is trying to replenish its depleted supply. However, in cats and certain breeds of dogs (i.e., Cavalier King Charles), it can be a relatively normal finding.

American College of Veterinary Internal Medicine (ACVIM) Consensus Statement

Thrombocytopenia is established when a manual platelet estimate is less than 100,000/μl. A blood smear is made from a fresh blood sample and evaluated at the feathered edge and monolayer (where cells are not overlapping each other) at ×100 (oil lens). Thrombocytopenia can be false if

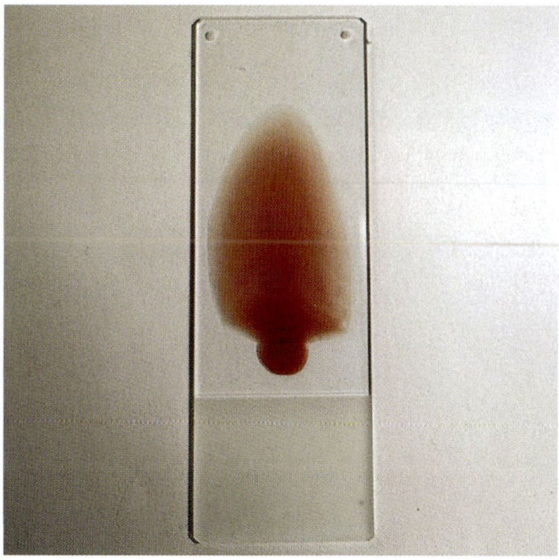

Image 11.1 Unstained blood smear provided by Vera Ortiz.

platelets are clumping together, so it is important to get a fresh sample and reevaluate the slide. To perform a platelet estimate, you need to count the number of platelets in each field for 10 fields. Then divide that total by 10 and multiply by 10,000–20,000. I personally multiply by 15,000 (smack dab in the middle of the recommended multiplication factor). What is important is for each repeat evaluation to use the same methodology. You can have platelet estimates lower than 50,000/μL, but you must establish that it is not due to consumption from acute or severe blood loss or disseminated intravascular coagulation (Image 11.1).

Once thrombocytopenia is established, diagnosis is a game of rule-outs. Before establishing if this is a primary or secondary form of IMTP, you must rule out other reasons for thrombocytopenia. For instance, if your patient has evidence of sepsis, disseminated intravascular coagulation (DIC), myelofibrosis, or bone marrow toxin, then IMTP is unlikely the cause for a low platelet count. Performing coagulation tests such as activated partial thromboplastin time (aPTT) and prothrombin time (PTT) can help differentiate thrombocytopenia due to an intrinsic cause, such as liver disease, or an extrinsic cause, such as bromethalin (anticoagulant) toxicity. While not a diagnostic factor for IMTP, it is important to run a chemistry panel and complete blood count. According to studies referenced in the ACVIM's consensus statement, an elevated blood urea nitrogen (BUN) and low hematocrit were indicative of greater disease severity in dogs with primary IMTP. These baseline values will also be beneficial for deciding what type of blood product to use if a transfusion is necessary for your patient. For most cases, a diagnosis of primary IMTP is considered "probable" or "possible." The only definitive way to prove IMTP is through ruling out underlying causes for IMTP and having a positive platelet/megakaryocyte-associated antibody screening via flow cytometry or radioimmunoassay. This is often cost-prohibitive and not necessary to come to the conclusion of IMTP. In practice, if a patient has low platelets and no other evidence (via diagnostic screening) of underlying causes, that is good enough for a diagnosis of primary IMTP (Image 11.2).

The ACVIM has listed six potential causes for IMTP with either low, intermediate, or high evidence that there is a causal relationship between the disease process and IMTP. Some causes, such as drug-induced, specific types of neoplasia, vaccination, toxins, and non-IMHA inflammatory disease, aren't even touched on in the consensus statement because there isn't enough data to prove these agents can or cannot cause IMTP (Huang 2012). There have been little to no studies

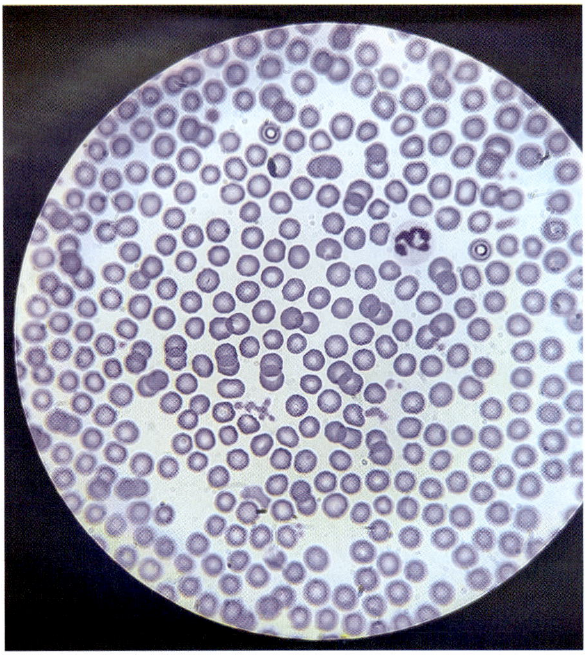

Image 11.2 100× oil lens blood smear with mild platelet clumping present. *Source:* Courtesy Danielle Schuler, RVT.

conducted in these areas, meaning that future research needs to be done. That being said, there has been evidence that specific drugs like cefazedone, gold salts, and sulfonamide drugs can cause IMTP in dogs, and hyperthyroid cats receiving propylthiouracil can have immune-mediated disease syndrome. Unfortunately, research across the board has been minimal or not conducted at all, so there is not enough data to identify causes in feline patients for any comorbidity causing IMTP. More commonly, we can see comorbidities such as infectious agents, either vector-borne or viral infections, as the cause for secondary IMTP. *Ehrlichiasis*, *leishmaniasis*, and *rangeliasis* all have high levels of evidence that they can cause IMTP in dogs. Other vector-borne diseases that have intermediate to low levels of evidence that they cause IMTP are *Anaplasma* spp. and *Babesia* spp.

So now that we know what IMTP is and the causes behind it, let's talk about diagnostics a little bit more. It may not seem like it, but getting a detailed patient history is one of our greatest diagnostic tools. As technicians, we are the first people who get our hands on these patients and get their history. This should include confirmation of vaccine history, current medications, and any concerns the owner might have noted at home. If the patient is already established at your practice, it will be easy to confirm previous history, including recent lab work or exposure to vector-borne diseases via ticks. This is also a good opportunity to make sure they are giving the appropriate monthly preventatives. If the patient is new to the clinic, getting previous medical records will go a long way in filling those knowledge gaps about that patient.

So, the great news is if you find your patient newly diagnosed with IMTP, you have the answers to a lot of important questions to rule out whether they have a primary or secondary form of IMTP. And the answers you don't have quite yet will come with the results of diagnostic testing. If you read the previous chapter, you're going to be running pretty similar tests. Most likely, you've already run a complete blood count (CBC) (and potentially a chemistry) for some baseline values. The low platelet count should tip you off into making a blood smear before your doctor even asks for one. It's a good rule of thumb to scan your smear for all cell abnormalities (including red and white cells), but your primary focus should be on the platelets. You should be performing a platelet estimate but also looking at if those platelets are large or normal size. Once you have confirmation of decreased platelets, it's running other diagnostics to rule out a secondary cause for IMTP. An easy test to confirm or run is a heartworm/4Dx to look for tick-borne pathogens. Testing for Babesia, Leishmania, and Rangelia should also be considered based on your regionality or if that patient has traveled to a location that has these diseases recently. Radiographs +/− ultrasound will be helpful in ruling out neoplasia and other consumptive causes. While radiographs, three views of the chest and abdominal cavity, with radiologist review, should easily be done at your practice, and diagnostic ultrasound should be done by a specialist (i.e., internist, radiologist, ultrasonographer, etc.).

Treatment (Transfusion Guidelines, Treatment, and Hospitalization)

We talked a lot about what IMTP is and how to diagnose it, but let's face it – as technicians, our primary focus is on how to effectively help our patients. We're all looking out for their best interests, right? So how do we accomplish that? The first step is discovering the problem. The second step is doing what you can in the here and now. And the third is getting them the specialized care that they need. Now, with that thinking, not all IMTP cases theoretically need to see an emergency room (ER) or internal medicine facility. Sometimes these cases are managed solely by their primary care provider. But this book is explicitly talking about cases that need us (the ER team) and internal medicine care. So, what do you need to do to prepare this case for a potential transfer? First things first, before you give any medications, make sure you have all the blood samples you need. While we can draw extra labs if needed at the ER, it's best practice if we are going to send out more comprehensive testing to the lab to have blood taken before any treatments are administered. Blood tubes I would love to see your patient transfer with are a ethylenediaminetetraacetic acid (EDTA) lavender top, tiger/gold top (serum), and/or a green top (lithium heparin for plasma) and a blue top (citrated). At least one of each tube, but if you can grab it, sending over or keeping hold of an additional lavender (EDTA) and tiger/gold (serum) top tube for outside reference lab testing is always a good idea. Second is getting a catheter in place. Like I mentioned earlier, bigger is not always better. Especially in our platelet-challenged friends. A regular "short" catheter is perfectly fine, but if you have one of those 2" 20 g or 18 g catheters and your patient is a large breed, go ahead and don't be afraid to throw that in there. Personally, I like a 2" catheter in dogs with long legs like great danes, cane corsos, etc. I do think they last a little longer and aren't as prone to falling out like a shorter catheter would in these guys. Don't go fishing in the vein; be gentle with your pokes. And please, if you value your ER team, please leave us a fresh leg to work with. We will appreciate your foresight in the most probable case that, at some point in their hospitalization, we will need to replace the catheter. We can see more complications with our thrombocytopenic patient's catheters blowing than in normal circumstances (Images 11.3 and 11.4).

So what will we do at the ER? Once they are transferred to use with all of your helpful records and diagnostics, we'll triage them to get another set of baseline vitals as well as note any bruising, petechiae, and/or ecchymosis. This can be formally assessed with a novel IMTP bleeding assessment for dogs, otherwise known as the DOGiBAT (Makielski 2018). This system is based on the human immune thrombocytopenia bleeding scale (IBLS) scoring to assess and grade bleeding symptoms in IMTP patients. This can be done daily to monitor the severity of bleeding and response

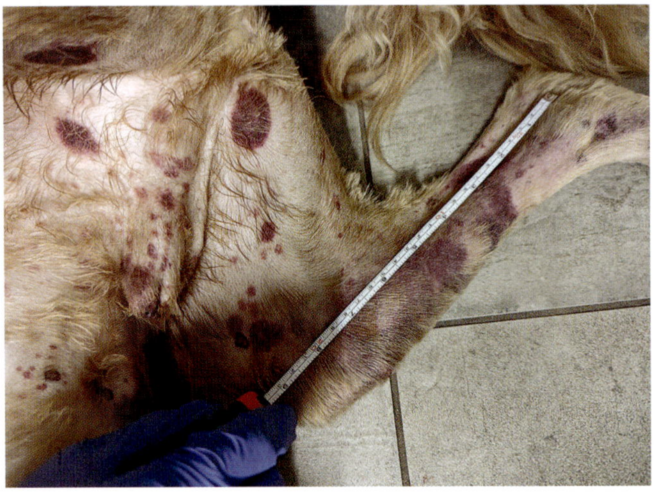

Image 11.3 Petechia noted in a golden doodle with IMTP. *Source:* Courtesy Danielle Schuler, RVT.

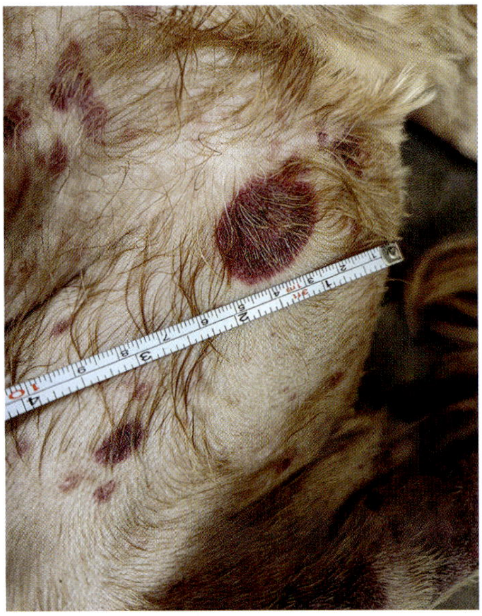

Image 11.4 Petechia noted in a golden doodle with IMTP. *Source:* Courtesy Danielle Schuler, RVT.

to treatment. There are nine anatomic sites that are given a score of 0–1 with the highest score being 18 (severe bleeding). Zero scoring means no presence of bleeding. A score of one indicates minimal bleeding, while a score of two indicates major bleeding. What may seem obvious is the lower the platelet count of the patient, the higher the DOGiBAT score (Figure 11.2).

After the initial triage is done by the technician and the doctor has done their physical exam, we'll make recommendations for hospitalization and treatment options. Something that can be done prior to transfer is starting a glucocorticoid at an immunosuppressive dose. This can be given as an injection in the form of Dexamethasone sodium phosphate, or if your patient is eating, it can be given as Prednisolone orally. This is the standard starting point and treatment therapy for immune-mediated disorders. Beyond that, treatment plans are created based on specific patient needs and doctor's preference. Keep in mind that once you have started steroids, it will interfere

Site	Bleeding grade 0	1	2
Skin	No	Petechiae/ecchymoses single site	Petechiae/ecchymoses >1 anatomic site
Catheter/venipuncture/ other cutaneous bleed	No	Self-limiting and <5 minutes	>5 minutes and/or intervention to control
Oral mucosa	No	Petechiae	Frank hemorrhage
Intraocular	No	Funduscopic	Hyphema
Epistaxis	No	Unilateral and <5 minutes	Bilateral or >5 minutes
Gastrointestinal	Occult blood (−); (Hema-chek™, Siemans Healthcare Diagnostics Inc., Tarrytown, New York)	Occult blood (+); (Hema-chek™, Siemans Healthcare Diagnostics Inc.)	Hematemesis, hematochezia, melena
Urinary	No	Microscopic (dipstick)	Macroscopic
Pulmonary hemorrhage (suspected/observed)	No	N/A	Yes
Intracranial hemorrhage (suspected/observed)	No	N/A	Yes

Each anatomic site receives a grade of 0 (none), 1 (mild), or 2 (severe), as detailed above. The grades at each site are totaled to give a maximal DOGIBAT of 18.

Figure 11.2 DOGiBAT novel bleeding score. *Source:* Makielski (2018) / with permission of John Wiley & Sons.

with future diagnostic testing, so make sure you have all the samples you may need before administering medications.

Oftentimes, a patient's platelet levels are so low and/or their signs of hemorrhage are so great that they will need some type of transfusion. Platelet-rich plasma would be the preferred product to infuse to increase platelets, while whole blood is a close second. Whole blood straight from a donor should be considered if your patient is both anemic and thrombocytopenic. Unfortunately, platelet-rich plasma is not readily available, and whole blood requires your facility to have on-call donors that match your patient's blood type. A whole blood transfusion may not be applicable if your patient's packed cell volume (PCV) isn't low, not requiring the transfusion of red blood cells that will come with a whole blood transfusion. The next best thing is a platelet-poor plasma in the form of fresh frozen plasma (FFP) or frozen plasma (FP). This is much more readily available, and your local ER most likely has it in stock. The downside of utilizing FFP/FP is that those transfused platelets are rapidly destroyed and usually require multiple transfusions. Plasma transfusions are administered like a blood transfusion, and patients should be monitored for adverse reactions while receiving it.

Vincristine is a chemotherapy drug commonly used to treat lymphoma, among other cancers, in cats and dogs. It has also been shown to rapidly increase platelet production in conjunction with steroid use in IMTP patients. Vincristine has a narrow safety margin with common side effects such as GI distress, including vomiting and diarrhea, and bone marrow suppression. One paper by Dr. Poirier et al. described neurotoxicity in an accidental overdose case. This is all to say that vincristine, like any chemotherapeutic drug, needs to be handled extremely carefully, for your and your patient's safety. It should be drawn up using a closed syringe system with technicians in full personal protective equipment (PPE), including gown, mask, safety eyewear, and chemotherapy-rated gloves underneath a chemotherapy hood. The patient's catheter needs to be patent, so for the sake of safety, a new one might be placed (depending on the patient's bleed risk) to avoid extravascularization. Chemotherapy agents need their own dedicated fridge and biohazard disposal unit. A lot of general practices don't have this equipment, making transfers to an ER with a specialty service like internal medicine and/or oncology worthwhile.

While steroids are the first line of treatment for primary IMTP, they may not be the only treatment they need. Adjunct treatments should be considered if platelet counts are not increasing after the first couple of days. Like I mentioned earlier, vincristine can be given as a single dose in conjunction with steroids to increase platelet production. However, if platelet numbers are not improving, other medications such as azathioprine, modified cyclosporine, or mycophenolate can be considered. It is recommended to start with a single secondary immunosuppressive, with little evidence that using three immunosuppressive medications did not have an increased effect on increasing platelet numbers while increasing the chance of negative side effects associated with each medication. All these medications come with their own side effects, such as GI upset, including anorexia, vomiting, and diarrhea, so choosing which drug best fits your patient should be considered. I have personally seen fewer side effects when patients are on modified cyclosporine, and the side effects are decreased when you keep it frozen. Some patients can't tolerate prednisone's long-term side effects, so transitioning them from a steroid to another immunosuppressive drug may be necessary.

Treating patients with confirmed secondary IMTP may not even need long-term immunosuppressive treatment. If you can treat the root cause and clear the infection with antibiotics, the body's attack on its own platelets should cease. Depending on the infection type will determine which antibiotic is best, but commonly, doxycycline is started in the hospital with continued use at home.

At the ER, we can provide round-the-clock care, and a patient's stay is determined by how well they are doing once treatment starts. We're not only addressing their primary illness but also the problems that often coincide with said primary illness. Besides giving the potential plasma transfusion, we will continue to monitor bleeding signs and provide supportive care while in the hospital. These patients can be hypovolemic due to blood loss and will be started on intravenous (IV) fluids. These patients will oftentimes have melena due to GI bleeds, so we will start gastroprotectants like sucralfate.

To summarize our patient's stay, let's start from the beginning to when they are ready to leave. Once they leave your hospital and arrive at the ER/specialty facility, they will be triaged by a nurse and seen by a doctor. If you sent them with a catheter, we will assess it for patency. During the initial assessment, we'll make the determination if a transfusion is necessary and admit to the hospital. During their hospital stay, we'll keep them on intravenous fluid therapy, administer steroids, and give a vincristine injection if needed. If indicated, we'll start antibiotics and continue to monitor for GI signs such as vomiting, diarrhea, and anorexia. All of these things we can monitor and treat symptomatically with drugs like maropitant, ondansetron, proviable, mirtazapine, and capromorelin. We'll continue to monitor their CBC and manual platelet estimates. It's especially important to monitor a CBC if vincristine is used. Even with a single dose, neutropenia can be seen. If patients are neutropenic, we can use antibiotics like ampicillin-sulbactam to intervene and prevent infection. If platelet response is not high enough, secondary immunosuppressive medications can be considered. Once patients are responding well to treatment, we can discharge them home!

Follow-Up Care

Once discharged from the ER, our patient's journey is far from over. Patients will need follow-up care that can be managed by their primary care physician or internal medicine specialist. The ACVIM remission algorithm states that a complete response is when platelets are greater than

100,000, and there is no evidence of bleeding. At that point, a weaning trial can be performed while monitoring platelet counts to ensure they don't decrease. It is possible for these guys to be off medication completely. There is up to a 47% relapse rate, which commonly happens during the weaning period, so figuring out a schedule to have them reevaluated, including a PE, CBC, and manual platelet estimate, is crucial for monitoring (LeVine 2024). Working in internal medicine, I have been fortunate enough to see a lot of these patients recover and live a good life.

Evans Syndrome

Now that we have discussed IMHA and IMTP separately, I wanted to touch on cases where these guys have both problems concurrently. While rare, patients who have decreased platelets and red blood cells due to an immune process have Evans syndrome. While we can see cases of IMTP with concurrent anemia, those are typically because of hemorrhage. Conversely, you can have patients with IMHA who have decreased platelets due to consumption from the hemorrhage. Evans syndrome means that the body is rejecting both platelets and red blood cells. Luckily, treatment is the same, but their survival rates decrease if both autoimmune diseases are present.

Works Cited

Cornell University. (2023). Secondary Hemostasis. From eclinpath.com: eclinpath.com/hemostasis/physiology/secondary-hemostasis

Huang, A.M.-M. (2012). Idiopathic immune-mediated thrombocytopenia and recent vaccination in dogs. *Journal of Veterinary Internal Medicine* 142–148. https://doi.org/10.1111/j.1939-1676.2011.00850.x.

Jandrey, K. (2012). Assessment of platelet function. *Journal of Veterinary Emergency and Critical Care* 81–98. https://doi.org/10.1111/j.1476-4431.2011.00707.x.

LeVine, D.G. (2024a). ACVIM consensus statement on teh treatment of immune thrombocytopenia in dogs. *Journal of Veterinary Internal Medicine* 1982–2007. https://doi.org/10.1111/jvim.17079.

Levine, D.K. (2024b). ACVIM consensus statement on the diagnosis of immune thrombocytopenia in dogs and cats. *Journal of Veterinary Internal Medicine* 1958–1981. https://doi.org/10.1111/jvim.196996.

Makielski, K.B. (2018). Development and implementation of novel immune thrombocytopenia bleeding score for dogs. *Journal of Veterinary Internal Medicine* 1041–1050. https://doi.org/10.1111/jvim.15089.

12

Not So Simple: AHDS

Simone Conwell[1,2]

[1] *VeG ER for Pets, 1858 Reisterstown Road, Pikesville, MD, USA*
[2] *Veterinary Emergency and Critical Care Society Member, USA*

Diarrhea. Sometimes it happens. Sometimes it's coming, and pet parents know it's coming because that happened the last time Bella got into cheese. According to the American Veterinary Medical Association (AVMA) (n.d.), vomiting/diarrhea are consistently among the top 13 veterinary emergencies each year (AVMA, n.d.). I know almost everyone reading this book has had a pet parent call about vomiting or diarrhea, and a lot of you have had owners then elaborate that there is blood in the diarrhea and they want to be seen as soon as possible, since, in emergency medicine anyway, they're about to go on vacation. But the bloody diarrhea. Is it a little frank blood from straining too hard? Or is it the jam of hematochezia? Or is it straight bloody liquid diarrhea? Are the gums pale? When is it acute diarrhea syndrome (AHDS), and when did we stop calling it hemorrhagic gastroenteritis (HGE)?

AHDS vs Anaphylaxis

It is tempting to call every case of hematochezia AHDS, especially in the warmer months, but AHDS is more of a cooler-month disease (Mortier 2015). Weather doesn't exclude AHDS as a diagnosis, but it can hide anaphylaxis. Anaphylaxis is a hypersensitized immune reaction of immunoglobulin E (IgE) to a previously exposed antigen (Drobatz 2012). Mast cells have 500,000–1,000,000 IgE molecules on their cells' surfaces, and only 200 bound receptors are needed to degranulate a mast cell (Smith 2023). Unfortunately, these receptors can also be activated by multiple potential allergens that usually would only cause moderate reactions, converging to cause anaphylaxis (Smith 2023). Unlike in humans and cats, whose anaphylaxis reactions tend to be related to cardiorespiratory symptoms, dogs tend to have anaphylaxis symptoms expressed through the gastrointestinal tract (GIT) since histamines are released from GI mast cells. From there, they move to the liver through the portal vein, which results in dilation of the hepatic artery and a subsequent increase in hepatic blood flow (Smith 2023). Then venous constriction occurs, and hepatic vein constriction concomitant with hepatic artery dilation results in hepatic congestion, as there is limited option for venous drainage (Smith 2023). This is an incredibly acute increase of almost 300% blood volume, and that pressure starts to feed backward, which results in gallbladder edema formation (Smith 2023). The congestion causes constriction of the hepatic vessels, resulting in a decrease of 30% of cardiac output from splanchnic vasculature not returning

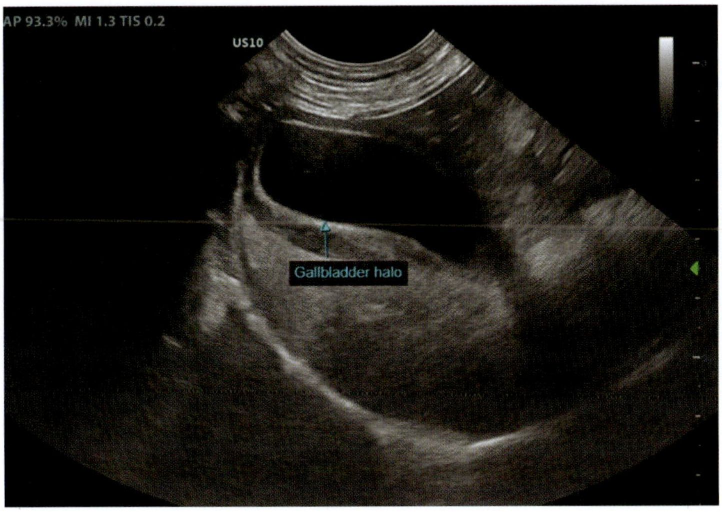

Image 12.1 Gallbladder wall edema, "gallbladder halo" in a dog with anaphylaxis.
Source: Photo courtesy of Simone Conwell, RVT, VTS (ECC).

circulation and causing a massive fluid shift in the resulting distributive shock (Drobatz 2012; Smith 2023). Distributive shock is a maldistribution of blood flow due to a decrease in systemic vascular resistance (vasodilation) (Smith 2023). While cardiac function may appear clinically normal, hypovolemia and cardiac compromise exist and worsen the state of shock, which will require the underlying cause to be addressed and the use of alpha-adrenergic agonists, namely epinephrine (Drobatz 2012). Since the GIT is the shock organ in dogs, anaphylaxis will often result in GI signs such as vomiting and diarrhea, prompting a visit to the vet (Drobatz 2012) (Image 12.1).

Activated mast cells also affect the clotting cascade at multiple steps. The activated mast cells release not only histamine but also heparin, tryptase, antithrombin, and anti-Xa (Smith 2023). All of these factors degrade thrombin, plasmin, and factor XIII, which stabilize fibrin clots (Smith 2023). They also activate factor XII, which activates the intrinsic system and disables fibrinogen while activating tissue plasminogen activator and urokinase, resulting in fibrinolysis (Smith 2023). Platelet-activating factor is also activated, and while that induces platelet aggregation, it can result in endothelial dysfunction and leakage (Smith 2023). The overall effect in blood work is most often an increase in prothrombin time/activated partial thromboplastin (PT/aPTT) and thrombocytopenia, with the aPTT affected earlier and more noticeably (Smith 2023). Why is this relevant? Because that leakage has to come out, and often does so through the GIT in the form of bloody diarrhea that looks like strawberry/raspberry jam. Anaphylaxis is a look-alike for AHDS and is treated very differently. A point-of-care ultrasound (POCUS) performed by a skilled technician or doctor can help monitor for gallbladder wall edema, which would point to anaphylaxis, and pulling blood to run PT/aPTT can save time later and help rule out disease processes.

Diagnostics

Because our patients cannot speak to us, diagnostics are imperative in making a treatment plan and healing those same patients. The first, and often overlooked, diagnostic will be the vitals check and tech exam. Yes, our doctors will do their own exam, sometimes on their own, sometimes with us, but we are usually touching the patient significantly more than the doctor because we do the nursing care, draw blood, take radiographs, and perform the treatments. For example, my doctors do not stand nearby to watch over my shoulder when I'm giving a patient calcium gluconate, even though the patient could become bradycardic, because they trust me to read the electrocardiogram (ECG) and watch the heart rate and alert them as I am stopping the medication if the patient reacts poorly. So take ownership of your knowledge and skills, and remember your vitals check is an important diagnostic tool.

So back to basics and what a normal TPR (temperature, pulse, and respiration rate) looks like in dogs.

Normal vitals in dogs.

Parameter	Normal Range
Temperature	99.5–102.5°F/ 37.5–39°C
Heart rate (beats per minute, bpm)	70–160 bpm
Respiratory rate (respirations per minute, rpm)	8–20 rpm
Mucous membrane color	Pink
Capillary refill time (seconds)	<2 s

Values from Sirois (2019).

Auscultate the thorax – listen for murmurs, muted heart sounds, "sneakers in the dryer" that can indicate atrial fibrillation, crackles, wheezes, and loss of sound. If you hear a murmur on the right side, it's over the tricuspid valve. As for the others, remember PAM 345: pulmonary, aortic, and mitral (PAM) valves at intercostal spaces 3, 4, and 5 (Pace) (Image 12.2).

The level of consciousness should also be evaluated. There is a difference in a laterally recumbent chihuahua with a heart rate of 40 bpm and a greyhound walking in the door with the same heart rate.

Assessment of level of consciousness.

Signs	LOC
Fully conscious, alert, and engaged	Bright, alert, responsive (BAR)
Fully conscious and alert, but not engaged – may be fearful – generally subdued	Quiet, alert, responsive (QAR)
Aware of surroundings and can be roused with tactile or verbal stimuli, but withdrawn/depressed	Lethargic, dull/depressed
Very depressed and uninterested in surroundings. Not fully rousable with tactile or verbal stimuli	Obtunded
Sleeplike state, nonresponsive to verbal stimuli. Only responds to noxious tactile stimuli	Stuporous
Unrousable	Comatose

Table pulled from Sirois (2019).

You may also want to obtain a blood pressure reading on your patient on presentation. It can be used as an indicator of pain/discomfort, indirectly as a measure of cardiovascular status, and again

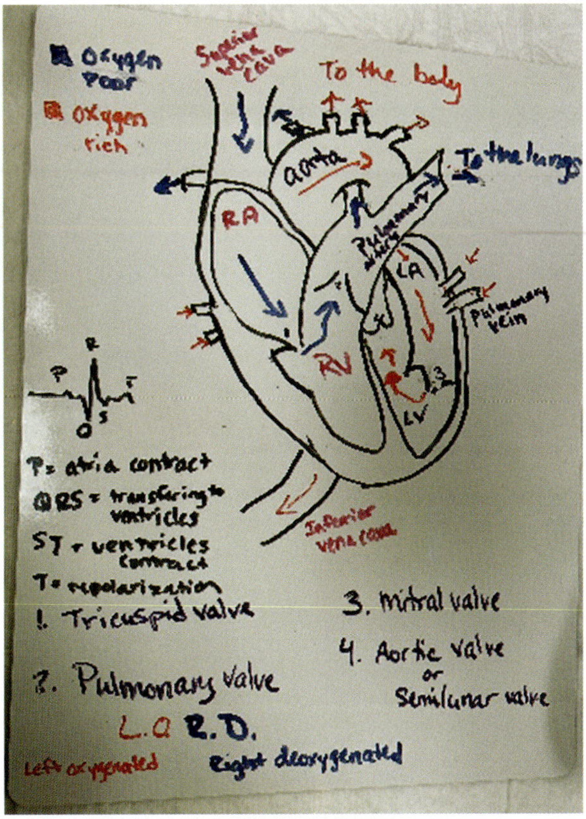

Image 12.2 A drawing of the anatomy of the heart and some of its structures, with an ECG tracing. *Source:* Courtesy of Simone Conwell, RVT, VTS (ECC).

indirectly as an indicator of shock. While no validated noninvasive measurement device exists, a skilled technician can use a doppler blood pressure unit or oscillometric device to estimate the systolic blood pressure. The American College of Veterinary Internal Medicine (ACVIM) has no direct consensus statement on taking blood pressure readings, but the consensus statement on the identification, evaluation, and management of hypertension in cats and dogs does offer a protocol and observes that the skill of the operator can have a drastic effect on the results (Acierno 2018) (Image 12.3).

Ideal Guidelines for Obtaining Non-Invasive Blood Pressure (NIBP) Readings **(Acierno 2018)**

- Be in a calm, quiet environment where the patient is acclimated.
- Ideally, have the patient calmly resting in ventral or lateral recumbency for ease of placing the limb at heart level.
- Cuff width of 30–40% of limb/tail circumference.
- The same individual should perform all readings using a standardized protocol that they have been thoroughly trained on.
- Measurements should be taken while the patient is motionless.
- Discard the first measurement and repeat five to seven times until the blood pressure is consistent.
- Average the readings.

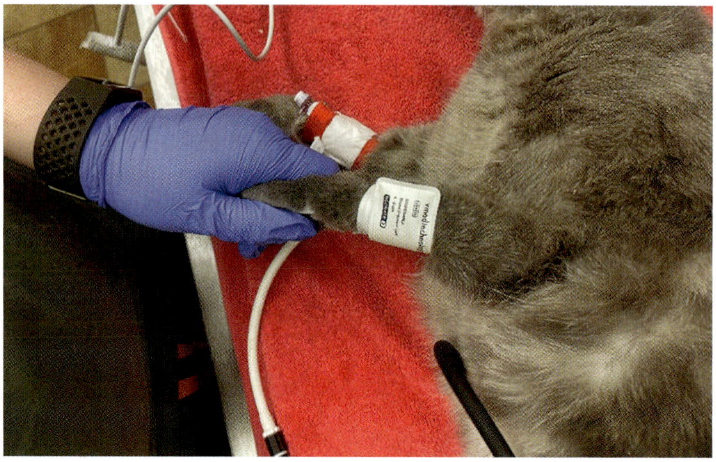

Image 12.3 Image of a cat in lateral recumbency where a Doppler blood pressure is being obtained on a forelimb. *Source:* Photo courtesy of Simone Conwell, RVT, VTS (ECC).

Normal NIBP ranges in dogs in millimeters of mercury (mmHg).

Size	Average heart rate (bpm)	Systolic/doppler	Diastolic	Mean arterial pressure (MAP)
Small	90–140	100–160	60–90	80–120
Medium	80–120	100–160	60–90	80–120
Large	60–100	100–160	60–90	80–120

Values from Sirois (2019).

It is also useful when using a Doppler to obtain the blood pressure to retake the heart rate by counting the number of beats heard. It is important to monitor trends as much as individual numbers to see the whole picture. If the patient is hypotensive, the crystal for the Doppler can be taped to the pulse point for convenient monitoring not only of the blood pressure but also of the heart rate itself. Some readers may have heard of permissive hypotension, and while that is a valid tool in certain situations, this is not one of them. That topic will not be covered in this book.

If there is significant hypotension or the patient looks sufficiently dull, it is often protocol in an emergency vet to place an intravenous (IV) catheter. From there, a blood panel including a complete blood count (CBC), biochemistry panel, and electrolytes is often pulled. If your hospital has the capability to run them in-house, coagulation (PT/aPTT) tubes should also be pulled. These tests do not need to be performed immediately and can be set aside, though centrifuging the lithium heparin/serum tubes should be performed in a timely manner, and the PT/aPTT should be run after 15 minutes. However, a lactate, blood glucose, and packed cell volume/total solids (PCV/TS), also known as a "big four," should be run (see chapter 1 "Bloodwork basics" for further information). Lactate is a measurement of cellular metabolism through the production of lactic acid, and is often seen in hypovolemic shock (Randels-Thorp 2017; Sirois 2019). Hypoglycemia is often an indicator of sepsis or other metabolic abnormalities in adult animals (Sirois 2019). The PCV/TS will be the most obvious of the big four to indicate AHDS. There will usually be hemoconcentration >60% and a normal to decreased total solids (Collier 2025; Drobatz 2012). But sometimes the values will appear normal due to hemoconcentration from dehydration (Morrison 2019). Anytime a patient loses fluids through vomiting and diarrhea, there is a massive risk of hypovolemic shock, and the blood loss in AHDS increases that risk (Peck 2022). As mentioned in chapter 1's Bloodwork Basics, memorizing normal values relies on the specific machine being used, and rather, being able to recognize values as abnormal for your machines is more important than the values themselves. As PCV is a percentage, remember that normal is generally between 35 and 45% (Lee n.d.).

Other abnormalities that may occur in bloodwork include panhypoproteinemia, increased blood urea nitrogen (BUN), hypokalemia, hyponatremia, increased hematocrit, and potentially a hypochloremia if hematemesis has started, most of which are to be expected to some degree in any vomiting/diarrhea case due to ongoing losses and hypovolemia (Morrison 2019). For AHDS, it's really the hemoconcentration and hematochezia +/− hematemesis that make the diagnosis (Morrison 2019). But let's discuss the consequences of a panhypoproteinemia for a moment. All proteins include albumin. Why is albumin important? Because it makes up 50% of plasma protein concentration, aids in hemostasis, and maintains microvascular permeability and colloid osmotic/oncotic pressure (COP) (Spurlock). COP prevents unnecessary fluid shift from the intravascular space to the extravascular space by application of Van't Hoff's law (Holowaychuk). The large size of albumin and their associated cations (mostly sodium intravascularly) provide 60–70% of COP, while globulins comprise the rest (Spurlock). When these molecules are compromised through hemorrhage into the GIT, symptoms of AHDS can progress to the point that fluid boluses will not be sufficient resuscitation, and colloids are needed to maintain COP (Dibartola 2012).

Another set of potential diagnostic bloodwork can include D-dimers and thromboelastography to monitor for disseminated intravascular coagulopathy (DIC) (Morrison 2019). DIC occurs when intravascular thrombosis overwhelms anticoagulant pathways and leads to a consumptive and decompensated coagulopathy (Drobatz 2012). Unfortunately, most places do not have access to tableside thromboelastography units, and D-dimers are sent to an outside laboratory. DIC is a devastatingly uncommon complication that can lead to multiorgan failure, thrombosis, and ultimately death (Morrison 2019; Norkus 2019).

An ECG should be performed on any suspected AHDS patient due to hypovolemia and electrolyte imbalance (Morrison 2019; Norkus 2019). Ventricular tachycardia may occur secondary to hypovolemia due to decreased cardiac output and preload (Morrison 2019; Norkus 2019). Recall that cardiac output is defined as stroke volume times heart rate, and stroke volume is determined by contractility, afterload, and preload (Norkus 2019). Stroke volume, the volume of blood pumped by the heart, is decreased during hypovolemic shock due to fluid loss, resulting in a decreased cardiac output (Norkus 2019; Peck 2022). The heart rate, in turn, increases as a compensatory mechanism (Image 12.4 and 12.5).

Radiographs are perhaps not as useful as an abdominal ultrasound in suspected AHDS patients. Both should (hopefully) only show ileus and fluid-filled bowel loops, though ideally at least one is performed and interpreted by a boarded radiologist to rule out a GI foreign body or perforation (Collier 2025) (Image 12.6).

Hydration and Medication

AHDS needs fluids for treatment. A large amount of isotonic crystalloid fluids is imperative to mitigate the hypovolemic shock state (Collier 2025). The diarrhea and vomiting must also be controlled with antidiarrheals and antiemetic therapy (Collier 2025). The patients must also eat as soon as possible, as eating is associated with faster healing time (Busch 2022). Because of the large volume of fluid and the potentially already compromised electrolytes, monitoring electrolytes and

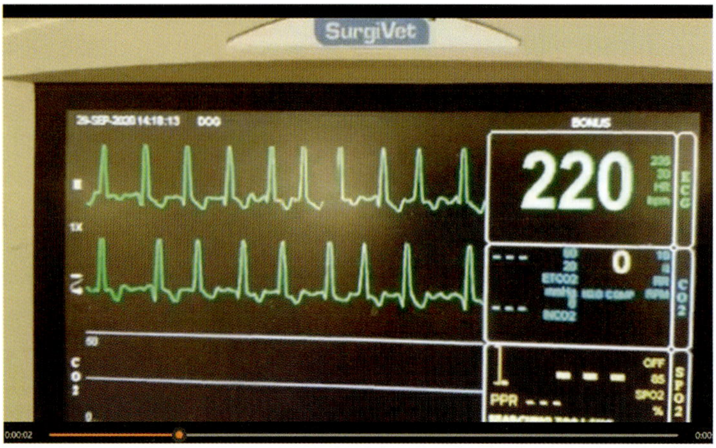

Image 12.4 Left: Still frame of ventricular tachycardia in a patient. *Source:* Photo courtesy of Simone Conwell, RVT, VTS (ECC).

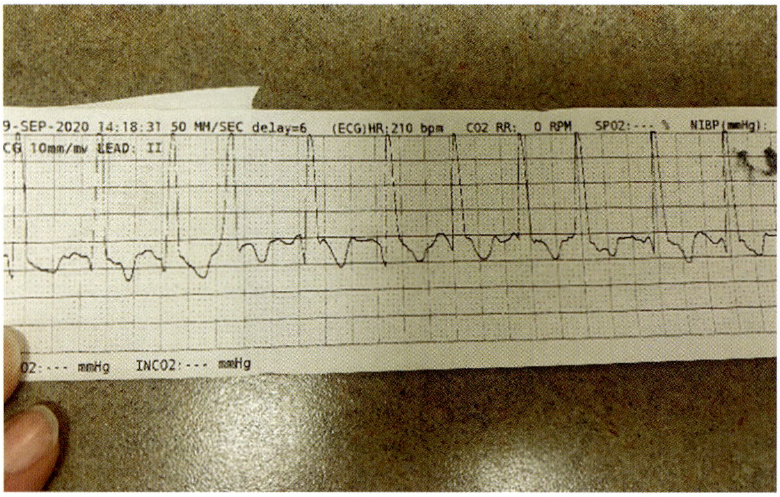

Image 12.5 ECG printout of ventricular tachycardia for the same patient. *Source:* Photos courtesy of Simone Conwell, RVT, VTS (ECC).

providing supplementation as indicated is necessary (Bush). If the panhypoproteinemia is severe enough to warrant treatment, colloids such as albumin, fresh frozen plasma/frozen plasma, and even synthetic colloids should be considered, provided there is no pre-existing kidney damage (Busch 2022, Holowaychuk). Prokinetic medications like metoclopramide are often indicated due to ileus, and as sloughing of the GIT is painful, pain medication should be administered (Busch 2022). Please see the chapters in section 2 for pain control suggestions. Lidocaine can also be administered for a twofold benefit; while providing visceral pain relief, it is an anti-arrhythmic for the patients whose ECGs show they have ventricular tachycardia (Norkus 2019). While it may be surprising to some, proton pump inhibitors are not recommended in cases of AHDS due to increased risk of dysbiosis (Busch 2022).

Image 12.6 A blanket with severe hematochezia soaking in. *Source:* Photo courtesy of Simone Conwell, RVT, VTS (ECC).

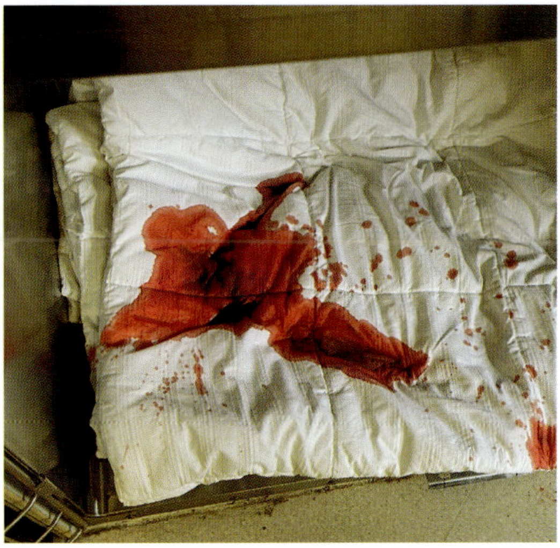

Maropitant is usually the first emetic chosen, though ondansetron may be needed if the patient seems nauseous still (Busch 2022; Collier 2025; Morrison 2019). Antidiarrheals can include probiotics and an increase in fiber intake, but depending on the severity of the dysbiosis and if there is evidence of infection, including sepsis, metronidazole, enrofloxacin, and ampicillin sulbactam may be indicated (Busch 2022; Collier 2025). The use of antibiotic therapy in AHDS cases is somewhat controversial in the time of multidrug-resistant pathogens, and there are studies showing that using antibiotic therapy in aseptic AHDS (Busch 2022). Septic cases will require antibiotic usage and should follow the surviving sepsis campaign.

As the patient improves, the fluid rate should be decreased and medications transferred from intravenous to oral. The patient should continue to be fed a palatable, bland diet in smaller, more frequent meals over the next several days to avoid unnecessary stress on the GIT (Busch 2022).

Nursing Considerations

These patients are going to produce large amounts of diarrhea. A rectal Foley can be used, provided that they will tolerate it and the diarrhea is liquid enough to pass through. Their fur and skin should be kept as clean and dry as possible to avoid skin infections. Copious pee pads over the bedding can minimize the need to change bedding, and frequent walks should be undertaken. Considering Kirby's Rule of 20 (see section 1), this patient is going to feel like they are only being touched to have something happen to them. Consider sitting with them and petting or talking softly to them, brushing them, etc., so they are not anticipating only having uncomfortable and potentially frightening experiences with you. Allow their owners to visit if your hospital is not open-concept, and encourage the owners to offer them food from their dishes from home if possible. While it may be impractical due to diarrhea to have bedding/toys from home directly in the kennel, consider having something nearby with the familiar scent. I had a patient whose owner told me she had been fed from a fork when she was sick while young, and that is how I got that patient to eat again. Talk to your patient's humans and get an idea of who their pet is, what commands they use when they go outside, and if they prefer fish instead of chicken when sick (that owner was a chef, and his dog had an expensive palate).

Works Cited

Acierno, M.B. (2018). ACVIM consensus statement: guidelines for the indentification, evaluation, and management of systemic hypertension in dogs and cats. *Journal of Veterinary Internal Medicine* https://doi.org/10.1111/jvim.15331.

American Veterinary Medical Association. (n.d.). 13 Animal Emergencies that Require Immediate Veterinary Consultation and/or Care. Retrieved from www.avma.org: https://www.avma.org/resources/pet-owners/emergencycare/13-animal-emergencies-require-immediate-veterinary-consultation-andor-care

Busch, K.U. (2022). Update on acute hemorrhagic diarrhea syndrome in dogs. *Advances in Small Animal Care* https://doi.org/10.1016/j.yasa.2022.06.003.

Collier, A. (2025). Acute Hemorrhagic Diarrhea Syndrome in Dogs. Retrieved from merckvetmanual.com: https://www.merckvetmanual.com/digestive-system/diseases-of-the-large-intestine-in-small-animals/acute-hemorrhagic-diarrhea-syndrome-in-dogs?autoredirectid=29916

Dibartola, S. (2012). *Fluid, Electrolyte, and Acid-Base Disorders in Small Animal Practice*. St. Louis, Missouri: Elsevier Saunders.

Drobtaz, K.M. (2012). *Manual of Small Animal Emergency and Critical Care Medicine*. Iowa: WIley-Blackwell.

Lee, J. (n.d.). The Importance of PCV/TP in Veterinary Medicine. Retrieved from vetgirlontherun.com: https://vetgirlontherun.com/veterinary-continuing-education-pcv-tp-big4-vetgirl-blog/

Morrison, J.A. (2019). *Small Animal Gastrointestinal Diseases*. Hoboken, NJ: Wiley-Blackwell.

Mortier, F.S. (2015). Acute haemorrhagic diarrhoea syndrome in dogs: 108 cases. *Veterinary Record* https://doi.org/10.1136/vr.103090.

Norkus, C. (2019). *Veterinary Technician's Manual for Small Animal Emergency and Critical Care*. Hoboken: John Wiley & Sons, Inc.

Pace, C. (2017). How to maximise your auscultation technique. *The Veterinary Nurse*. Retrieved from https://www.magonlinelibrary.com/doi/full/10.12968/vetn.2017.8.9.512

Peck, C. (2022, January). A Review of Shock. Retrieved from mspca.org: https://www.mspca.org/angell_services/a-review-of-shock/

Randels-Thorp, A. (2017). *Acid-Base and Electrolyte Handbook for Veterinary Technicians*. Ames, Iowa: John Wiley & Sons, Inc.

Sirois, M. (2019). *Mosby's Veterinary PDQ*. St. Louis, Missouri: Mosby.

Smith, M.R. (2023). *Anaphylaxis: Beyond Fluids and Epinephrine. VIN/VECCS Rounds.*

Spurlock, N. (2016). Alternative Plasma Protein Products : Albumin and Human Immunoglobulin Therapy. In: *Manual of Veterinary Transfusion Medicine and Blood Banking*, 83–102. Ames, Iowa: Wiley Blackwell.

13

Gasping for Breath – Feline Asthma

Danielle Schuler[1,2]

[1] *VeG ER for Pets, 1858 Reistertown Rd, Pikesville, MD, USA*
[2] *Veterinary Emergency and Critical Care Society Member, USA*

Have you ever been sitting on your couch, hanging out with your feline friend, and out of nowhere they kinda hunker down, extend their neck, and produce this short, dry cough like they've got something stuck in their throat? They do one or two good coughs, and then they look at you like 'What? I just had something stuck in my throat.' That is the best way I can think to describe what a stable asthma attack sounds like. Infrequent attacks like this can absolutely be managed by their primary care veterinarian. On the other hand, it's those cats who cough and wheeze, and now they are panting and can't breathe. These kids need to be seen as soon as possible as an emergency. In this chapter, we'll go over what feline asthma is, diagnostics, and how to treat these breathing-troubled friends.

So, what exactly is feline asthma? Feline asthma is bundled into a class of feline lower airway disease, including asthma and bronchitis, which affect the bronchi and bronchioles. Branching from the trachea into the left and right bronchus, each air passageway branches off into smaller and smaller pathways until ending in alveolar sacs – housing tiny alveoli. This is where carbon dioxide and oxygen are exchanged in external respiration (Colville 2008). Normal, healthy air passageways are unobstructed with inflammatory fluid or mucus with no signs of bronchoconstriction. Lungs that are suffering from lower airway disease often times are narrow (due to bronchoconstriction), look red or inflamed, and can have mucus or inflammatory fluid present.

An asthma attack is the lungs' hyperresponsiveness to inhaled allergens or antigens in the environment, causing inflammation to lung tissue (Johnson 2011). This causes a spasming, coughing fit that can sometimes lead to retching. In my experience, owners will come into the emergency room (ER) calm as can be because what they think they see is their cat vomiting white phlegm. Then, once you get them out of the carrier for triage, they are gasping for breath. This is a critical situation and should be addressed immediately. In some cases, the attack is acute and can be treated with light sedation and oxygen. In more chronic or severe cases, these cats will need full sedation and intubation before they go into respiratory collapse, and you initiate resuscitation efforts.

Oxygen Therapy

Now, these kids come in already tachypneic, dyspneic, and panicking. For reference, a cat's normal respiratory rate is between 15 and 30 bpm. These cats come in with abnormal rates and effort – but we don't know why yet. There are two causes of respiratory distress that most concern me in these situations – congestive heart failure and asthma. At first glance, they can present the same, so it's important to get a thorough history from the owner. Have they been diagnosed with a heart murmur or heart disease in the past? This will help your doctor, along with diagnostics, to know how to best treat them. While you're obtaining vitals, I would stick to the minimum noninvasive ones, including heart rate, respiratory rate, mucus membrane color, and capillary refill time (CRT). I will skip getting a temperature if it stresses them out more. While you are getting these vitals and your doctor is doing their initial assessment, someone should be holding flow-by oxygen near the patient's face, ideally 2 cm or less from the patient's nose (Silverstein 2023). Generally, flow by is set to 2 or 3 l/min, and that will provide an F_iO_2 of 25–40% (Silverstein 2023). Auscultating their lungs can help point you in the right direction. Cats with lower airway disease will commonly sound like they are wheezing and can have crackles or harsh lung sounds on auscultation (Loewen 2022).

If your patient isn't in too much distress, you can attempt to place an intravenous (IV) catheter to give a sedative. But if the patient is in too much distress – muddy or cyanotic gums, panting, and/or abdominal breathing – then it is more beneficial to get them into an oxygen chamber and give the sedative intramuscularly (Dietschel 2013). No treatment should delay getting these cats into oxygen. We don't need heavy sedation for these kids, and a major pain management component like a full μ-agonist opioid is not necessary because they are not in pain. Our best treatment option for a calming effect is butorphanol. This is a partial μ-agonist/antagonist, so there is some mild pain control, and it induces a light sedation effect to help them calm down. A dose of around 0.2–0.3 mg/kg is what my doctors commonly order for these patients (Dietschel 2013). Butorphanol has a short period of action and can be re-dosed every 4–6 hours regularly, or sooner if your patient is still in distress (Budde 2023).

Let's talk about oxygen. Back in the early 2000s, having a climate-controlled oxygen chamber at a general practice was not the norm. It was only until I started in emergency medicine that I had the luxury of having an oxygen chamber. These days it has become more commonplace, and I think that's great! If your practice does not have an actual oxygen chamber, you can jerry-rig a makeshift one easily with some cling wrap over the cage door with an oxygen line pumping oxygen in (Lynch 2022). Just make sure to have a ventilation flap on the top so it's not fully enclosed. This isn't a perfect solution because you can't control the percentage of oxygen in your makeshift cage, but it can be beneficial for the patient before you transfer them to an ER facility. With a proper oxygen cage system, you can control the percentage of oxygen in the cage, temperature, and see the humidity. Typically, we will start at 40% oxygen, but that number can be increased if needed (Image 13.1).

Radiographs

Once your patient is on oxygen, this is when you can think about further diagnostics. While blood work is important and can help rule out other causes, it is typically not the first thing my doctor will ask for. The most useful diagnostic your doctor will ask for in these cases is radiographs. Radiographs will be helpful in looking at the chest and lung space. There are several diagnoses that can be made from evaluating radiographs, which is why this imaging step is so important (Gareis 2023). Lungs that are suffering from pleural effusion and lungs that have chronic airway changes look different from each other (Gareis 2023). Lung space that is mostly whited out with little definition most likely has fluid accumulated in the chest. This can be verified by a quick scan with the ultrasound. Fluid on ultrasound is anechoic, or black in appearance. The easiest way I can think of is to describe it if you take an abdominal radiograph, and you can visualize the bladder because it is a nice round circle. A bladder on ultrasound will have a definitive hyperechoic

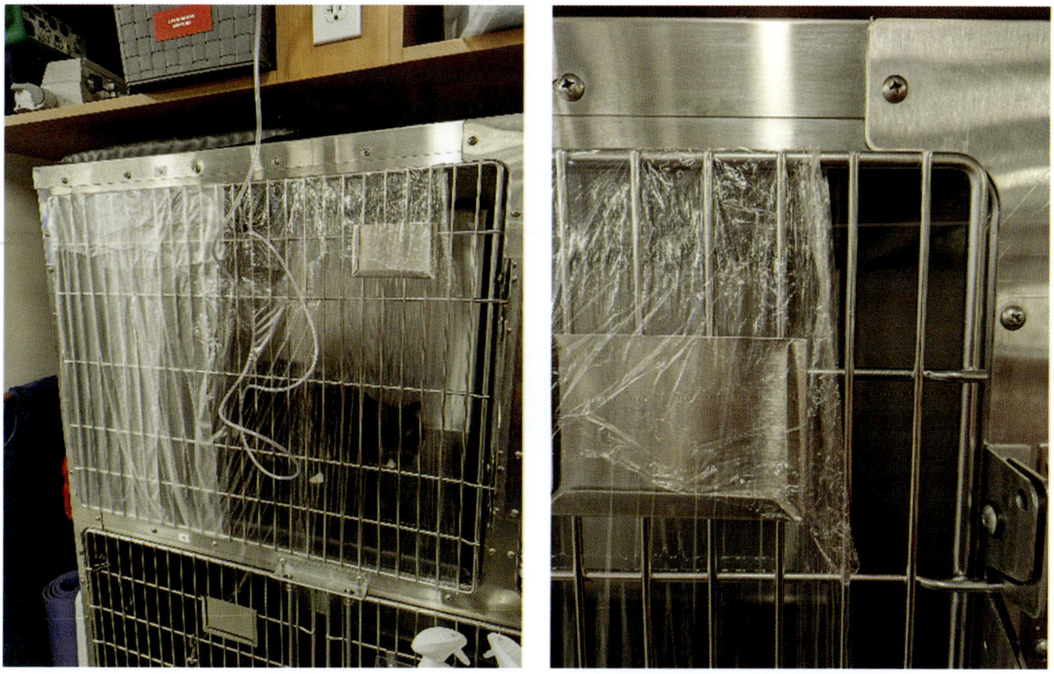

Image 13.1 Makeshift oxygen cage with Geordi, an asthmatic cat. *Source:* Courtesy Danielle Schuler, RVT.

(meaning brighter) outline, which is the bladder wall, and the fluid inside will be black. Pleural effusion would not be indicative of asthma and is more likely related to congestive heart failure or the effusive form of feline infectious peritonitis (FIP). Asthma on radiographs looks like a diffuse, busy pattern across the lung space as seen in Figure 13.1 below (Gareis 2023). At my current ER, and I believe it is industry standard, we send these images out for a 1 hour read with a board-certified radiologist. What we can glean can be verified and further expounded upon by a radiologist (Images 13.2 and 13.3).

Medications

I was listening to a lecture by Dr. Justine Lee (n.d.), a double-boarded veterinary criticalist and toxicologist and founder of VETgirl, on respiratory distress a couple of years ago, and something she said stuck with me, and I think about it any time I see a respiratory case come into the hospital. How I remember it is 'Nothing should die in radiology.' And I think that is one of the main takeaways from that lecture that really stuck with me, and I hope it sticks with you because it's true. Nothing should die because you are trying to take consecutive three-view chest and abdominal radiographs on an animal that can't breathe. Radiographs can be done piecemeal, taking one or two at a time, then giving your patient a break in oxygen until their color and breathing look better. If putting them on their back stresses them out, take a dorsoventral (DV) instead of a ventrodorsal (VD) view. Just label your sides appropriately. Additional butorphanol can be used if they are becoming excessively stressed again, and you can even give an albuterol puff if your doctor is confident it is asthma-related. Getting a full set of radiographs can be time-consuming but ultimately safer for your patient.

Assessment:

1. Moderate to marked bronchial pulmonary pattern is most consistent with lower airway disease such as feline asthma or bronchitis (infectious, inflammatory, toxic, etc.). Consider empirical therapy for lower airway disease, such as removing noxious stimuli from the patient"s environment, bronchodilator, anti-inflammatory and/or trial antibiotic treatments as clinically appropriate. If the patient does not respond consider referral for airway washing for cytology and culture for more definitive diagnosis.
2. Gastrointestinal material likely represents normal ingesta with normal postprandial changes.

Figure 13.1 Radiology report for the diagnostic imaging in Image 13.2 (Brody 2024).

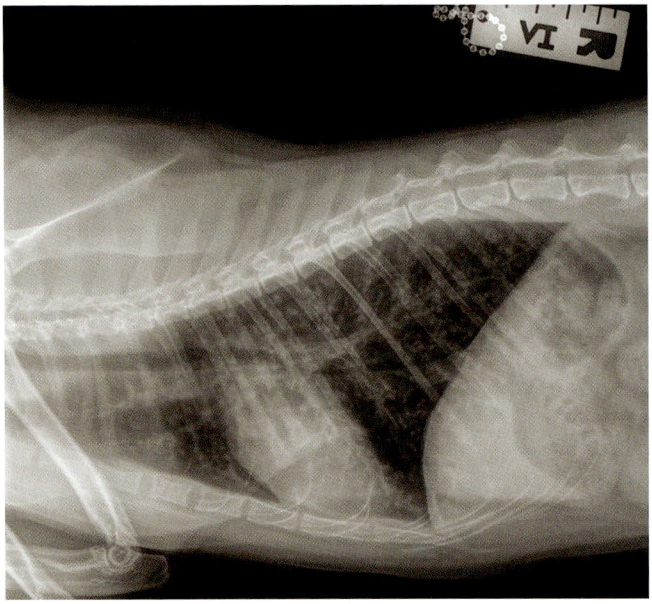

Image 13.2 Right lateral radiograph courtesy of Danielle Schuler, RVT.

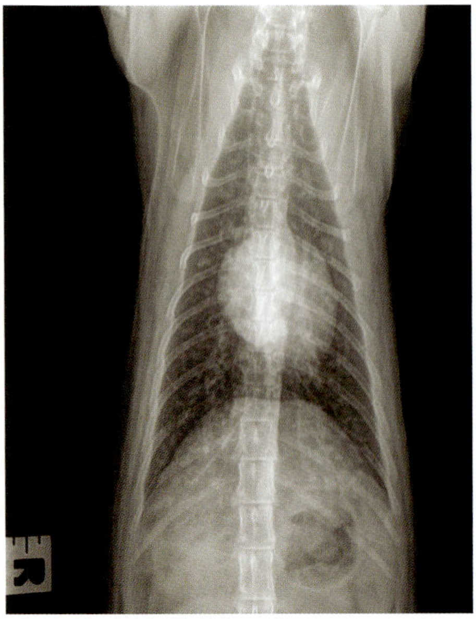

Image 13.3 Ventrodorsal (VD) radiographs courtesy of Danielle Schuler, RVT.

We've given a sedative, and yes, that will temporarily help calm our patient, but we haven't actually treated the problem. Sedation and oxygen therapy are our starting point in treatment, but that should be followed up with a bronchodilator to help open their airways. Our rescue drug of choice is albuterol as an inhalant. Albuterol is used as a rescue drug when these cats are experiencing an attack (Dietschel 2013). But have you ever spritzed something in your cat's face, and it ended well for you? I didn't think so. To ensure these guys get their dose and not stress them out more be sure to use a spacer chamber like an Aerokat. This has a soft mask to cover their face and an insert for the inhaler on the other end. Holding it there for 7–10 breaths will ensure they have breathed in the aerosolized albuterol. During hospitalization, we would continue this treatment as needed until their breathing normalizes. In more severe cases, we can also give terbutaline, which is another bronchodilator, IV, subcutaneously, or intramuscularly (Dietschel 2013). Terbutaline is a sympathomimetic drug that stimulates beta-2-adrenergic receptors in smooth muscle in the lungs (Budde 2023). All this to say it relaxes the smooth muscle of the bronchioles, allowing for better airflow (Image 13.4).

Now that we have helped open our patients' airways with a bronchodilator, we need to treat the inflammation that is happening as well. The best way to treat it is with steroids. Typically, we would start out with injectable dexamethasone sodium phosphate (dex SP) in the ER (Dietschel 2013). If able to do so, it is possible to do most of the diagnostics at a general practice – take the radiographs, provide oxygen, and confirm it is likely asthma – before transfer. If the patient is too oxygen dependent to immediately transfer, giving a mild sedative such as butorphanol at 0.2–0.3 mg/kg and calling your closest ER vet for advice is a viable option (Budde 2023). Oral prednisolone can be prescribed as well. Long-term steroid use should be targeted to the lungs. Because feline asthma is a lifelong disease, transitioning from an oral steroid to an inhaled one is preferred. Side effects of long-term systemic steroid use can cause weight gain, polyuria/polydipsia (PU/PD), and can even push some cats into diabetes mellitus. For continued use at home, we would

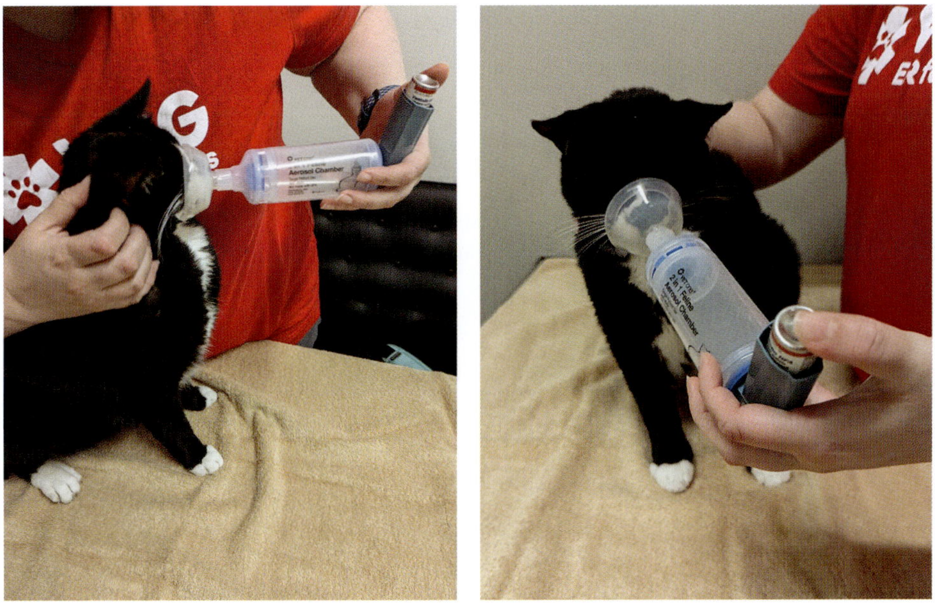

Image 13.4 Geordi receiving an albuterol dose with an aerosol chamber. *Source:* Image courtesy of Danielle Schuler, RVT.

prescribe a fluticasone inhaler (Dietschel 2013). This is given the same way as albuterol and is better at managing asthma symptoms.

Hospital stays for asthma attacks can be relatively short. Once the initial trigger is gone, we have them in a highly oxygenated environment and start medications; recovery time is relatively short. I've had patients who needed to stay on oxygen for 24 hours+, and I've had patients who just need a couple of hours and are ready to go. It really is all determined by the severity of the disease and attack. As patients' respiratory rate and effort decrease to normal, we will start to decrease the oxygen percentage by 5% every 1–2 hours. As long as they continue to breathe well, we will continue to drop the oxygen percentage until we reach 25%, which is a little over the percentage in room air. At that point, we trial them out of oxygen, and if they can continue to breathe normally, they get to go home.

Feline asthma is a lifelong condition. This will mean frequent follow-up visits with you, their primary care hospital, and maybe even a trip to a specialty internal medicine. A referral to an internist would be for our more complicated cases. Are we trying to rule out other causes of a cough/breathing issue? Performing a bronchoscopy to visually inspect the airways for inflammation, nodules, and mucus buildup. While performing a bronchial alveolar lavage (BAL) to acquire samples to send out for cytology, aerobic/anaerobic cultures, and fungal culture can point you to an underlying cause (Loewen 2022). Most of the time, asthma is triggered by an environmental cause. Lifestyle changes may need to happen to minimize future asthma attacks. Using low-dust cat litter, air purifiers, decreasing the use of strong/odious products, and not smoking (tobacco or marijuana) in the home will all decrease the chances of your patient experiencing an asthma attack.

Administering an inhaler to a cat is also a lifestyle change. Geordi belongs to the editor of this book and has had a plethora of other medical issues that will not be covered here; he is an exceptionally tolerant cat, and she is able to do almost anything to him with minimal stress and resistance. Aerokat is perhaps the most commonly used inhaler for cats in the vet hospital, and they have many useful resources for acclimating cats to using an inhaler, instructions on how to use it, and how to clean it on the following website: https://trudellanimalhealth.com/pages/cats/how-to-use?srsltid=AfmBOoq0fQQhWM3HnYfLdjlqPChin6b4jFiuvA-QCF_26cKXMj-161Mq.

Works Cited

Brody, A. (2024). Radiology report. Pikesville.

Budde, J.A. (2023). *Plumb's Veterinary Drug Handbook*. Hoboken, NJ: Wiley-Blackwell.

Colville, T. (2008). The respiratory system. In: *Clinical Anatomy and Physiology for Veterinary Technicians* (ed. T. Collville and J. Bassert), 254–257. St. Louis, Missouri: Mosby Elsevier.

Dietschel, S.A. (2013). Feline chronic bronchial disease (feline asthma). In: *Emergency Procedures for the Small Animal Veterinarian* (ed. S. Plunkett). St. Louis, Missouri: Saunders Elsevier.

Gareis, H., Hörner-Schmid, L., Zablotski, Y. et al. (2023). Correlation of clinical and radiographic variables in cats with lower airway disease. *Journal of Veterinary Internal Medicine* 37: 2443–2452. https://doi.org/10.1111/jvim/16874.

Johnson, L.V. (2011). Bronchoscopic findings in 48 cats with spontaneous lower respiratory tract disease (2002–2009). *Journal of Veterinary Internal Medicine* 236–243. https://doi.org/10.1111/j.193901676.2011.00688.x.

Lee, J. (n.d.). Dr. Justine Lee. Retrieved from https://drjustinelee.com

Loewen, J.M. and Bach, J.F. (2022). Respiratory distress in small animals: Pathophysiology and clinical approach. *Journal of Veterinary Emergency and Critical Care* 32: 3–15. https://doi.org/10.1111/vec.13121.

Lynch, A. (2022). Providing supplemental oxygen to patients. *Today's Veterinary Practice*. Retrieved from https://todaysveterinarypractice.com/respiratory-medicine/providing-supplemental-oxygen-to-patients

Silverstein, D.A. (2023). *Small Animal Critical Care Medicine*, 3e. St. Louis, MO: Elsevier.

14

Communication Across Cultures: How Language Helps

Máriam Ordoñez[1,2] *and Simone Conwell*[2,3]

[1] *Veterinary Technician Student, Columbia, MD, USA*
[2] *VeG ER for Pets, 1858 Reisterstown Road, Pikesville, MD, USA*
[3] *Veterinary Emergency and Critical Care Society Member, USA*

Working in veterinary medicine means more than just caring for animals; it means caring for people too. As a bilingual veterinary professional, I've come to appreciate just how powerful language can be, especially in moments of stress, urgency, and uncertainty. Speaking Spanish has not only been an asset in my career; it has been essential.

My name is Máriam, and I'm originally from Colombia, South America. Spanish is my first language, and I've been working in veterinary medicine since 2013. During this time, I've gained experience across general practice, various specialties, and most significantly, emergency medicine. The emergency room (ER) is where I've truly found my stride – those who know, know.

One of my most valuable assets in this field has been my fluency in Spanish, particularly medical Spanish. It may not seem like a big distinction, but the difference is substantial. Being able to communicate and, more importantly, to understand complex medical terms in a second language has a direct impact on the quality of care and client trust (Nishi 2023). It's a skill that bridges gaps and makes a real difference every day.

In many communities, particularly in regions with large Spanish-speaking populations, language can become a barrier to proper veterinary care. I've seen it time and time again: a concerned pet owner walks into the clinic, desperate for help, but unable to fully explain what's wrong. When communication falters, so does trust (Nishi 2023). That's where speaking Spanish changes everything.

As a fluent Spanish speaker, I'm able to step in and bridge that gap. I can ask the right questions, clarify medical histories, and offer reassurance in a language that feels familiar and safe. It's not just about translation; it's about connection. It's about giving clients peace of mind that their concerns are being heard and their pets are in good hands.

When I have a client who speaks or understands some English, it can certainly help, but there's a big difference between understanding something in a second language and hearing it in your native tongue. Communicating in your mother language brings a deeper level of clarity and comfort. Even when a staff member speaks Spanish, small translations can sometimes miss the mark. Fluency doesn't always guarantee the right words will be found to fully connect with the client or convey exactly what they need to hear.

Medical Spanish isn't the same as conversational Spanish. It involves a specific vocabulary, an understanding of clinical terms, and the ability to convey complex information clearly. For example, explaining something like "gastrointestinal obstruction" or "renal failure" requires more than just a literal translation – it requires context, empathy, and **cultural awareness**.

Over the years, I've developed the ability to shift fluently between medical and everyday language, depending on the client's comfort level. This skill has been especially vital in high-pressure settings like emergency medicine, where time is limited and clarity is critical.

Speaking Spanish in veterinary medicine also means being an advocate for the pet, the client, and even the veterinary team. I often find myself translating not just language, but emotion. I explain cultural nuances to my colleagues, help diffuse misunderstandings, and offer insights that improve the way we communicate as a team.

In a field where every detail counts, being bilingual gives me the ability to enhance patient outcomes, build client relationships, and contribute to a more inclusive and compassionate practice.

Technology has become a lifeline in many veterinary clinics where Spanish-speaking staff are not available. Tools like phone translators, video interpretation services, and search engine translations are commonly used, and in some situations, they can be helpful. But let me be honest, they have their limits.

Phone translators are often robotic, slow, and impersonal. The time it takes to connect, repeat information, and clarify details can feel endless when a pet is in critical condition. I've seen situations where every second counts, but everything stalls because the translator on the other end doesn't understand the medical context or misinterprets tone and urgency.

Then there's search engine translation. It can be a useful quick-fix for a basic phrase here and there, but veterinary medicine is full of nuanced terminology. "Seizure" might be translated as "ataque" (attack) or "convulsión," and depending on the region or country the client is from, even that might not be the clearest choice. Literal translations often miss medical or cultural subtleties, leading to confusion or even fear.

At my workplace, we rely on a translation service for communication with non-native-speaking clients and even deaf clients. However, I've witnessed multiple instances where the doctor's message is not accurately conveyed by the service. Often, the translation doesn't align with the doctor's intent, and I am left to step in and correct the errors. The issue seems to stem from the fact that the translation staff lacks training in medical Spanish, let alone specialized veterinary terminology, which can lead to misunderstandings and potential risks to patient care. In a fast-paced clinical setting, this can result in **errors, rushed translations**, or **missed cultural nuances**.

I've watched well-meaning staff use a well-known translation app, only to leave the client more confused than when they started. A conversation that should build trust ends up feeling clinical and disconnected. I usually end up going back in and editing the discharges or even the medication labels, so our client can understand and have the resources to look back at. For example, I had a doctor tell an owner she needed to get an E-collar for her pup, and the translation app interpreted a collar meant to prevent licking an incision as a "shock collar" instead. Thankfully, the mistake was caught, but that shows even the internet can be wrong.

This is where a bilingual veterinary professional becomes irreplaceable. I don't just translate – I interpret. I read body language, listen for unspoken concerns, and adjust my explanations based on the client's understanding. I can switch between technical and conversational Spanish as needed, and I tailor my tone to fit the situation – whether it's calming a panicked owner, delivering difficult news with empathy, or explaining medication instructions in a way that truly sticks.

What does help is hiring for your demographics. I live and work in the DC Metro area, where approximately 17% of our community is Spanish speaking (DataUSA 2023). We have areas that have dense concentrations – therefore, a larger base of Spanish-speaking clients who may not know or understand English. When new hospitals are being built continuously, it would be ingenious to hire for the demographics in your area; this will help not only the clients but, most importantly, the patients.

More than anything, I *care* – about the client, the patient, and the experience both are having. No app or device can replicate that.

Microaggressions

Many companies have diversity, equity, and inclusion (DEI) trainings in-house that are mandatory each year. It also almost always seems to be a white man who is doing the speaking about representation and discrimination, even though white preferences in employment still exist (Austin 2023). Even though Eddie Murphy played Dr. Dolittle in the late 90s, data from 2023 shows that black veterinarians make up only 2.2% of the field and Hispanic/Latinx doctors make up only 0.5% (Childers 2023, *It Takes a Village*). Hispanic/Latinx technicians make up 10% of the overall population, which is an improvement, but similarly to veterinarians, only 3% of vet techs are black (Childers 2021, *Practice Without Prejudice)*. Looking at the demographics for the DC Metro area, where 17% of the community is Hispanic, almost 25% of the same area is black (DataUSA 2023). It is possible to surmise that the demographics here are a little better than the national averages, but from my experience, it's likely not significantly different. So why aren't practices hiring to reflect their communities (Nishi 2023)?

Older white men have long been leaders in veterinary medicine, despite veterinary medicine having become a woman-dominated field in 2009 (Hopkins 2024). Leadership in veterinary schools – particularly the deans – is still largely comprised of men (Hopkins 2024). A 2021 study by Llorens et al. documents that men in leadership create barriers for women in science, technology, engineering, and mathematics (STEM) through their entire career, as positions with hiring, promoting, funding, and policymaking powers are still largely offered to men whose unconscious (or not so unconscious) biases impede the advancement of women (Hopkins 2024). Breaking that down by race shows that, in the medical and health sciences overall, black professionals with a bachelor's degree are twice as likely to be unemployed as white professionals with identical qualifications (Austin 2023).

A diverse, especially multilingual, staff can increase clientele and revenue (Childers 2023, *It Takes a Village*). I know of a clinic that hired a Korean-speaking doctor in an area that was close to a city with a heavy Korean-American population, and their Korean clientele population exploded to the point that these clients were leaving hospitals they had been going to for years and driving further because they knew this doctor was one of their own. That level of trust and sense of belonging to a client is invaluable, and something hospitals should foster, especially as the number of multicultural pet owners continues to rapidly increase (Childers 2023, *It Takes a Village*).

I have seen multiple instances over the years of clients being subtly or outwardly racist toward doctors and staff who didn't look like them, and seen management either ignore it or suggest the black, indigenous, and people of color (BIPOC) person it was directed to "be the bigger person" and disregard it. I worked with a wonderful doctor who had experienced so much racism that he often brushed it off and expected management to make excuses for why it was ok, which is ridiculous and not ok. I've had a coworker ask if a client "sounded black" after finding out they were unable to afford gold standard treatment, to the shock and silence of our other coworkers. I was not silent; I told her why her comments were ignorant and racist using my best Baltimore accent because I knew that would bother her more than the dressing-down. This is not something I would necessarily expect from my BIPOC coworkers, because everyone has an anecdote about a racist or sexist manager where they had to keep their heads down to keep their jobs. But silence from those who have the privilege to speak amounts to acceptance and agreement.

A Brief List of Affinity Groups within Veterinary Medicine that encourage and have resources for improving DEI (and belonging).

PrideVMC: pridevmc.org – LGBTQA+ allyship
Black DVM Network: blackdvmnetwork.com – networking for black veterinarians
National Association for Black Veterinarians: nabvonline.org – a nonprofit dedicated to providing mentoring and support to black veterinary professionals across the country
Latinx Veterinary Medical Association (LVMA): latinxvma.org – for Hispanic and Latinx veterinary students AND professionals in the field
Multicultural Veterinary Medical Association: mcvma.org – promoting diversity and cultural competency in veterinary medicine
American Association of Veterinarians of Indian Origin: aavio.org – networking opportunities and resources for veterinarians of Indian origin
Association of Asian Veterinary Medical Professionals: aavmp.org – space for Asian preveterinary/veterinary professionals for support, mentorship, scholarships, and networking
Women's Veterinary Leadership Development Initiative: wvldi.org – for women in veterinary medicine to learn leadership skills and network
Please consider reading DEI in Veterinary Medicine edited by Kemba Marshall, DVM, DABVP (avian medicine) for more about this topic.

Works Cited

Austin, A. (2023). The continuing power of white preferences in employment. Center for Economic and Policy Research. Retrieved from https://cepr.net/publications/the-continuing-power-of-white-preferences-in-employment/

Childers, L. (2021). Practice without prejudce. American Animal Hospital Association. Retrieved from https://www.aaha.org/trends-magazine/publications/practice-without-prejudice/

Childers, L. (2023). It takes a village. American Animal Hospital Association. Retrieved from https://www.aaha.org/trends-magazine/may-2023/ht-it-takes-a-team/

DataUSA. (2023). Washington-Arlington-Alexandria, DC-VA-MD-WV. Retrieved from datausa.io: https://datausa.io/profile/geo/washington-arlington-alexandria-dc-va-md-wv?

Hopkins, C. (2024). The state of women in vet med- according to the data. American Animal Hospital Association. Retrieved from https://www.aaha.org/newstat/publications/charts-the-state-of-women-in-vet-med/

Nishi, N.C. (2023). Miroaggressions in veterinary communication: what are they? How are they harmful? What can veterinary professionals and educators do? *Journal of the American Veterinary Medical Association* 262 (3): 1–6. https://doi.org/10.2460/javma.23.07.0412.

Part IV

Common Surgical Emergencies

15

Forbidden Snackies: There's No Way He Ate That!

Fernanda Flynn-Galicia

Veterinary Technician Student, VeG ER for Pets, Brooklyn, NY, USA

Overview

Foreign bodies are abundantly common in the veterinary world. As much as owners attempt to keep tasty foreign material out of reach, pets will find the most outrageous, often comical, objects to consume. This chapter hopes to cover the basics of what diagnostics are necessary to diagnose and manage a gastrointestinal foreign body, primary stabilization efforts, including ideal catheter placement, fluid therapy, medication recommendations, and finally, risks associated with various foreign body surgeries. At the end of this chapter is a brief overview of total intravenous anesthesia – also known as "total intravenous anesthesia" (TIVA) – and appropriate cases to consider alternatives to traditional inhalant anesthesia.

Imaging

Patients presenting with a wide variety of symptoms such as vomiting, diarrhea, lethargy, and anorexia should be considered for potential gastrointestinal obstruction. While it is generally associated with younger animals and repeat offenders, any pet is at risk for a mechanical or partial mechanical obstruction. It is important to remember that foreign material ingestion is not the only cause of obstruction, although it accounts for approximately 80% of them (Cole et al. 2023). There are conditions, such as intestinal neoplasia, that can lead to both partial and full mechanical obstructions (Cole et al. 2023). Radiographs can be a wonderful starting point to rule out gastrointestinal obstruction. According to Vet's Choice Radiology (n.d.), three-view abdominal radiographs offer the best possible view of the abdomen by minimizing potential artifacts and can increase confidence in diagnoses. However, a standard two-view abdominal radiograph is just as likely to yield a diagnosis of gastrointestinal obstruction (Mavromatis et al. 2018). Unfortunately, radiographs can only offer an approximate 70% accuracy in detecting foreign bodies (Sharma et al. 2011). Repeating radiographs after an 8–12 hour period of fasting can help to rule out normal food ("ingesta") in the stomach versus a foreign object or to track improvement in intestinal distension (Carrillo et al. 2024). In the case of the small intestine versus the colon, a pneumocolonogram can be an easy, relatively inexpensive additional view to capture to aid in determining the location of foreign material. Pneumocolonograms involve using a French red rubber catheter to push 4 ml/lb of air into the rectum to differentiate the colon from the small intestine (O'Brien 2010). If it is available, an abdominal ultrasound performed by a radiologist or internist is a helpful tool in ruling out a foreign body. Abdominal ultrasounds have an approximate 97% accuracy in detecting foreign bodies, making them an indispensable tool for diagnostic imaging (Sharma et al. 2011). There are times when a radiologist will recommend an abdominal ultrasound in place of repeat, fasted radiographs. It can significantly reduce the time between the initial radiographs and a definitive foreign body diagnosis, depending on the availability of abdominal ultrasound. Once you have a definitive diagnosis, it is time to prep the patient for either surgery or for medical management, depending on the opinion of the veterinary care team (Images 15.1–15.3).

Based on Images 15.1 and 15.2, this patient has ingested what appears to be three metal screws. Unfortunately, it is difficult to tell definitively if it is in the small intestine or the large intestine. When sent out to be read by a radiologist, the radiologist recommended an abdominal ultrasound but estimated that it would most likely be in the small intestine based on the dilation of the intestines. It was mentioned that the left lateral appeared to have an affected intestinal loop ventral to the descending colon, but an abdominal ultrasound was recommended to confirm. The radiologist additionally suggested that if an ultrasound were unavailable, a pneumocolonogram could be beneficial. The patient was placed in lateral recumbency for the pneumocolonogram, and an additional right lateral and ventrodorsal image was submitted for comparison. Ultimately, it was still not definitive with the additional views. The patient was then transferred from an urgent care facility to an emergency room, where an abdominal ultrasound was available on the same day. The abdominal ultrasound confirmed the presence of a small intestinal obstruction; therefore, surgery was recommended. The patient had a single-site enterotomy and was discharged the next day after weaning off fentanyl and readily consuming two meals.

As previously stated, if ultrasound is not available, repeat fasted radiographs can be compared typically over an 8–12-hour period to monitor the patient for increased/decreased intestinal dilation, movement of ingesta, and to minimize artifact (Carrillo et al. 2024). While a patient is waiting for repeated radiographs, it is recommended that the patient be hospitalized with IV fluid therapy

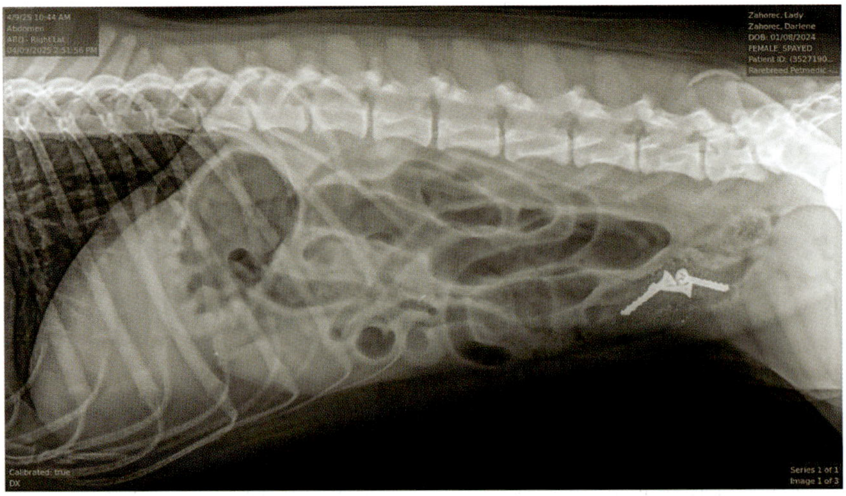

Image 15.1 Right lateral abdominal view of a canine patient with suspected metal foreign material ingestion. *Source:* Photos courtesy of Fernanda Flynn-Galicia.

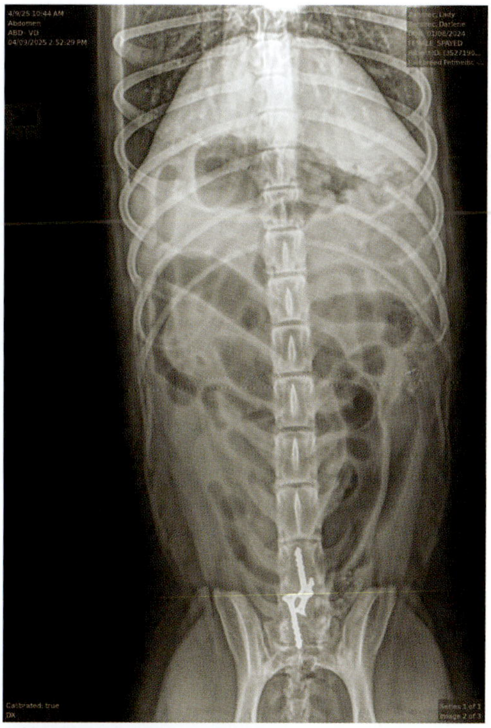

Image 15.2 Ventrodorsal abdominal view of a canine patient with suspected metal foreign material ingestion. *Source:* Photos courtesy of Fernanda Flynn-Galicia.

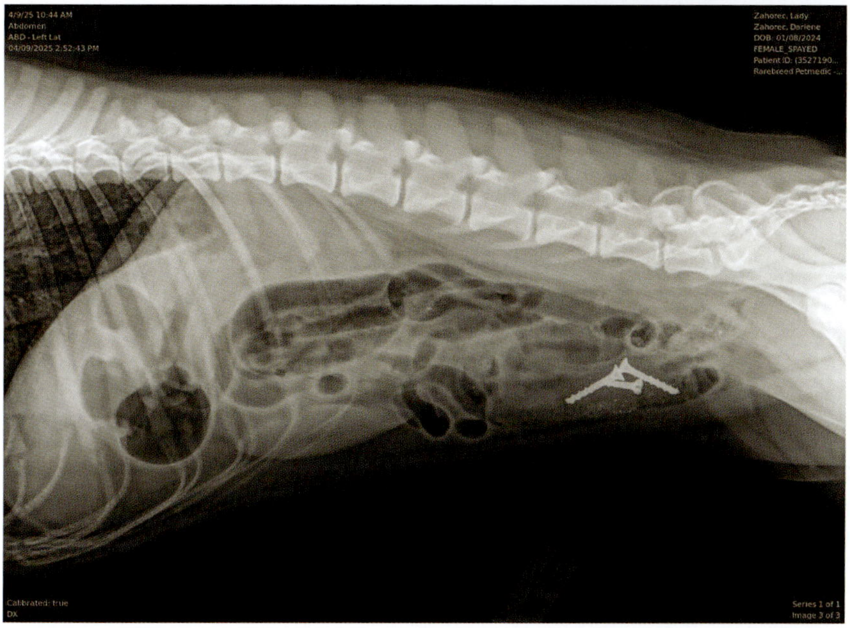

Image 15.3 Left lateral abdominal view of a canine patient with suspected metal foreign material ingestion. *Source:* Photos courtesy of Fernanda Flynn-Galicia.

to correct any dehydration or electrolyte abnormalities in the event that the patient requires surgery following the repeated radiographs (Bryant 2010).

As seen above (Images 15.4 and 15.5), the patient has a considerable increase in intestinal dilation. The initial set of radiographs was submitted to a radiologist, revealing suspected fabric foreign material in the small intestine. At the time, a full mechanical obstruction was not likely, and repeated radiographs with medical management were considered for the patient. Due to some unforeseen events, the patient was not re-evaluated for 30 days. The repeated radiographs

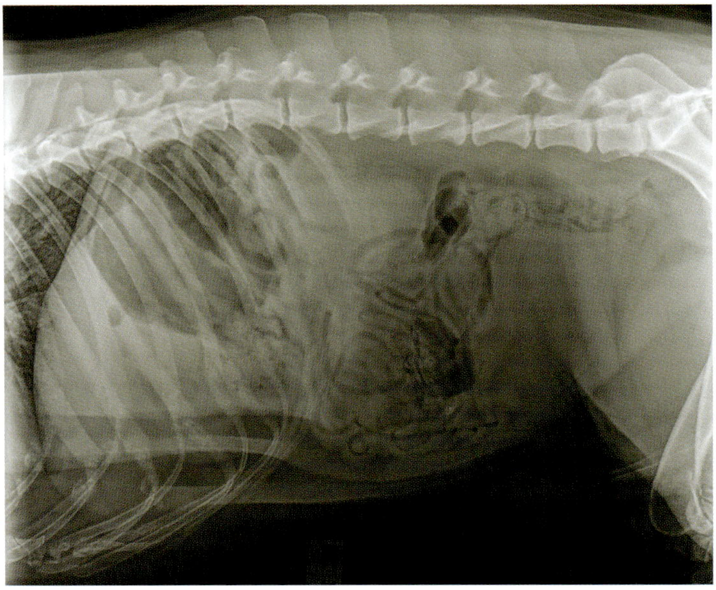

Image 15.4 Right lateral abdominal view of a canine patient who presented with vomiting and diarrhea. Per the radiologist, a cloth-like structure was seen in the small intestine. *Source:* Photos courtesy of Fernanda Flynn-Galicia.

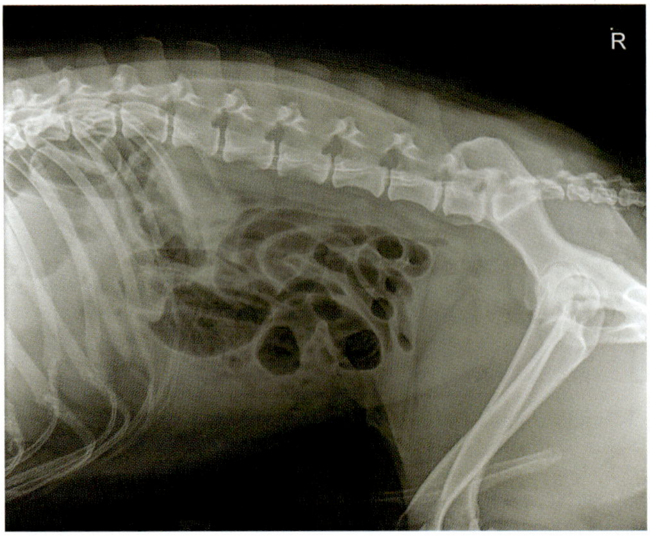

Image 15.5 Right lateral abdominal view of the same canine patient approximately 30 days later. *Source:* Photos courtesy of Fernanda Flynn-Galicia.

confirmed a mechanical obstruction, and surgery was recommended. Additional diagnostics revealed multiple comorbidities typical of chronic foreign bodies, such as sepsis, electrolyte abnormalities, azotemia, and severe dehydration. The patient was transferred from an emergency facility to a specialty facility with an anesthesiologist, criticalist, and board-certified surgeon.

Catheters

Whether considering surgical intervention or hospitalized medical management, the patient will require an intravenous catheter. While previously it was believed that larger bore catheters were always the way to go, the increased flow rate is not always worth the additional trauma to the vein. The intravenous catheter should still be placed within reasonable ranges based on patient size, but not every canine patient requires an 18G.

If invasive blood pressure (IBP) capabilities are available for surgery, an arterial catheter should be considered. IBPs allow for a gold standard of monitoring blood pressure intraoperatively. IBP is helpful for monitoring sudden drops in blood pressure as well as confirming non-invasive blood pressure (NIBP) readings. Readings are real-time and offer a wider insight into anesthetic depth when titrating analgesic medications. It can also be useful in determining the efficacy of vasopressors and fluid boluses if required to treat hypotension during a surgery. Additionally, placement of an arterial catheter will allow for intraoperative arterial blood gases that can help monitor for appropriate ventilation of the critical patient (Bryant 2010).

Due to their relatively low flow rates, a patient who is unable to receive other methods of catheterization and relies on an intraosseous catheter (IO) should not be considered for general anesthesia unless deemed absolutely necessary. As IO catheters are meant to be part of initial stabilization efforts, consider proceeding with general anesthesia once intravenous access has been acquired (Shelby 2024). Potentially, the patient may need a central line before undergoing anesthesia to offer the best possible outcome. Higher doses of vasopressors carry a reduced risk of extravasation when administered through a central line (Bryant 2010). Additionally, the sampling line offers a way to quickly check a patient's blood glucose, venous blood gas, and more during surgery and in recovery. These parameters may aid in determining medications required to safely maintain the patient under anesthesia (Sidari and Carter 2025).

Following the surgery, it would be reasonable to place a sampling line, such as a PICC (peripherally inserted central catheter) or a multi-lumen central line placed at the jugular, while the patient is anesthetized. It is helpful to continue monitoring blood work postoperatively to adjust fluid type, rates, and additives. The ability to run medications, fluids, and sample blood is indispensable to the critical patient (Sidari and Carter 2025).

Fluid Therapy

Surgical fluid rates are generally calculated by the veterinarian performing the surgery. As recommended by the 2024 AAHA fluid therapy guidelines, most veterinarians will calculate a rate that falls between 3 ml/kg/hr for feline patients and 5 ml/kg/hr for canine patients, with some exceptions for patients with cardiac disease or other comorbidities that may be susceptible to fluid overload. The type of fluid will also be selected by the veterinarian, but suggestions could be made based on patient needs. Most patients will generally benefit from crystal colloids; therefore, fluid therapy should be started as soon as possible to minimize complications during surgery. Clinically dehydrated patients are at risk of hypovolemia-induced tachycardia, hypotension, and subsequently poor perfusion under anesthesia. Patients who have been suffering from a foreign body are at risk for certain bloodwork abnormalities, such as electrolyte imbalances, hypoglycemia, and acute kidney injuries secondary to dehydration (Bryant 2010). If possible, patients should be left on fluids until they have been stabilized and any abnormalities have been corrected. Depending on the severity of the patient's condition, surgery may be necessary prior to correction with fluid therapy. In these cases, a pre-induction bolus may help to avoid the worst of intraoperative complications (Grubb et al. 2020). Reasons to take a patient suffering from gastrointestinal obstruction to surgery rather than waiting will be covered later in this chapter.

In addition to fluid therapy, patients with chronic foreign bodies may need additional supplements to correct secondary issues such as hypoglycemia. A hypoglycemic patient should be started on dextrose supplementation and have blood glucose values checked frequently to adjust supplementation. Dextrose supplementation may be required intraoperatively, especially if the patient is septic. In the case of dextrose supplementation, it is recommended to have a sampling line available prior to induction to ensure ease of monitoring while on the surgical table (Bryant 2010). When supplementing a patient using their fluid bag, it is imperative to bring another bag of fluids that contains no additives in the event that a fluid bolus is required. Hypotension is an unfortunately common side effect of many of the medications used for general anesthesia, and it is best practice to prepare for it.

Gastric Versus Intestinal Foreign Body

A gastric foreign body is foreign material in the stomach of the patient. If the object is large enough, it can cause an outflow obstruction. Occasionally, intermittent symptoms will be observed as the object adjusts away from the pylorus. These foreign bodies have the option to be potentially retrieved using endoscopy instead of a traditional gastrotomy. It is important to always prepare owners for the very real possibility that an endoscopy may end with the need to perform a gastrotomy if the object is too difficult to grab or if time under anesthesia begins to run long (Shuler and Tobias 2006). Below is an example of a gastric foreign body. The images are of a canine patient that presented for suspected corncob ingestion. This was confirmed with a standard abdominal radiograph study, and the corn was retrieved with a flexible gastroscope (Images 15.6 and 15.7).

An intestinal foreign body is foreign material in the intestinal tract of the patient. Surgical intervention is the most common recommendation for duodenal and jejunal foreign bodies. Medical management has a higher rate of success for foreign material that has reached the ileum when compared to duodenal and jejunal foreign bodies. Once foreign material has reached the large intestine, it is generally considered best practice to treat the patient supportively with IV fluid therapy and any medications required to manage the patient's symptoms, such as nausea (Carrillo et al. 2024). While a patient is being treated for a foreign body in the large intestine, consider walking the patient frequently to help with gastric motility.

While a large intestine foreign body may be the best-case scenario, a gastric foreign body is better than an intestinal one. Gastrotomies generally have a lower rate of surgical complications when compared to enterotomies. Surgery time tends to be shorter, incisions made to the stomach are less prone to dehiscence, and stomach tissue has a lower chance of requiring resection than the small intestine. The stomach has a greater ability to stretch than the small intestine and therefore can avoid the worst of injuries (Schuler and Tobias 2006). Gastrotomies may even be able to be performed as an outpatient procedure, depending on the patient's overall status and their recovery. This is not to say that gastrotomies are without their share of risks.

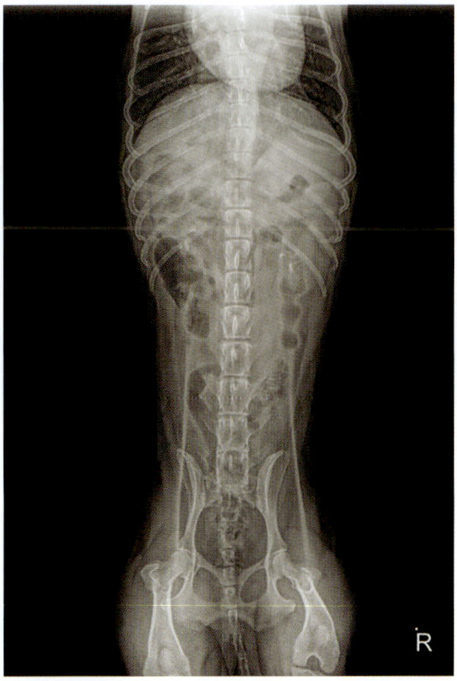

Image 15.6 Ventrodorsal abdominal view of a canine patient with a known corncob ingestion. *Source:* Photos courtesy of Fernanda Flynn-Galicia.

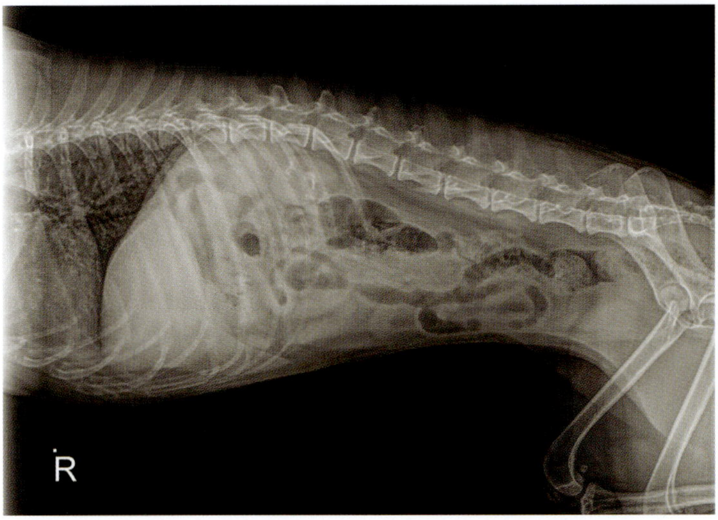

Image 15.7 Right lateral abdominal view of a canine patient with a known corncob ingestion. *Source:* Photos courtesy of Fernanda Flynn-Galicia.

Depending on the object itself, as previously mentioned, endoscopy can be considered for the retrieval of the foreign material for gastric foreign bodies. Endoscopy has the unique advantage of retrieving the material while avoiding any incisions, thereby minimizing the majority of risks associated with traditional surgery (Schuler and Tobias 2006). Many patients who have successful endoscopies performed for foreign body retrievals are able to go home as soon as they have

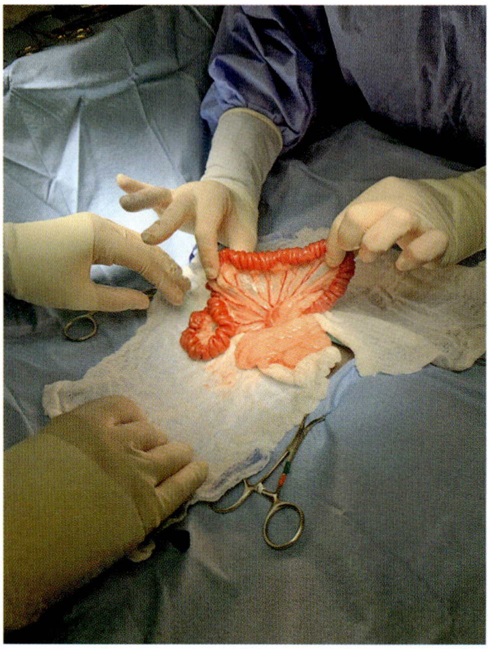

Image 15.8 Intestinal plication in a feline patient with a linear foreign body. *Source:* Photo courtesy of Fernanda Flynn-Galicia.

recovered. Objects that may damage the esophagus when brought back up should be avoided for endoscopic retrieval when possible. For example, multiple glass shard fragments may be more safely removed through a gastrotomy than an endoscopy (Schuler and Tobias 2006). Such decisions are up to the veterinary care team and vary from patient to patient.

Small intestinal foreign bodies place the patient at increased risk for perforation and subsequent sepsis. The more time that has passed since the initial ingestion, the higher the risk (Tobias and Ayres 2006). Generally, it is common for patients to be hospitalized following a foreign body surgery involving the small intestine to ensure the patient is eating and to monitor for free fluid immediately following the surgery. In some cases, it is possible to "milk" the object from the ileum to the colon by gently massaging the intestines. These cases minimize the risk of intestinal dehiscence by eliminating the intestinal suturing process. Small intestinal obstructions that involve longer, flexible objects, such as string, pose the risk of "bunching" the intestines. This bunching is called plication (Image 15.8) and increases the risk of tissue damage as blood flow to the area is compromised (Cole et al. 2023). These kinds of small intestinal foreign bodies will be detailed in the section below.

Linear Foreign Bodies and R&A

Linear foreign bodies can occur if any material becomes anchored in the stomach or the pylorus, as well as if linear material, such as string, is ingested (Cole et al. 2023). Linear foreign bodies tend to be a lot more time-sensitive with regard to avoiding additional complications such as perforation with subsequent sepsis. Additionally, the pressure built up from the foreign body can cause damage to the tissue that may ultimately result in a need for a resection and anastomosis, often referred to as an R&A for short. An R&A can significantly increase your surgical complication rate as well as increase anesthesia time (Tobias and Ayres 2006). Whether or not the intestines will need to be

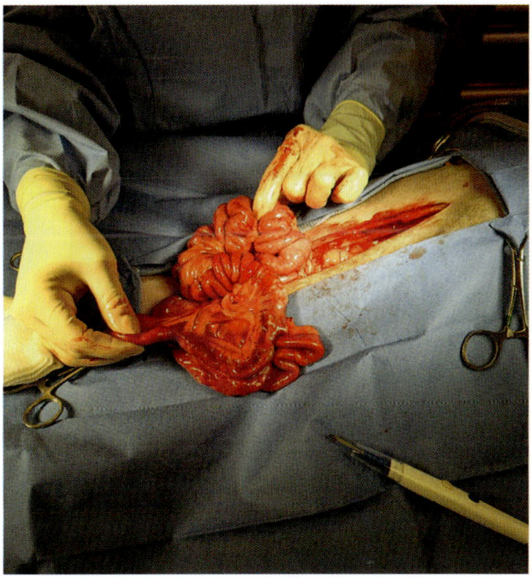

Image 15.9 Intestinal plication in a canine patient with a linear foreign body. *Source:* Photos courtesy of Danielle Schuler, RVT.

resected is difficult to tell prior to the surgery (see images below for examples of healthy versus damaged intestinal tissue). The best thing to do is to prepare a surgical protocol and to prepare the surgical suite in the event that an R&A becomes necessary.

Pictured in Image 15.9 is an example of plicated intestines commonly seen with linear foreign bodies. In this patient, the intestines continue to have an appropriate pink appearance. During the surgery, the veterinary team was able to determine that the mesenteric window continued to have strong pulses. An important factor in whether or not a section of damaged tissue will heal appropriately instead of continuing to deteriorate is the blood supply (Tobias and Ayres 2006). If the pulses are strong, it is receiving an adequate blood supply and will most likely improve. If the pulses are weak, the blood flow is dwindling, and there is a risk that the tissue will deteriorate and dehisce. For example, in Image 15.10, the intestines are not as pink in appearance. Usually, the intestines begin to improve in appearance after the pressure from the foreign material has been removed. In Image 15.11, after the foreign body has been removed, it is still questionable if the intestines will recover based on their appearance. After their assessment, the veterinary team proceeded with removing approximately 6 inches, as seen in Image 15.11.

Multimodal Anesthesia

The basics of anesthesia involve monitoring and managing a patient for ECG abnormalities, hypoxia, hypo- or hypertension, hypo- or hyperthermia, and hypo- or hypercapnia (Sidari and Carter 2025). The greatest tool in the arsenal of an anesthetist is their own five senses. Observe and assess the patient as frequently as the numbers on the monitor or more. Remember to take the occasional manual measurement to confirm that the monitor is capturing vitals accurately (Bryant 2010). Anesthesia safety begins the moment a patient walks through the doors. Full diagnostics aid in adjusting an anesthetic protocol to the individual pet and guide any necessary supplementations or corrections prior to induction. The time prior to induction is the key to good patient preparation. Pre-oxygenating a patient helps to avoid hypoxia when intubating.

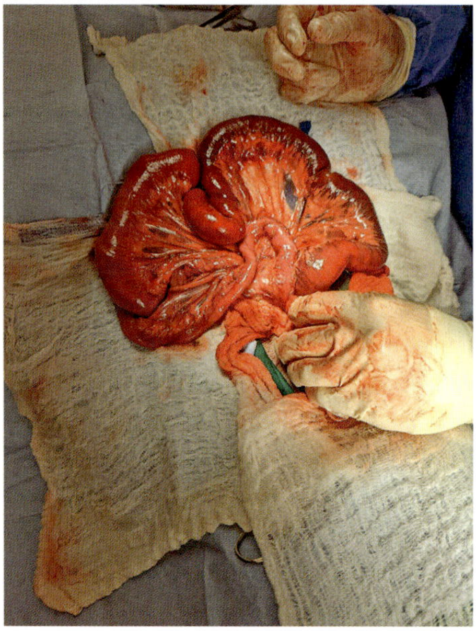

Image 15.10 Appearance of the same intestines from Image 15.9 following foreign body removal. *Source:* Photos courtesy of Danielle Schuler, RVT.

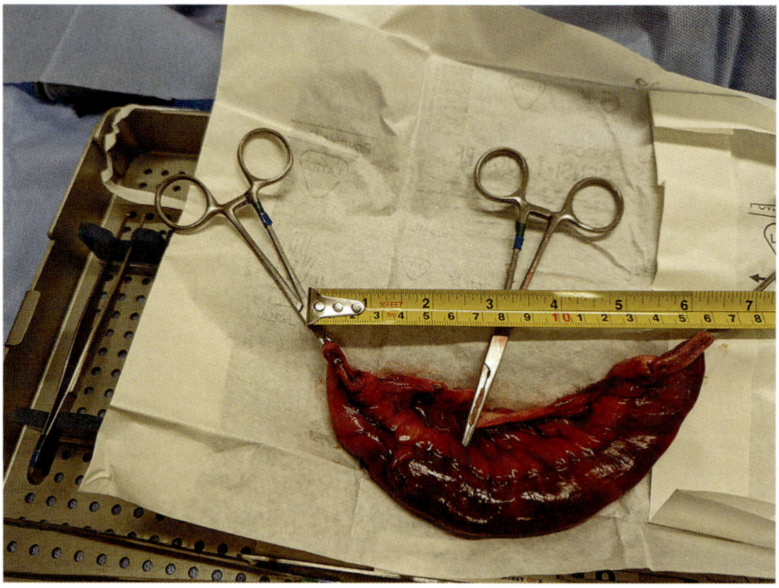

Image 15.11 Resected portion of the small intestine from Images 15.9, 15.10, measuring approximately 6 inches. *Source:* Photos courtesy of Danielle Schuler, RVT.

Pre-warming equipment to begin heat support immediately can help to avoid hypothermia (Sidari and Carter 2025). It is these little adjustments that can elevate the standard of care for everyone.

During the preparation period, it is important to discuss an anesthetic protocol that will prioritize patient comfort and safety. Multimodal anesthesia focuses on appropriate depth and pain management using a varied approach that aims to reduce the quantity of each individual medication in an effort to reduce side effects. It is important to recall that as the dose of a medication increases, so do side effects (Bryant 2010). Most medications used in anesthesia have what is known as a minimum alveolar concentration (MAC). This is defined as the minimum concentration of anesthetic required to maintain appropriate anesthetic depth for 50% of patients despite noxious stimuli (Bryant 2010). Generally, when being used alone, medications will require higher concentrations than their MAC to maintain an anesthetic depth. When used in combination with each other, the synergistic relationship of medications can aid in reducing the MAC of each individual component. Most commonly, general anesthesia involves the use of inhalant medications such as sevoflurane and isoflurane. Inhalants can cause a plethora of side effects that affect perfusion, such as hypotension, bradycardia, and hypothermia (Sidari and Carter 2025). While there are remedies for each complication, prevention is key.

Certain medications, such as opioids, will offer a high MAC reduction of inhalants, making them an indispensable part of a surgical anesthetic protocol. Other medications, such as dexmedetomidine, will also reduce an inhalant's MAC but should be avoided in patients with certain comorbidities, such as heart disease (Bryant 2010). Ideally, a patient would receive premedication that would allow them to be shaved prior to induction to reduce anesthesia time. Premedications can also reduce the dose required of induction medications by reducing the risk of hypotension, bradycardia, and apnea, as is noted with the use of large volumes of propofol or alfaxalone at induction (Sidari and Carter 2025). Additionally, using a variety of constant/continuous rate infusion (CRI) medications in an anesthetic protocol can aid in titrating doses based on frequent patient assessments to reduce inhalant use as much as possible while also avoiding large concentrations of any one specific medication.

Some medications may offer additional benefits other than reducing inhalant use. For example, lidocaine has been documented to reduce gastrointestinal inflammation, leading to increased patient comfort when managing a foreign body (Bryant 2010). It also couples nicely with fentanyl and ketamine in what is commonly referred to as an "FLK CRI." Ketamine by itself can reduce inhalant use significantly when used intraoperatively (Solano et al. 2006). An FLK CRI combines the pain management of fentanyl and ketamine with the anti-inflammatory and pain management properties of lidocaine. High doses of fentanyl and ketamine can cause apnea, so it is important to monitor a patient closely and to adjust each individual component as needed. If using an FLK CRI correctly, inhalant use should be greatly reduced, thus improving patient comfort and safety while anesthetized.

Anesthesia safety begins with assigning a safety rating from the American Society of Anesthesiologist (ASA), referred to as the ASA status. The ASA physical status is a classification system developed to assess anesthesia candidates for risk. A healthy patient with no underlying comorbidities may be a 1, while a severely compromised patient with multiple unmanaged comorbidities that is expected to pass away with or without surgical intervention is a 5. Inhalants such as isoflurane and sevoflurane should be used with caution in patients who have an ASA physical status of 4 or 5 (Grubb et al. 2020). Depending on what the underlying comorbidities are, the veterinary team may opt to forego inhalant medications altogether to avoid the threat to homeostasis that they pose. In cases where inhalants should be avoided, total intravenous anesthesia may be considered as detailed below.

Total Intravenous Anesthesia ("TIVA")

For patients with severe comorbidities or with sensitivities to traditional inhalant anesthesia, total intravenous anesthesia should be considered. Inhalant anesthetic gases disrupt the autoregulatory processes of the body and can exacerbate underlying conditions even in lower concentrations

(Sidari and Carter 2025). As previously discussed, multimodal anesthesia relies on the synergistic relationship between certain medications to reduce side effects by lowering each individual drug's dosage. It is worth mentioning that as a patient's ASA physical status goes up, the required dosages of many medications will be reduced due to the patient's compromised status. These comorbidities may include, but are not limited to, severe cardiovascular disease, endocrine diseases, diabetes, advanced renal disease, and liver dysfunction, in addition to any secondary issues due to foreign bodies (Sidari and Carter 2025). It is important to tailor any anesthetic protocol to the patient's specific needs and to avoid medications that are directly contraindicated due to one of the patient's underlying disease processes.

Due to the acuity of a patient requiring TIVA, the ideal scenario would include a surgical ventilator and multiple intravenous catheters, such as a central line, in addition to a peripheral catheter. As discussed earlier in this chapter, IBP is ideal to compare with NIBP to maintain adequate perfusion, as severely compromised patients may have been hypotensive prior to induction and may need vasopressors. If a patient is confirmed to be septic and is hypotensive despite fluid resuscitation, consider a norepinephrine CRI and possibly a dopamine CRI in tandem if the response is not enough with one alone. It is important to ensure that the patient has had IV fluids to correct dehydration; otherwise, perfusion will not improve even though the blood pressure value will read as normal (Sidari and Carter 2025). When monitoring a patient on a vasopressor such as norepinephrine, a total assessment should be completed to confirm adequate perfusion. One of the signs that the blood vessels are constricting without adequate rehydration is if the mucous membranes become pale (Bryant 2010).

As previously discussed, the exact protocol will be determined based on the individual patient. For the purpose of discussing TIVA as it relates to a foreign body, a patient could be adequately anesthetized with an FLK CRI in conjunction with a propofol CRI for maintenance. Low doses of dexmedetomidine can be considered if the patient's history allows. For inducing a critical patient such as this, consider midazolam as a coinduction agent. Preference should be given to midazolam, fentanyl, lidocaine, ketamine, and dexmedetomidine over propofol, as propofol can cause a multitude of complications, as previously discussed.

While electrocardiograms (ECG), pulse oximetry (SPO_2), blood pressure (NIBP or IBP), and temperature are important, end-tidal CO_2 ($ETCO_2$) should be closely monitored while using a TIVA protocol to confirm the patient is perfusing appropriately. Many of the medications used in TIVA protocols can cause hypoventilation and even apnea. Perfusion begins with adequate gas exchange to oxygenate tissues and remove excess carbon dioxide. If the patient is hypercapnic or hypoxic, consider titrating their medications to start them on a surgical ventilator without the patient breathing against the ventilator. Whether or not a patient is breathing against the ventilator can be assessed by their capnogram.

It is important when preparing a patient for a TIVA protocol that multiple intravenous access points are available. Consider inserting a central line or a PICC line in addition to a standard peripheral IV catheter to minimize the risk of extravasation of any of the medications used. When transferring a critical patient to surgery, there is no such thing as too many catheters, as there are medications that do not play nicely with each other.

Not every patient requires a TIVA protocol for surgery, but what TIVA can show us is that it is possible to reduce inhalant use to zero. Multimodal anesthesia offers the ability to minimize common surgical complications and expedites patient recovery time without compromising patient comfort and safety.

Works Cited

American Animal Hospital Association. (2020). 2020 AAHA Anesthesia and Monitoring Guidelines for Dogs and Cats. Retrieved from www.aaha.org: www.aaha.org/resources/2020-aaha-anesthesia-and-monitoring-guidelines-for-dogs-and-cats

American Animal Hospital Association. (2024). 2024 AAHA Fluid Therapy Guidelines for Dogs and Cats. Retrieved from www.aaha.org: www.aaha.org/resources/2024-aaha-fluid-therapy-guidelines-for-dogs-and-cats

Bryant, S. (2010). *Anesthesia for Veterinary Technicians*. Hoboken, NJ: Wiley-Blackwell.

Carrillo, A.J., McCord, M.A., and Dickerson, V.M. (2024). Clinical features and outcomes of dogs with attempted medical management for discrete gatrointestinal foreign material: 68 cases (2018–2023). *Journal of the American Veterinary Medical Association* 262 (9): 1251–1258. https://doi.org/10.24.0/javma.24.01.0050.

Cole, Robert, et al. (2023, June). Inestinal mechanical obstruction. *Today's Veterinary Practice*. Retrieved from https://todaysveterinarypractice.com/radiology-imaging/radiographic-diagnosis-of-small-intestinal-mechanical-obstruction/

Grubb, T. et al. (2020). *2020 AAHA Anesthesia and Monitoring Guidelines for Dogs and Cats. AAHA*, 12 Feb www.aaha.org/resources/2020-aaha-anesthesia-and-monitoring-guidelines-for-dogs-and-cats/.

Mavromatis, M.V., Solano, M., and Thelen, M.Y. (2018). Utility of two view vs three view abdominal radiography in canines presenting with acute abdominal signs. *Veterinary Radiology & Ultrasounds: The Official Journal of the American College of Veterinary Radiology and the International Veterinary Radiology Association* 59 (4): 381–386. https://doi.org/10.1111/vru.12611.

O'Brien, R. (2010). Constrast radiography made simple: GI tract (proceedings). *Fetch dvm360*. dvm360. Retrieved from www.dvm360.com/view/contrast-radiography-made-simple-gi-tract-proceedings

Schuler, E. A. (2006). Key gastrointestinal surgeries: gastrotomy. *Dvm360*. Retrieved from www.dvm360.com/view/key-gastrointestinal-surgeries-gastrotomy

Sharma, A., Thompson, M.S., Scrivani, P.V. et al. (2011). Comparison of radiography and ultrasonography for diagnosing small-intestinal mechanical obstruction in vomiting dogs. *Veterinary Radiology & Ultrasounds: The Official Journal of the American College of Veterinary Radiology and the International Veterinary Radiology Association* 52 (3): 248–255. https://doi.org/10.1111/j.1740-8261.2010.01791.x.

Shelby, A. M. (2024). A Comprehensive Guide to Intraosseous (IO) Catheter Insertion Techniques. Retrieved from www.zoetisus.com: www.zoetisus.com/petcare/blog/io-catheter-placement

Sidari, H. A. and Carter, H. (2025). Anasthesia and analgesia for patients with comorbidities. *Today's Veterinary Nurse*. Retrieved from https://todaysveterinarynurse.com/anesthesiology/anesthesia-and-analgesia-for-patients-with-comorbidities

Solano, A.M., Pypendop, B.H., Boscan, P.L., and Ilkiw, J.E. (2006). Effect of intravenous administration of ketamine on the minimum alveolar concentration of isoflurane in anesthetized dogs. *American Journal of Veterinary Research* 67 (1): https://doi.org/10.2460/ajvr.67.1.21.

Tobais, K. A. (2006). Key gastrointestinal surgeries: intestinal anastomosis. *Dvm360*. Retrieved from www.dvm360.com/view/key-gastrointestinal-surgeries-intestinal-anastomosis

Vet's Choice Radiology. (n.d.). Benefits of Obtaining Three Views of the Abdomen. Retrieved from vetschoiceradiology.com: www.vetschoiceradiology.com/benefits-of-obtaining-three-views-of-the-abdomen

16

Don't Flip Over a GDV

Puja Wright

BluePearl Pet Hospital, 1 Taft Ct., Rockville, MD, USA

What the flip is happening? What does a bloat mean? But why is bloating such a big deal? Why is everyone getting so twisted? (Okay enough with the puns ...)

Terminology

The acronym GDV stands for gastric dilatation-volvulus. Dilatation refers to the excessive expansion of the stomach with either air, fluid, or other materials. Pets may have a simple dilatation without having the stomach twist as well. Volvulus refers to the twisting of the stomach into a malposition. These malpositions, depending on the severity, can occlude the esophageal sphincter, the pyloric sphincter, and even include the spleen in the torsion. A volvulus can occur in a clockwise direction up to 360° or a counterclockwise direction up to 90°. A GDV is commonly referred to as "bloat"; however, this term can be confusing as it can be used to refer to a simple gastric dilatation (e.g., "food bloat") as well. Simple dilatation is still an emergent condition that is very uncomfortable and painful for an animal, but it is not a surgical emergency like gastric dilatation with volvulus is. "Stomach torsion" is another term used for GDV that refers to the version of bloat with volvulus.

Presentation to the Veterinary Clinic

When the pet walks into the clinic, they will seem highly uncomfortable. Most times, GDVs occur in large and giant breed dogs with deep chests, such as Labrador Retrievers, Great Danes, Saint Bernards, German Shepherd Dogs, Weimaraners, Irish and Gordon Setters, Standard Poodles, Doberman Pinschers, Bernese Mountain Dogs, and Basset Hounds (Mazzaferro 2021; Radlinsky 2013). While it is rare, this disease has been documented in smaller breed dogs, cats, guinea pigs, and even humans; a large breed dog having these symptoms should cause suspicion. Do not write off animals that have these symptoms but fall outside the typical signalment (Mazzaferro 2021). Diagnosis of GDV is largely based on clinical signs, history, radiographs, and physical exam.

Clinical Signs

On presentation, these pets will have acute abdominal pain or discomfort, which may show as an arched back. They may also have abdominal distension, unproductive vomiting/retching, abdominal stretching, drooling, lethargy, weakness, and acute collapse (Mazzaferro 2021). Occasionally, they will sometimes also be straining to defecate. Care needs to be taken to make sure when owners report vomiting, that it isn't just retching with the production being clear, frothy saliva. Some of these animals present with hypersalivation and agitation; this saliva is unable to pass the volvulus and pass into the stomach, so it is brought back up, which is what some owners may report as vomiting (Mazzaferro 2021). Some animals may only present with vague signs of lethargy and anorexia (Drobtaz 2012).

History

When collecting a history on a possible GDV, be aware that the risk of GDV increases with age. There is a correlation between increased laxity in the hepatogastric ligament and the occurrence of a GDV (Monnet 2012). Normally, this ligament attaches the lesser curvature of the stomach to the liver; it is theorized that this laxity allows the stomach to move and twist instead of staying in its place (Monnet 2012). This ligament can relax with age and repeated overdistension of the stomach (Monnet 2012).

The risk of GDV also increases significantly with a first-degree relative who has had a GDV (Radlinsky 2013). In many studies, correlations have been made between larger meal sizes and gastric dilatation. It is often recommended to feed dogs at a higher risk for GDV smaller, more frequent meals instead of one large meal. Reduction of stress at mealtimes, not feeding out of raised food bowls, and limiting exercise surrounding mealtimes can help prevent the aerophagia that may lead to GDV (Radlinsky 2013).

A retrospective study in Australia looked at presentation times for GDV patients. Presentation times correlated with the idea that owners were getting home from work, feeding an evening meal while providing exercise for the pet before or after the meal. Presentation of GDV cases increased starting at 7 p.m. and peaked between 8 p.m. and 1 a.m., in correlation with this idea (Drobtaz 2012). Often, these pets will present symptoms after being fed a meal. It is important to note the last time the pet ate, what they ate, symptoms, what (if anything) the pet is vomiting up, if the pet has had similar episodes prior, and if the pet has a history of prophylactic gastropexy.

Prophylactic gastropexies are often recommended in high-risk dogs; however, an animal that has had a gastropexy may still develop a simple gastric dilatation, which is still an emergent situation. Occasionally, gastropexies, based on various factors, may fail to scar down, in which case stomach torsion is still possible. While knowing if a gastropexy has been done is important, the presence of one should not deter the pet from being treated as an emergency.

Physical Exam

On a physical exam, a variable degree of a distended abdomen with a tympanic area would be noted. On very deep-chested animals and obese animals, it can be harder to assess the amount of distention or tympany present. Animals with GDV can present standing and acting minimally uncomfortable (to where discomfort may be missed or misinterpreted as anxiety), in a particular hunched stance showing significant abdominal discomfort, or laterally recumbent. It can be highly dependent on how severe GDV is and how long the pet has been sick.

Depending on the severity and length of the GDV, the patient can present in a variation of cardiovascular system compromise. The pet may present in various stages of hypovolemic shock, causing other physical signs to vary. Early-stage hypovolemic shock may show sinus tachycardia with normal femoral pulses and tachypnea, as the body is still trying to compensate for a lower circulating blood volume by driving the heart rate and respiratory rate higher. Blood pressure may be slightly low but close to normal as the body drives the heart rate higher to compensate (Monnet 2012). The body will also try to compensate for the loss of circulatory volume by vasoconstricting peripheral vessels that will show as slowed capillary refill times, pale mucous membranes, and cold extremities (Monnet 2012).

Animals presenting in later stages of shock can be in a combination of hypovolemic and obstructive shock due to the gross hindrance to circulation from the GDV (Standl 2018). Occasionally, when a patient also has bacterial translocation from the disease or when tissue compromise leads to a systemic inflammatory response, distributive shock can play a role as well (Standl 2018). These sicker patients may show cardiac arrhythmias (particularly ventricular arrhythmias) on an ECG and femoral pulse deficits on palpation. These pulse deficits are indicative of a decrease in cardiac output, since they are created when the ventricles are pumping too fast to fully fill with blood before contracting. When these half-filled ventricles contract, they send a decreased amount of blood out of the body and lungs, creating less blood for the lungs to oxygenate, as well as weak or absent pulses. This decrease in cardiac output leads to cardiac arrhythmias. These patients' bodies are still in a compensatory phase of shock, so they would have a tachycardia and tachypnea (Monnet 2012). The systemic response from endotoxemia can lead to a fever and red and injected mucous membranes; however, the compromised circulatory function leads to slowed capillary refill times (Monnet 2012). The pressure put on the caudal vena cava and other abdominal vasculature by the distended stomach also lends to obstructive shock by causing a physical barrier that keeps the blood from returning to the heart. This shock is unable to be resolved without surgery to derotate and deflate the stomach.

Depending on the pressure on the vagus nerve and if a late stage of hypovolemic shock is present, patients may be bradycardic instead of tachycardic (Mazzaferro 2021). In these instances, the bradycardia should not be taken as a sign that the pet is not painful. Instead, there are outside forces (such as increased vagal tone or decompensated hypovolemic shock) at play that are influencing the heart rate beyond the pain. These patients are likely to be the ones presenting laterally recumbent with bradycardia and severe hypotension (Monnet 2012). When the animal is in decompensated shock, their mucous membranes may be blue-gray to white with prolonged capillary refill times (Macintire; Monnet 2012).

Diagnostics

Abdominal Radiographs

Most commonly, radiographs will be the diagnostic tool that provides a definite diagnosis of a volvulus, differentiating the GDV from the gastric dilatation patient. As the first point of contact with a potential GDV, when receiving a history and symptoms from an owner that point to a GDV, the technician needs to be prepared to take abdominal radiographs.

Unlike most abdominal radiograph series, the two most important views for a potential GDV are going to be a dorsoventral radiograph and a right lateral radiograph. Often times a dorsoventral view is preferred over the standard ventrodorsal orthogonal view due to the fact that when these patients are put in ventral recumbency, they often decompensate since the position puts even more pressure on their large vessels and nerves (vena cava, aorta, and vagus nerve) as well as increased pressure on their diaphragm, which already has restricted movement from the gastric dilatation. This can cause them to go into respiratory distress very quickly, even during the fastest radiographs.

The right lateral radiograph is more important as opposed to the traditional left lateral radiograph, as the right lateral will be where the inversion of the pylorus is seen and the appearance of "double bubble" or a backward "C-shape" is seen (Herring 2014). In a 360° clockwise rotation of the stomach, the backward "C-shape" may not be seen, as the pylorus is usually back where it is expected ventrally on the right lateral radiograph instead of dorsally like a classic GDV. These cases may be difficult to diagnose on radiographs, as they look similar to gastric dilatation. Radiographically, the pylorus may look like a smaller gas-distended bubble ventrally, while the body of the stomach looks like a larger gas-distended bubble dorsally. The distension of the pylorus, along with malposition of the spleen, can help distinguish a 360° GDV from a gastric dilatation on radiograph (Li et al. 2022). Further distinction of a gastric dilatation can be made by the presence of both dilated stomach and dilated jejunal loops (Monnet 2012) (Images 16.1 and 16.2).

If a radiologist needs to be consulted, the reading of the radiographs needs to be immediate. Oftentimes, if the patient is going to a referral center, the better option may be to send the radiographs ahead of the patient while in communication with the referral center. If the center has a radiologist, they may be able to get a read faster than a typical "stat" read on a web-based platform. If they do not have a radiologist on staff, their surgeon would at least be able to confirm if the case is indeed a surgical emergency or not, and in turn be prepared.

Thoracic Radiographs

Chest radiographs can screen for metastatic disease in older patients, aspiration pneumonia, as well as abnormal heart silhouettes seen with extreme disease (Herring 2014). If chest radiographs are

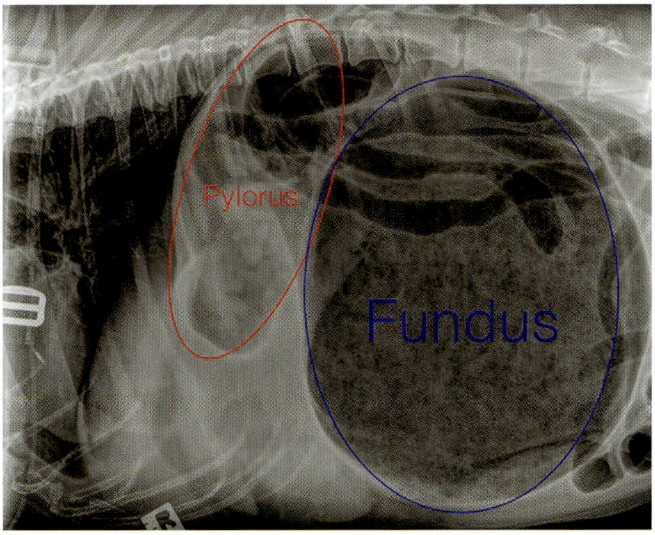

Image 16.1 Right lateral photograph of a GDV; note the pylorus is dorsal. *Source:* Photo courtesy of Simone Conwell, RVT, VTS (ECC).

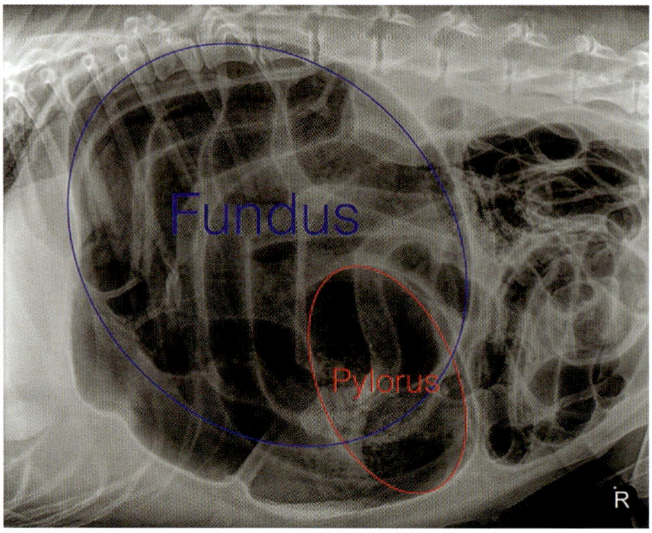

Image 16.2 Right lateral radiograph of a gastric dilatation in the same patient 6 weeks later. Note how the pylorus is ventral, as this pet was gastropexied during surgical correction of the GDV. He did not develop a volvulus. *Source:* Photo courtesy of Simone Conwell, RVT, VTS (ECC).

done, care needs to be taken with placing these patients in dorsal recumbency. This can increase pressure on an already compressed caudal vena cava and portal vein, decreasing return volume to the heart even more. It can also further impinge on the diaphragm of an animal already in respiratory distress (since the distended stomach keeps the patient from fully utilizing its diaphragm muscles). These patients can decompensate and crash quickly in dorsal recumbency! Placing these animals in dorsal recumbency can also cause them to aspirate. Consideration should be given to taking a dorsoventral thoracic view in place of the traditional ventrodorsal view, especially in less stable patients.

Bloodwork

For a GDV, a recommended minimum database includes a packed cell volume and total solids, lactate, blood glucose level, and blood gas if available (Herring 2014). These would show if the patient is hemorrhaging, dehydrated, or in shock, as well as some clues to prognosis. Some studies correlate a lactate of >6 mmol/l with worse prognosis. This finding can be associated with an increased likelihood of the need for a gastrectomy (Gibson 2020). Other sources say that the lactate level response to fluid therapy is a better indicator of prognosis. If available, a complete blood count (CBC) and chemistry panel can also help determine the extent of systemic damage (Herring 2014). If further available, coagulation panels can give insight into if coagulation cascades have been activated, and there is prolonged coagulation time.

What Does All This Mean? An Anatomical Deep Dive

The stomach is divided into four sections. The part where the esophagus enters the stomach is called the cardia. The fundus is the pouch-like part of the stomach that flares out to the right-hand side (from the surgeon's viewpoint). The main portion of the stomach that then leads to the left is called the body. The last portion of the stomach that leads to the small intestine is the pylorus. There are sphincters where the esophagus attaches to the stomach, and the pylorus goes into the small intestine. These are called the esophageal sphincter and pyloric sphincter, respectively. The lesser curvature refers to the shorter curved border, or convex surface, of the stomach that travels from the right side of the cardia to the pylorus on the cranial side of the stomach. Along this side is where the hepatogastric ligament attaches the stomach to the liver. The greater curvature is the longer curved border, or concave surface, that goes from the left side of the cardia, outlining the fundus and the caudal border of the stomach, and ends at the pylorus. Along the greater curvature in the fundus are the short gastric vessels that span between the stomach and the spleen. Other normal vasculature is found all along the surface of the stomach (Figure 16.1).

The dilatation of the stomach takes place mainly through the fundus and body of the stomach. It can occur with excessive accumulation of food, water, or air in the stomach. As the stomach becomes larger, pressure is placed on all the vessels along the surface of the stomach as the distended surface presses against the other surfaces inside the abdomen. This pressure can impede blood flow, much like when placing pressure on a wound to stop bleeding. The increased size of the stomach can also lead to pressure on the caudal vena cava and portal vein.

This impedance leads to blood volume stagnating in the stomach vessels instead of returning to the greater circulatory volume and the heart, decreasing the venous return to the heart. A decrease in circulating volume leads to a decrease in cardiac preload. Lower cardiac preload decreases stretch to the ventricular myocytes, in turn decreasing the force of the ventricular contraction (King 2025). All of this lends to a decreased stroke volume (King 2025). This, in turn, drives the patient's blood pressure downward and decreases the amount of oxygenated blood that is reaching bodily tissues. The stagnant blood in the gastric vasculature can also start to diffuse out into adjacent tissues and the stomach itself, further compromising tissues and adding to the fluid volume in the stomach. This expanded stomach can also apply pressure cranially on the abdominal side of the diaphragm, leading to the pet's inability to fully expand their lungs to intake an appropriate

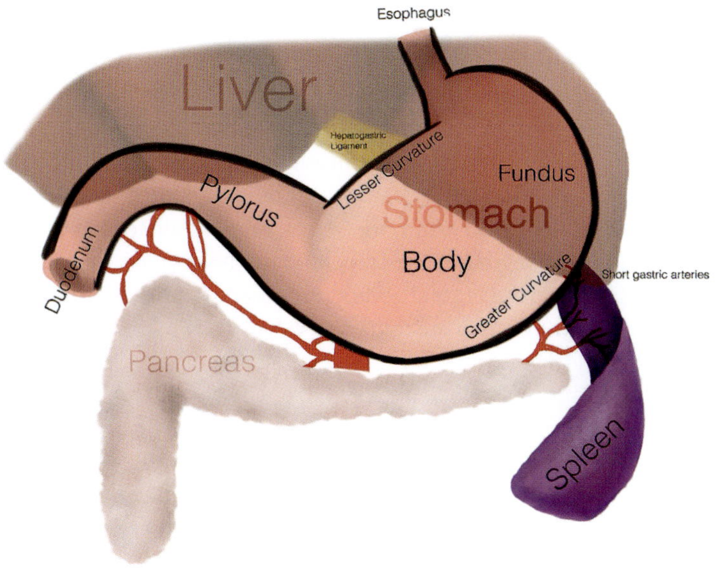

Figure 16.1 Diagram of normal stomach placement and relative anatomy. *Source:* Drawing courtesy of Puja Wright, RVT.

amount of oxygen. The forced shallow breaths combined with lowered circulatory volume can lead to hypoxemia in the patient as well. These issues combined occur in even a simple gastric dilatation, which is why it is considered an emergency.

It is suspected that volvulus occurs prior to dilatation and impedes the pylorus, which impedes the normal outflow from the stomach into the rest of the gastrointestinal (GI) tract, causing this accumulation to stay in the stomach (Gibson 2020). Some theorize that the laxity in the hepatogastric ligament allows for the extra movement that leads to a volvulus. This laxity could be attributed to intrinsic causes, such as genetics and age, or extrinsic causes like a continued history of larger meals contributing to the stretching of the ligament with consistent stomach stretching (Monnet 2012). During a gastric dilatation with volvulus, the esophageal sphincter and pyloric sphincter can be occluded depending on the degree of the volvulus. Rotation of the stomach is categorized by how far the stomach has rotated in a clockwise fashion. A stomach that has rotated greater than 180° is where occlusion of the distal esophagus happens; until then, in a mild volvulus of less than 180°, the pyloric sphincter is the only one affected (Gibson 2020). As such, pets with mild volvulus may continue to try to pant or drink water or eat to try to alleviate discomfort, thereby distending the stomach further. This in turn raises pressure in the stomach, which impedes the duodenum and pyloric sphincter even further by entrapping it against the body wall as the stomach twists (Gibson 2020). This becomes a vicious cycle for the patient as the pyloric sphincter and the esophageal sphincter both become more occluded; the excess stomach contents are unable to evacuate from either direction.

The volvulus of the stomach can cause further impedance of the blood supply to the stomach. This further interruption in blood circulation can cause necrosis to the stomach wall, leading to the need to partially resect the stomach. This necrosis is often related to the amount of time the blood circulation is interrupted, making the time to surgery incredibly important. The necrosis and injury can be mitigated by techniques used to reduce the dilatation of the stomach before surgery.

In a GDV, the stomach is not the only organ affected by the dilatation and volvulus. Trauma also occurs to the short gastric vessels from the rotation. These vessels can become avulsed during the GDV, which can lead to bleeding and free fluid in the abdomen. Hemostasis may occur on its own by the time the pet is in surgery, but bleeding may continue in some patients and needs to be ligated to prevent further blood loss. The volvulus cannot only avulse some of the vasculature between the stomach and spleen; it can also involve the spleen in the volvulus, since the spleen is connected to the stomach with short ligaments. This can cause the spleen to become injured to various degrees. The volvulus of the vessels to the spleen can cause hypoperfusion, leading to a splenic thrombus, or clot, causing the blood supply to the spleen to become compromised. In these cases, a splenectomy would be indicated. On a physical exam, the spleen may feel distended due to the blood supply that is backed up in the parenchyma of the spleen. Sometimes GDV can lead to splenic torsion as well. When the blood supply in the cranial abdomen becomes this compromised, other sensitive organs that may share vasculature can sustain injury too, such as the pancreas. Often, postoperative GDV patients will need to be treated for pancreatitis.

As perfusion becomes impeded from multiple points during GDV, the patient develops an obstructive shock (Drobtaz 2012). This lack of perfusion can cause tissue death in many body parts. Parts of the stomach itself can suffer from ischemic injury, which can require resection of the dead tissue for the pet to survive. If not, this dead tissue may become perforated and cause sepsis in the patient. Similarly, necrosis can occur in the spleen if the blood supply is interrupted for long enough, requiring a splenectomy. Lack of adequate perfusion to other vital organs, due to the reduced venous return to the heart, can cause hypoxic injury to other organs like the heart, liver, and kidneys, leading to endotoxemic shock. These injuries can show up on our diagnostics as

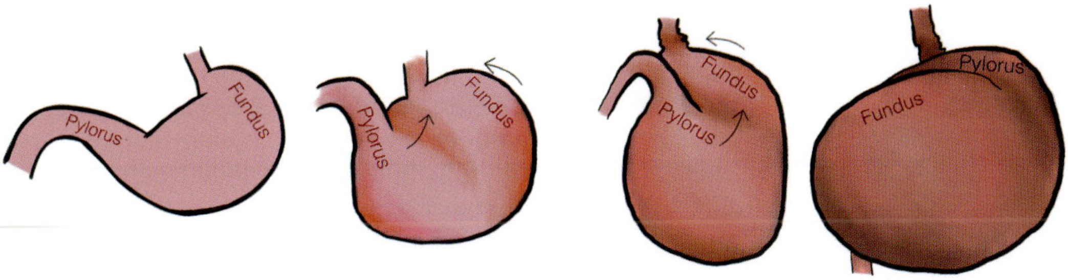

Figure 16.2 Progression of a normal stomach, twisting clockwise to the "typical" 180° GDV on the right. *Source:* Drawing courtesy of Puja Wright, RVT.

arrhythmias on ECG and elevated liver values and elevated kidney values on blood work. The blood that is accumulated in the torsion also has a tendency to activate clotting factors, which can sometimes lead to clotting cascade problems like disseminated intravascular coagulopathy (DIC) (Drobtaz 2012) (Figure 16.2).

A Race Against the Clock

Emergencies are often a rush against the clock, so to call a GDV a race against the clock seems redundant. However, in GDVs, this idiom is multiplied. Increased time to treatment, i.e., surgery, is one of the biggest factors in increased mortality rates in patients with a GDV (Song et al. 2020). With timely intervention, the survival rate of GDV treatment is quite high – with only a 10%–18% mortality rate. Most of the deaths occur in patients requiring concurrent splenectomy or gastrectomy (Mazzaferro 2021). This makes sense, as these cases are likely to be the ones that have had a longer wait time for surgery, which would lead to increased tissue necrosis. This would make the patient more unstable both anesthetically and postoperatively, making them more likely to have complications. A retrospective study found that pets with greater than 3 hours from admission to completion of surgery had higher mortality rates than those that were admitted and through with surgery before 3 hours (Song et al. 2020). This finding highlights the need for expedience in this process for better patient outcomes. Not only is timeliness needed once the patient presents to the veterinary clinic, but any client whose pet is showing symptoms of GDV should be encouraged to seek veterinary evaluation immediately.

Decision to Pursue Surgery

Once a pet has presented to your clinic and a diagnosis of a gastric dilatation with volvulus is made, what needs to be done now? Treatment of GDV is surgery. If surgery is not an option, then humane euthanasia is the second option available to clients. The first decision a client needs to make is whether to pursue surgery or opt for euthanasia. Because time is such a determining factor in this disease and the success of treatment, trying to medically manage is unsuccessful, not only because the treatments themselves are not fixing the anatomical issue but also because of the time wasted in pursuing those treatments if the client then decides to do surgery.

The very next decision that needs to be made is if this case will be referred to the nearest emergency and surgical center or if it will be kept in-house. A conversation needs to be had with owners in very frank terms. Owners are often overwhelmed in an emergency situation and feel like they cannot make a decision right away. However, in this case, the client needs to know a decision needs to be made immediately, especially if treatment is to be pursued.

If they want to give their pet the best chance for a positive outcome, time is of the essence. If referral to a surgical specialist is available, this is the preferred option. One study shows a 90% survival rate when the surgery is done by boarded or residency-trained surgeons (Song et al. 2020). Another shows that surgeries done by someone other than a boarded surgeon (a general practitioner, residents, etc.) have a 2.03 times higher mortality rate than those operated on by boarded surgeons (Song et al. 2020). This same study, however, showed a survival rate of 81.7% for general practitioners and 88.7% for specialist surgeons (Song et al. 2020). To further interpret these studies: if referral is available in a timely manner, then that would be the ideal option. However, if referral is a distance away, consideration should be given to doing surgery in-house and transferring afterward if the veterinarian is confident in doing the surgery and the practice has the equipment necessary for an abdominal exploratory surgery and passage of an orogastric tube.

Consideration should also be given to postoperative hospitalization. Emergency and specialty centers often have 24-hour care, which these patients need after surgery. If this is not available at your location, then referral should be made after surgery is performed, once the patient is stable. These patients have the risk of postoperatively arrhythmia, as well as needing continued intravenous fluids and medications – they should not be left overnight without direct observation by a veterinary professional (Radlinsky 2013).

Fluid Resuscitation

As this treatment discussion is being had with the clients, stabilization for the GDV needs to be started as soon as possible. Once the decision to pursue treatment is made, there are three major priorities with stabilization that need to be focused on, whether the pet is referred to a specialist or stays at the general practice.

The first priority is rapid fluid resuscitation to replace the blood volume that is trapped within the volvulus of the GDV. Ideally, two large-bore intravenous (IV) catheters need to be placed in the cephalic veins. If these are not viable options, jugular veins can also be used (Monnet 2012). These catheters need to be cranial to the impedance of blood circulation in the GDV; otherwise, these shock fluids will just become trapped within the volvulus. Large volumes given in the hind half of the body would not help with the pet's hypovolemia but may contribute to making the congestion in the compromised tissues worse. While an IV catheter is being placed, it is a good idea to gather bloodwork prior to starting fluids. Large bore catheters refer to ideally 18-to-16-gauge catheters, with 20 gauge being the minimum in large dogs. Since most of these patients tend to be large or giant breed dogs, they will need very large volumes of fluids quickly.

For example, a 35+ kg dog could need up to 90 milliliters per kilogram (ml/kg) of shock boluses. That would be 3150 milliliters (ml) at a time. When time is of the essence, trying to get 3 liters of fluids into a patient over 15 or 30 minutes is faster than most fluid pumps are able to handle. As a result, these fluids should often be given with a squeeze bag to deliver them as quickly as possible. If trying to get these fluids into the patient within the hour, the flow rate needs to be around 52 milliliters per minute (ml/min) (which would be around 3120 milliliters per hour or ml/hr). For a 20-gauge catheter, the maximum flow rate is roughly 60 ml/min, which is why this is the smallest catheter that would be acceptable in one of these patients (Pedagogy 2025). As many of the giant breed dogs can be even bigger (a Great Dane can easily be 40–45 kg), a 20-gauge catheter would not be sufficient to get the appropriate volume of fluids into the patient quickly enough to stabilize them for anesthesia.

Fluid boluses for the GDV patient should be 20 ml/kg, up to 90 ml/kg, of isotonic crystalloids in dogs. Isotonic means that the IV fluids have the same amount of solutes as a cell, making these fluids neutral in osmotic movement from intravascular to extravascular spaces (Lopez 2023). They are equally available to stay intravascularly or diffuse out into the tissues as normal blood. This allows for appropriate rapid volume replacement of the circulating blood volume. Examples of these types of fluids would be lactated Ringer's solution (LRS), plasmalyte-A, normosol-R, normal saline 0.9%, and dextrose 2.5% in 0.45% saline. While all of these are isotonic, care needs to be given to the other additives and electrolytes in these fluids.

After giving crystalloids, reassessment of the patient through changes in decreased tachycardia, increased blood pressure, and improved mucous membrane color would indicate the patient's response to fluid resuscitation. If there is only minimal improvement to circulatory status with crystalloid boluses, consider colloids 5 ml/kg over 15–20 minutes (Herring 2014). Synthetic colloids, such as vetstarch or hetastarch, would increase the osmolarity intravenously, encouraging the volume from the earlier crystalloids to stay in the vasculature instead of diffusing out into the tissues. If indicated by bloodwork and coagulation profiles, fresh frozen plasma (FFP) is a natural colloid that can also replenish patient coagulation factors.

Gastric Decompression

The second priority is gastric decompression. Gastric decompression can help temporarily relieve the effects of obstructive shock. There are two main ways that gastric decompression is achieved: passage of an orogastric tube and percutaneous trocarization of the stomach.

Passage of an orogastric tube requires a large-bore smooth gastric tube that needs to be measured from the pet's nose to the last rib. Not all general practices may have this particular type of tube. Even if an orogastric tube is not placed at this point, one will be needed if surgery is attempted at the facility. A mouth gag needs to be in place to keep the pet from biting down on the tube and can be made from a 2-in. roll of tape. The pet needs to be heavily sedated or anesthetized to pass the gastric tube, which would require the patient to be more stable. This may be more complicated in higher-acuity patients. Sometimes, changing the patient's position from lying to standing is recommended to help with tube passage (Monnet 2012). Once the patient is adequately sedated, the roll of tape is placed in the mouth, holding it open, and the lubed gastric tube is passed through the tape roll, down the throat, into the esophagus. Resistance can be felt at the end of the esophagus when trying to pass the tube into the cardia of the stomach. A gentle twisting motion can be used to try to pass the gastric tube through into the stomach (Monnet 2012). However, care needs to be taken with the amount of force used. Depending on the severity of the volvulus, the esophageal sphincter and cardia may be pinched down, as well as have compromised tissue from the lack of blood flow. Care must be taken to not advance the tube too far into the stomach and puncture through any compromised areas of gastric tissue. This method can be combined with percutaneous gastric trocarization to try to increase the chances of successful gastric intubation.

Once the gastric tube is in the stomach, it can be used to remove excess air, fluid, and even some solid material from the stomach. However, to continue to keep the stomach deflated instead of reinstating, the orogastric tube needs to be kept in place, which requires keeping the patient under sedation or anesthesia (Monnet 2012). If the patient is being stabilized to then be transported to another facility, this could cause difficulty. If an orogastric tube is passed, it would need to be removed before transportation for the safety of the patient, and they would need to go directly to the referral facility in case they need decompression again on arrival.

The other method of gastric decompression is percutaneous trocarization. This method needs no specialized equipment and needs little to no sedation, making it more accessible to all practitioners. All this method needs is a 14- to 20-gauge IV catheter. This method can be quicker than passing an orogastric tube and can be done with little to no sedation. An area for trocarization is chosen by locating the most tympanic or distended area on the flank on either side of the body. This area is clipped and prepped aseptically. A large-bore catheter is then punctured through the skin, body wall, and into the stomach. The stylet needle is then removed from the catheter, and pressure can be applied to the body wall to help facilitate the removal of gas and fluid from the stomach. Rarely, there is a risk of lacerating the spleen. In one study comparing the two methods of decompression in 116 dogs, only one case of splenic laceration was identified in 85 dogs that were trocharized, of which the spleen had stopped bleeding by the time the pet was in surgery (Goodrich et al. 2013). This can be done multiple times to continue to decompress if the stomach re-dilates. The same study shows that there was no notable difference in mortality between the two methods of decompression or a combination of the two methods. This method of decompression is just as successful as passing an orogastric tube and generally more accessible and quicker to do (Goodrich et al. 2013).

Pain Control, Anti-Nausea, and Drugs

The third priority really needs to be done simultaneously with the first two. Pain management is very important; this condition is very painful. Dogs may present as very stoic or obtunded, but pain management is still needed. There are multiple reasons for pain in the GDV patient. There is visceral pain, or deep organ pain, from the stretching of visceral tissues in the torsion (from the stomach, spleen, omentum), stretching of the capsule of an organ (in the spleen with splenic swelling), inflammation, and invasion or compression of nerves (can happen with torsion on the vagus and other nerves) (Matthews 2012). Care needs to be taken to avoid medications with profound cardiovascular effects, such as acepromazine, tilatemine/zolazepam, ketamine, and dexmedetomidine. Acepromazine can have profound vasodilatory effects. In a GDV patient that is already hypotensive, vasodilation is going to lower the blood pressure. Dissociative anesthetic drugs such as tiletamine and ketamine work by releasing catecholamines from the adrenal glands. In a system that is already stressed, such as the GDV patient, the body will already be low on catecholamine reserves, so using these drugs would add stress to an already stressed system. Alpha-2-agonist drugs like dexmedetomidine cause peripheral vasoconstriction and, in turn, increased blood pressure and decreased heart rate. In a system where there is already a large amount of circulatory compromise, dexmedetomidine can complicate matters. The increased peripheral vasoconstriction would also be unwelcome in these patients who are already attempting to peripherally vasoconstrict to deal with hypovolemic shock. Further constricting the peripheral vessels could cause tissue injury due to hypoperfusion in these peripheral tissues.

Ideal pain medications in a GDV are pure mu-agonist opioids. The most commonly available of these are fentanyl, methadone, hydromorphone, and morphine. Non-lipophilic opioids, such as morphine and hydromorphone, are likely to reach the chemoreceptor trigger zone (CRTZ) that can induce vomiting before they reach opioid receptors. Lipophilic opioids like fentanyl are likely to reach the vomiting center before or at the same time as the CRTZ (Drobtaz 2012). For this reason, opioids need to be paired appropriately with anti-nausea medications, particularly hydromorphone and morphine. The last thing the patient who is trying to unproductively vomit needs is to try to vomit more. Maropitant should be given prior to the administration of the opioid or help lessen the vomiting and nausea associated with it. Ondansetron can be used as well to help lessen nausea associated with opioid usage (Burke 2022). These patients are going to have symptoms of nausea and vomiting anyway from the disease process, so anti-nausea medications are only going to help them.

If buprenorphine is the strongest opioid that is available in the facility, recall that it is only a partial mu-agonist (Budde 2023). Buprenorphine will have only mild to moderate pain control; it lasts about 8 hours and has a great affinity for the mu-receptor (Budde 2023). Buprenorphine is not going to be strong enough for surgical pain control. If this is the strongest pain medication available, then referral to another facility should be strongly considered. While butorphanol technically falls into the opioid category, it is a partial mu-antagonist and kappa-agonist, making it good for sedation but not appropriate for pain control for this population of patients (Budde 2023). There are some studies that point to butorphanol for visceral pain in canines, but it does nothing of somatic (superficial) pain and only has a duration of an hour max and requires redosing every 2 hours. Butorphanol also has a high affinity for the mu-receptor even after the two-hour window and will continue to interfere with any possible pure-mu opioids that the referral center would try to use in the next couple hours (Budde 2023). While nonsteroidal anti-inflammatory drugs are excellent for surgical pain, with the high chance of gastric tissue compromise, they should be avoided in GDV patients to prevent further gastrointestinal problems.

There are other drugs that can be helpful for usage in GDV patients. If sedation is needed, a benzodiazepine, such as midazolam or diazepam, is a good option. These drugs have minimal cardiovascular effects compared to other sedatives like acepromazine, tiletamine/zolazepam, or dexmedetomidine. If additional pain control is needed or the patient is having tachyarrhythmias on ECG, a lidocaine continuous rate infusion can help. Lidocaine has also been shown to have analgesic, prokinetic, and anti-inflammatory effects in addition to antiarrhythmic effects, all of which would be helpful to the GDV patient (Johnson 2022). Local anesthesia can be considered if going directly to surgery. While a local block like an epidural could be helpful, the extra time taken to perform these procedures should be considered, especially if the staff is not well trained to do them quickly. According to some sources, a lumbosacral epidural is only going to affect the caudal abdomen (Campoy 2013). However, if an epidural is used as adjunct pain control, a mixture of preservative-free opioids, like morphine (also called Duramorph), and a preservative-free longer-acting local anesthetic, like bupivacaine, would be ideal. If only preservative-free lidocaine is available, this is a fair choice as well. Keep in mind, however, that the lidocaine would last closer to 1–2 hours, while the bupivacaine lasts closer to 2–5 hours (Campoy 2013).

If a local block is necessary, an epidural should possibly be considered over a procedure like TAP (transverse abdominis plane) blocks, since the positioning for an epidural would be less stressful for the GDV patient, and the ultrasound guidance for the TAP block would be uncomfortable on the cranial abdomen for the GDV patient. However, if the technical ability is available and the patient is well stabilized, a TAP block provides excellent local coverage for abdominal exploration. As another venue of pain control, surgeons will use liposomal bupivacaine (brand name, Nocita) on closure of the abdominal incision. This bupivacaine is encased in lipid molecules, which the body has to break down to release the local anesthetic; it can last up to 72 hours.

For induction, hypnotic agents like alfaxalone or propofol are good choices. They can also be titrated to effect sedation if needed (Budde 2023). However, if used for sedation, the ability to induce and intubate should be available immediately, just in case. Induction agents like tiletamine and zolazepam or ketamine and midazolam should be avoided when possible due to the catecholamine release they would cause in an already stressed system, as previously discussed. Additionally, nausea control is important in these patients due to the gastric compromise, as well as their tendency to have pancreatitis after resolution of the GDV. Maropitant and ondansetron are helpful anti-nausea medications; additionally, prokinetics like metoclopramide can be helpful postoperatively to encourage gastrointestinal movement. However, they should not be given preoperatively as they can put extra pressure on an already compromised GI tract.

If the ECG is showing ventricular tachyarrhythmia, it should be treated with anti-arrhythmics (such as lidocaine) to preserve cardiac output. An intravenous bolus of 2 mg/kg of lidocaine can be given to test the response to the drug (Radlinsky 2013). If the patient does not respond, procainamide or sotalol can be tried (Radlinsky 2013). Bradycardia and hypotension should be treated appropriately with an anticholinergic (such as atropine or glycopyrrolate) to increase heart rate, or various vasopressor or inotrope therapies (such as dopamine, norepinephrine, dobutamine, ephedrine, etc.) to further support cardiovascular depression.

What Does Surgery Entail?

Whether the GDV patient ends up transferring for surgery or ends up in surgery at the current facility, it is important to know what surgical treatment of a GDV entails. There are three main concerns in a GDV surgery: derotation, abdominal assessment, and gastropexy.

Gastric Derotation and Abdominal Assessment

Derotation is the primary goal of surgery. Once the stomach is derotated, an orogastric tube is passed, and stomach contents are emptied. Gastric lavage used to be recommended at this point; however, there is no evidence supporting this practice as beneficial to postoperative recovery compared to simply emptying the stomach contents via orogastric tube. After this, a pause needs to be taken to assess the rest of the abdominal contents. The vasculature and the spleen need to be assessed for hemorrhage. If the volvulus involves the spleen, vessels can be torn loose when the organs are displaced, causing this hemorrhage. If this has not been resolved, it needs to be fixed by ligature or by removal of the spleen. If the spleen is intact but involved in the volvulus, it needs to be carefully evaluated for signs of necrosis or thromboemboli, in which case a splenectomy is indicated. If the spleen itself is torsed, it needs to be removed without derotating it to keep the toxins and thromboemboli trapped within the spleen from re-entering the general circulatory system prior to removal. Splenectomy can be done by hand ligature, stapling device, or vessel-sealing device. This is another area where referral to a specialist is preferable, as they tend to have stapling and vessel sealing devices that make splenectomies easier and less prone to hemorrhage. The rest of the abdominal contents need to be evaluated as well. If there is a splenic torsion as well, then the pancreas should be evaluated for involvement as well (Images 16.3–16.6).

Once the abdominal exploration is completed, the tissues of the stomach mucosa need to be evaluated. Derotating the stomach and letting it sit while the rest of the abdomen is explored gives the stomach mucosa a chance to reperfuse. The tissue should be allowed several minutes of reperfusion before being evaluated for necrotic tissue. If, after 10–15 minutes, these devitalized tissues do not show any improvement, a partial gastrectomy should be considered to prevent gastric perforation later in recovery. This tends to be where surgeons may consult with the owner and choose to euthanize intraoperatively. However, referral practices tend to have surgeons who may both be more likely to attempt a partial gastrectomy as they are more familiar with them, and they have advanced staplers, like the TA or EndoGIA staplers, to make this a more viable option (Image 16.7).

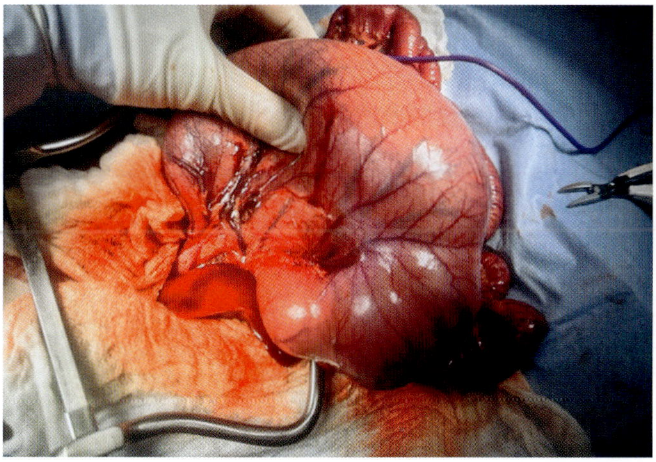

Images 16.3 Stomach where the volvulus has been relieved; however, the stomach is still dilatated. *Source:* Photo courtesy of Raphael Repellin, DVM.

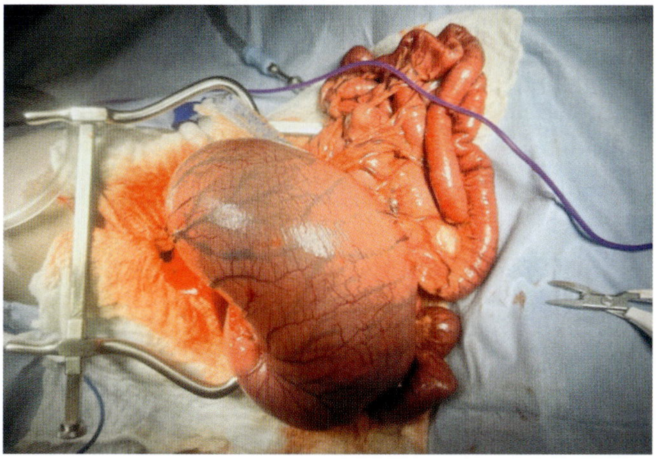

Image 16.4 The stomach from the previous image showing healthy and pink mucosa showing adequate perfusion and no grossly evident areas of necrosis or perforation. *Source:* Photo courtesy of Raphael Repellin, DVM.

Gastropexy

After abdominal organs are all cleaned up, the last step is a gastropexy to anchor the stomach and prevent a future volvulus. The two most common procedures for gastropexy tend to be incisional and belt-loop gastropexies. Both have been shown to be equally effective in the literature (Goodrich et al. 2013). A dog that has had a GDV but has not been gastropexied has an 80% chance of developing a GDV again (Goodrich et al. 2013). A GDV patient that had a gastropexy at the time of surgery has a 10% recurrence rate, largely dependent on the gastropexy procedure used (Goodrich et al. 2013). A gastropexy is a must during GDV surgery, as there is an extremely high chance of the pet having a recurrent GDV (Images 16.8 and 16.9).

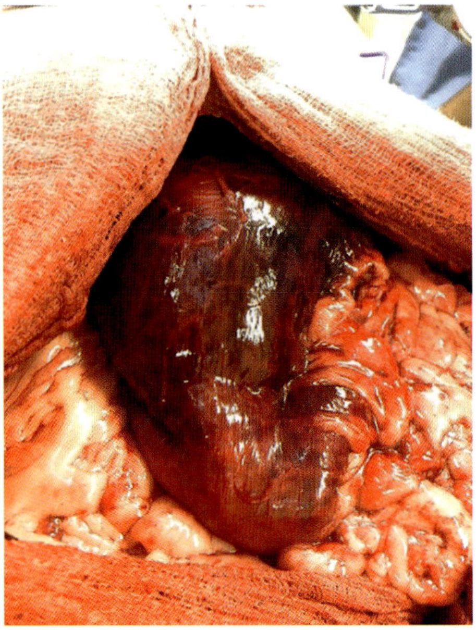

Image 16.5 This gastric mucosa continues to be devitalized even after letting it sit. *Source:* Photo courtesy of Raphael Repellin, DVM.

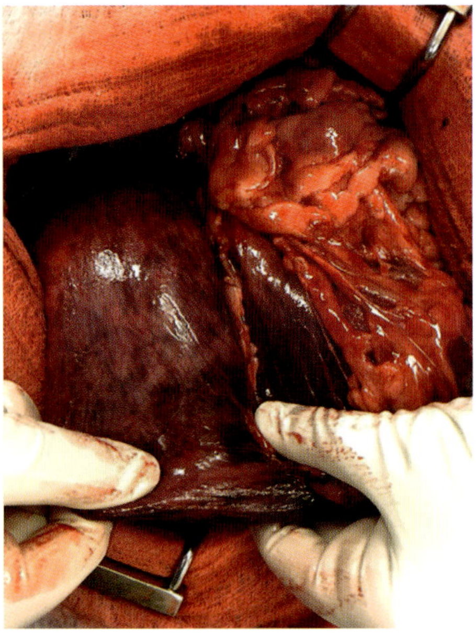

Image 16.6 This mucosa lacks elasticity, requiring a gastrectomy to remove the devitalized gastric tissue. *Source:* Photo courtesy of Raphael Repellin, DVM.

Prophylactic gastropexies are becoming more routinely performed in high-risk dogs at the time of their spay or neuter. As such, there is an increased movement to minimally invasive laparoscopic gastropexies. While these procedures do not tend to have the same aggressive scar tissue lesion created by open abdominal methods, there are studies that demonstrate they are as effective at creating adhesions to the body wall as open gastropexies due to the barbed suture used (Song et al. 2020). So, while any prophylactic gastropexy should be questioned on its success if the patient is showing the signs of a GDV, a laparoscopic gastropexy is not necessarily any less effective at preventing GDV than an open version.

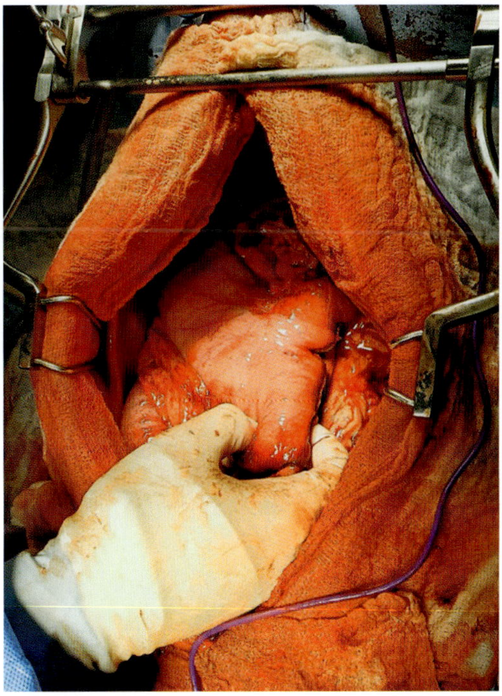

Image 16.7 Example of a stapled gastrectomy done with an EndoGIA stapler. *Source:* Photo courtesy of Raphael Repellin, DVM.

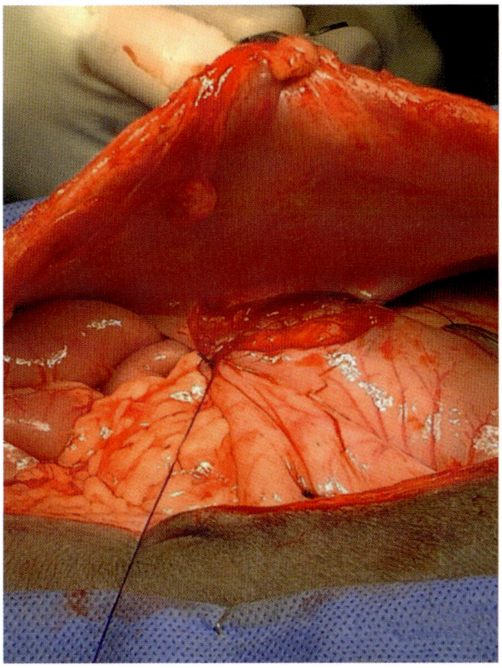

Image 16.8 Example of an incisional gastropexy where the mucosal layer of the stomach is incised. *Source:* Photo courtesy of Raphael Repellin, DVM.

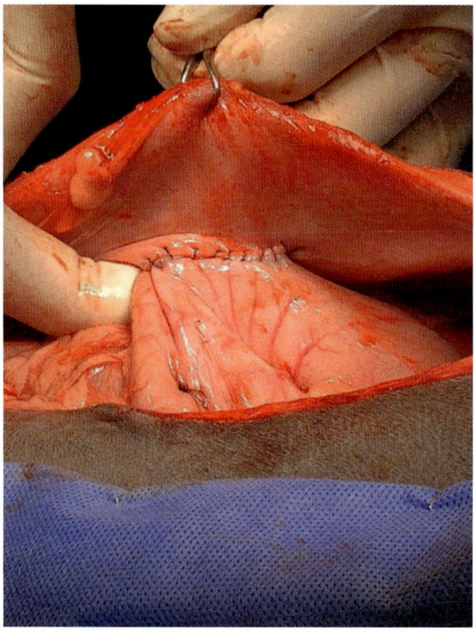

Image 16.9 Mucosal layer of the stomach attached to an incision made in the transverse abdominis muscle. *Source:* Photo courtesy of Raphael Repellin, DVM.

What Happens Next?

Overnight hospitalization for postoperative GDV cases is a must; one night in the hospital is a best-case scenario, while multiple nights are often more realistic. These patients can be very unstable upon arrival and throughout surgery. Even the ones that appear stable preoperatively need to be monitored closely postoperatively. These patients need to be on an appropriate amount of IV fluids to continue to support the patient's hydration status until they are able to hydrate appropriately on their own. Anti-nausea medications, such as maropitant and ondansetron, and prokinetic medications, such as metoclopramide, can be started to encourage the pet to eat. The pet needs to be offered frequent, small meals to encourage peristalsis and get the gastrointestinal tract moving again. Acid-reducing medications, such as famotidine, ranitidine, omeprazole, and pantoprazole, can be helpful in reducing gastric acidity and the chance of gastric ulceration (Radlinsky 2013). With partial gastrectomies, oral feeding may be delayed. Nasogastric tube placement needs to be considered in these patients for both feeding purposes and to empty the stomach of excessive stomach acid if ileus develops.

These patients will need to continue to be on injectable opioid pain medications to keep them comfortable for at least one night postoperatively. Once they are reliably eating, the transition can be made to oral medications. Nonsteroidal anti-inflammatory medications should continue to be avoided in these patients postoperatively.

Postoperative GDV patients may need to be on continuous ECG monitoring to keep an eye on any concerning ventricular arrhythmias, as up to 45.5% of patients can develop these (Radlinsky 2013). Ventricular arrhythmias can occur 12–36 hours after surgery, usually resulting from myocardial injury or an electrolyte imbalance. Such arrhythmias include ventricular tachycardia, multiform premature ventricular complexes (VPC or PVC), and R-on-T phenomenon. These can be treated with lidocaine as a first line. If that is unsuccessful, procainamide or sotalol can be considered. Electrolytes should be checked and corrected for if imbalanced; oftentimes, GDV patients will become hypokalemic postoperatively and need supplementation in their IV fluids (Goodrich et al. 2013).

These patients should also be monitored for signs of sepsis or DIC postoperatively. Sepsis can occur if the stomach perforates or a partial gastrectomy fails, generally 3–5 days after surgery. If this happens, another surgery is needed for correction of the perforation, as well as prolonged hospitalization and antibiotic therapy for treatment of sepsis. If clotting times are prolonged, the patient may benefit from a FFP transfusion to try to replenish clotting factors that may have been used up.

Once a patient is eating and drinking on their own, can be transitioned to oral medication, and no longer has ECG abnormalities, they can be released to go home. The following 10–14 days should have strict activity restriction at home while the abdominal wall incision heals and the gastropexy has a chance to scar down. Short leash walks are permissible for bathroom purposes only. Oral sedatives may be needed by the clients to help keep the postoperative patient quiet at home, particularly high-energy breeds. Clients should continue to feed multiple small meals throughout the day, rather than one or two large meals. After the recovery period is over, clients should continue to try to prevent patients from eating their meals too quickly, using feeding aids and slow-feeder bowls as necessary. They should also prevent vigorous exercise directly before or after a meal to prevent the pet from swallowing excessive amounts of air on top of a food-filled stomach. While a pet with a gastropexy is highly unlikely to develop a gastric dilatation with volvulus again, they can most certainly develop a simple gastric dilatation, as was seen in Image 16.2.

Works Cited

Budde, J.A. (2023). *Plumb's Veterinary Drug Handbook*. Hoboken, NJ: Wiley-Blackwell.

Burke, J.H. (2022). Effectiveness of orally administered maropitant and ondansetron in preventing preoperative emesis and nausea in healthy dogs premedicated with a combination of hydromorphone, acepromazine, and glycopyrrolate. *Journal of the American Veterinary Medical Association* 260 (S1): S40–S45. https://doi.org/10.2460/javma.21.02.0082.

Campoy, L.A. (2013). *Small Animal Regional Anesthesia and Analgesia*. Hoboken, NJ: Wiley-Blackwell.

Drobtaz, K.M. (2012). *Manual of Small Animal Emergency and Critical Care Medicine*. Iowa.

Gibson, T.W.G. (2020). Gastric dilation and volvulus in small animals (bloat). In: *Merck Veterinary Manual Professional Version*, 11e. Rahway: Merck&Co.

Goodrich, Z.P., Powell, L.L., and Hulting, K.J. (2013). Assessment of two methods of gastric decompression for the initial management of gastric dilation-volvulus. *Journal of Small Animal Practice* 54. https://doi.org/10.1111/jsap.12019: 75–79.

Herring, J. (2014). Gastrointestinal emergencies. In: *Handbook of Canine and Feline Emergency Protocols* (ed. M. McMichael), 45–63. Iowa: Wiley.

Johnson, R.S. (2022). *Canine and Feline Anesthesia and Co-Existing Disease*, 2e. New Jersey: Wiley-Blackwell.

King, J. L. (2025). Pysiology, cardiac output. *StatPearls [Internet]*. Retrieved from www.ncbi.nlm.nih.gov/books/NBK470455/

Li, W.W., Wu, R.S., Liu, P.C. et al. (2022). What is your diagnosis? *Journal of the American Veterinary Medical Association* 259: 1–4.

Lopez, M. H. (2023). Physiology, osmosis. *StatPearls [Internet]*. Retrieved from www.ncbi.nlm.nih/gov/books/NBK557609/

Matthews, K.S. (2018). *Analgesia and Anesthesia for the Ill or Injured Dog and Cat*, 1–7. Hoboken: Wiley-Blackwell.

Mazzaferro, E. (2021). Gastric dilatation-volvulus: the twisted truth. *dvm360,* 52. Retrieved from www.dvm360.com/view/gastric-dilatation-volvulus-controlling-crisis

Monnet, E. (2012). Gastric dilation-volvulus: controlling the crisis. *dvm360*. Retrived from www.dvm360.com/view/gastric-dilation-volvulus-controlling-crisis

Peripheral IV Catheter Chart 2025. (2025). From pedagogyeducation.com. Retrieved from https://pedagogyeducation.com/resources/infusion/peripheral-IV-catheter-chart

Radlinsky, M. (2013). Surgery of the digestive system. In: *Small Animal Surgery* (ed. T. Fossum), 482–487. St. Louis Missouri: Elsevier Mosby.

Song, K.G., Goldsmid, S.E., Lee, J., and Simpson, D.J. (2020). Retrospective analysis of 736 cases of canine gastric dilation volvulus. *Australian Veterinary Journal* 98: 232–238. https://doi.org/10.1111/avj.12942.

Standl, T.A. (2018). The nomenclature, definition, and distinction of types of shock. *Deutschmark Ärzteblatt*, Dtsch Arztebl Int. 2018 Nov 9 115 (45): 757–768. https://doi.org/10.3238/arztebl.2018.0757.

17

Trauma Llama

Allison Snow

BluePearl Pet Hospital, 1 Taft Ct., Rockville, MD, USA

Bite Wounds, Gunshot Wounds, Penetrating Foreign Body Wounds

Don't Panic

No exclamation point required. If panic ensues, thinking through the assessment process effectively becomes challenging. Time is likely of the essence so ... don't panic.

First, We Assess

Bleeding and respiratory distress must be managed first. These two factors are the most serious in determining the patient's compatibility with life. Things to consider are:

- Use of tourniquets, pressure bandages, Yunnan Bai Yao
- Sterile dressings over any wound which may communicate with the thorax
- Placement in an oxygen chamber or use of masked or flow-by oxygen supplementation

Once those two items are stabilized, you may move on to a basic orthopedic exam, as well as a neurological exam. Some items of particular note:

- Can the patient ambulate?
  - Are there fractures to be stabilized before transfer?
- Are the wounds easily identifiable?
  - This may require clipping the hair around the wounds for visualization
- Can the patient see?
  - Does the patient have PLR, menace response, and field of vision?
- Can the patient move at all?
  - Does the patient have deep pain?
- Is the patient vocalizing?
  - Pain response?
  - Neurological?

If the patient is otherwise stable at this point, it is appropriate to administer pain medication and collect venous blood samples. When possible, a well-placed peripheral IV catheter is appreciated prior to transfer. Please avoid exhausting venipuncture sites of all four limbs for placement, though your emergency room (ER) team will thank you if you can get a 20/22 g IV catheter in a medial or lateral saphenous that they can turn into a sampling line.

If homeostasis has been achieved and the patient is mildly to moderately hypovolemic, it is appropriate to administer a small to moderate bolus of 5–20 ml/kg of fluids intravenously prior to transfer. Please facilitate this bolus over 20–30 minutes. This will improve the likelihood that emergency staff will be able to place additional sampling lines or arterial catheters for invasive blood pressure monitoring if surgery is required.

Diagnostic work-up should be tailored to the patient. Be sure to choose the most comprehensive blood panel warranted for the patient's presentation. For trauma cases, a serum chemistry (or superchemistry) and a complete blood count will suffice. This will not only save your client money in the long run but will also give insight to baseline values and evidence of organ compromise secondary to the traumatic injury, systemic inflammatory response syndrome (SIRS), or sepsis. It is understandable that all clinics do not have access to blood gases; however, blood gases give insight into the extent of tissue damage through lactate values and creatinine kinase. Alternatively, if your chemistry analyzer has the capability of running these values, that provides a sufficient baseline (Image 17.1).

Good quality, appropriately collimated, orthogonal radiographs of the injured area can give some insight into the extent of injury. A primary complaint of veterinary surgeons is the poor quality of radiographs submitted from general practitioners. Here is your opportunity to shine! Take the time to educate your staff on proper radiographic technique and positioning. Techs, nurses, and assistants – advocate for your patient and yourself.

Hands-free radiography is the best way to ensure staff and patient safety. Veterinarians are responsible for providing the appropriate pain control and sedation to achieve diagnostic radiographs. This is a gold standard of medicine that every practice with radiography can achieve.

An adjacent pertinent discussion is the choice of analgesia. Traumatic injuries surpass the pain control achieved by butorphanol. Butorphanol is not to be considered a pain medication in trauma cases. Though more effective at providing sedation, butorphanol will prevent better analgesics

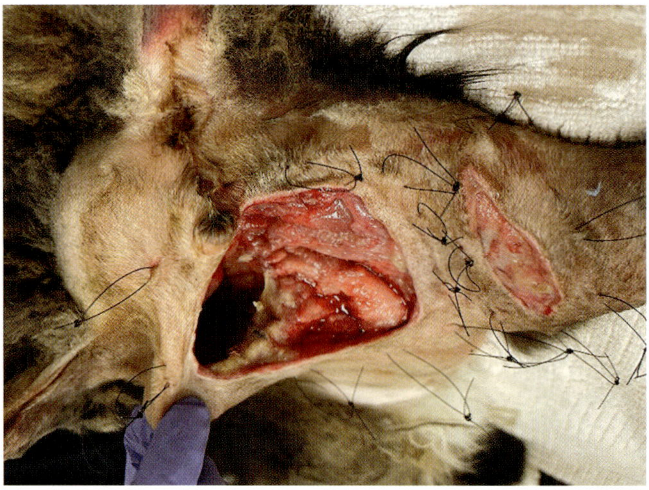

Image 17.1 Photograph of a healing wound in a cat caused by unknown trauma. The sutures are for a tie-over bandage. On initial presentation to the ER, the femoral artery, urethra, and colon were visible in the large wound. Somehow, none of that was torn. This cat was transferred to the surgery department for assessment, and this is at a recheck approximately 2 weeks after the initial assessment. *Source:* Photo courtesy of Simone Conwell, RVT, VTS (ECC).

from accessing pain receptors. This will, in turn, delay surgical treatment until it has worn off enough to administer another analgesic.

Penetrating Trauma

Bite Wounds, Gunshot Wounds, and Foreign Bodies, Oh My!

Advanced imaging will be required to determine the pathway of a penetrating object. There is still plenty of good information to be gained from acquiring radiographs. Conditions such as pleural effusion, atelectasis, and ascites can all be appreciated radiographically. Patients with severe trauma to the trachea will experience significant subcutaneous emphysema (which can often also be palpated) in the surrounding tissues. Pneumothorax or pneumomediastinum can also be appreciated radiographically. Primary care practices possessing ultrasound technology can use thoraco/abdominocentesis to further assess ascites or pleural effusion (Image 17.2).

Secondarily, educating the client on the limitations of imaging available to you is also of utmost importance. Almost universally, additional imaging will be required for the most serious cases. Computerized tomography (CT) or magnetic resonance imaging (MRI) may be necessary to locate foreign bodies deeply embedded in tissues. This is especially true regarding entry and exit of firearm projectiles, as entry and exit wounds must be identified and reconciled during treatment. Imaging alone cannot rule out or assess the severity of damage done to deep tissues in trauma cases, and most certainly, the wounds require surgical exploration under general anesthesia (Images 17.3–17.10).

Many significant structures within the cervical region are at risk in penetrating traumas of the neck, the spinal cord, trachea, and esophagus being the primary concerns. If your images appear obscured by fluid accumulation, there may be hemorrhage happening. The severity of the hemorrhage will indicate what is needed immediately. Severe hemorrhage could mean damage to the carotid artery or jugular vein, which must then be ligated before transfer. In canine patients, both

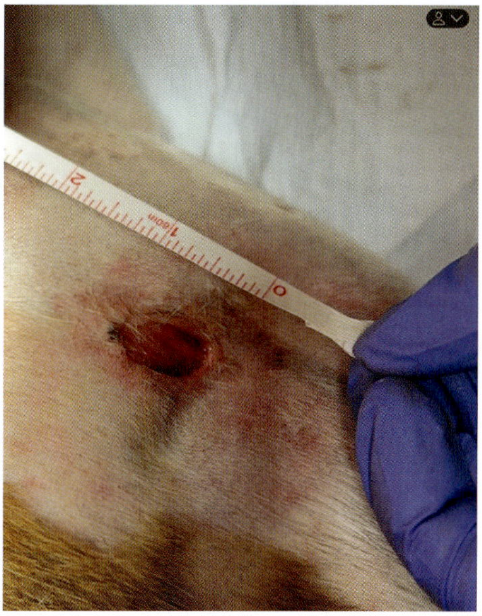

Image 17.2 Flail chest after a dogfight. *Source:* Photo courtesy of Simone Conwell, RVT, VTS (ECC).

THORAX: There is mild to moderate cardiomegaly with the appearance of left atrial enlargement and mild widening on the ventrodorsal projection. There is also a leftward mediastinal shift. There is mild fluid opacity within the pleural space. No definitive evidence of pneumothorax is identified. There are multiple regions that have rounded gas lucencies and a mottled appearance such as the cranial mediastinum in the caudoventral thoracic cavity which may be due to pulmonary pathology versus summation of the subcutaneous emphysema and soft tissue swelling. The diaphragm is unremarkable.

ABDOMEN: The abdominal and retroperitoneal serosal margin detail are adequate. Summating with the cranioventral liver on the left lateral projection there is mottled gas opacity. No other regions of gas are seen within the abdomen. The liver, spleen, kidneys and urinary bladder are otherwise unremarkable with normal silhouettes in size. The abdominal body wall appears intact. The stomach is mildly distended with gas and wispy soft tissue opacity. The small intestinal tract is in a normal location and normal opacity with no evidence of mechanical obstruction or herniation. The colon contains soft formed fecal matter.

CONCLUSIONS:
1. Multiple rib fractures along the ventral aspect of the left caudal thorax/cranial abdomen (ribs 7, 8, 9 and likely 10). Most of these appear to be short oblique with mild dislocation and 1 appears to be segmental with moderate dislocation.
2. Mild pleural effusion may be hemorrhage and/or serosanguineous.
3. The mottled appearance of the cranial mediastinum, caudal ventral thorax and over the liver is suspected to be artifact from summation of subcutaneous emphysema and soft tissue swelling of the skin summating with these regions however pulmonary bulla, mild pneumothorax and mild gas in the region of the liver are not entirely excluded. Pulmonary contusions may also be present. No definitive evidence of pneumothorax is identified.
4. Extensive subcutaneous/fascial plane emphysema and soft tissue swelling surrounding the neck, thorax and dorsal abdomen are consistent with reported trauma. Entrance into the thoracic cavity seems likely although not definitive. No definitive evidence of tracheal or esophageal tears although small tears may still be present.
5. Possible mild to moderate cardiomegaly (i.e. left atrial enlargement +/- biventricular, mild dilation or mild pericardial effusion). Correlate with any heart murmur if present. No evidence of congestive heart failure is identified.
6. Leftward mediastinal shift may be due to mild obliquity versus atelectasis or pulmonary contusions.
7. He 1213 IVDD.

COMMENTS:
Proceed as planned with supportive care and stabilization. Consider computed tomography of the neck and thorax if further evaluation may be useful such as for surgical planning. Endoscopic evaluation of the trachea and esophagus could also be performed to evaluate for patency if indicated.

Image 17.3 Radiology report of the dog in Image 19.2 illustrates the usefulness and limitations of radiology in diagnosing trauma. CT was not performed on this patient but would have provided a more definitive answer of whether the thoracic cavity had been penetrated. *Source:* Image courtesy of Simone Conwell, RVT, VTS (ECC).

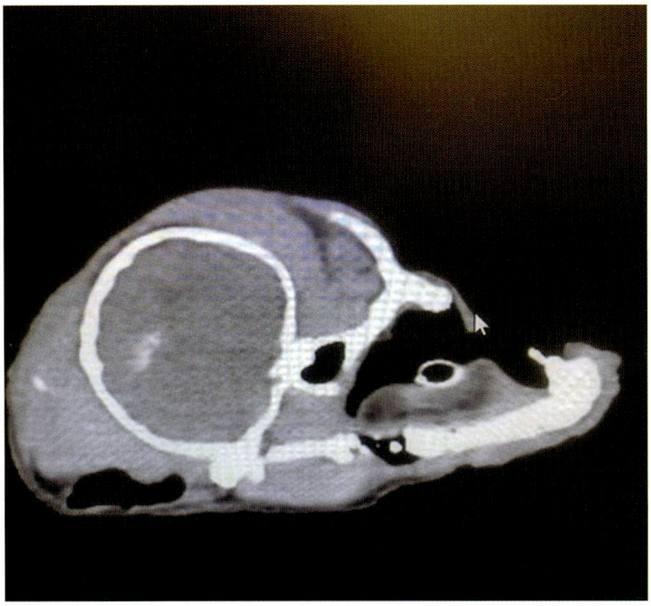

Image 17.4 Stills from a CT of a dogfight where the patient's skull was proven to not be intact, despite the dog still breathing and aware on his own. *Source:* Photos courtesy of Simone Conwell, RVT, VTS (ECC).

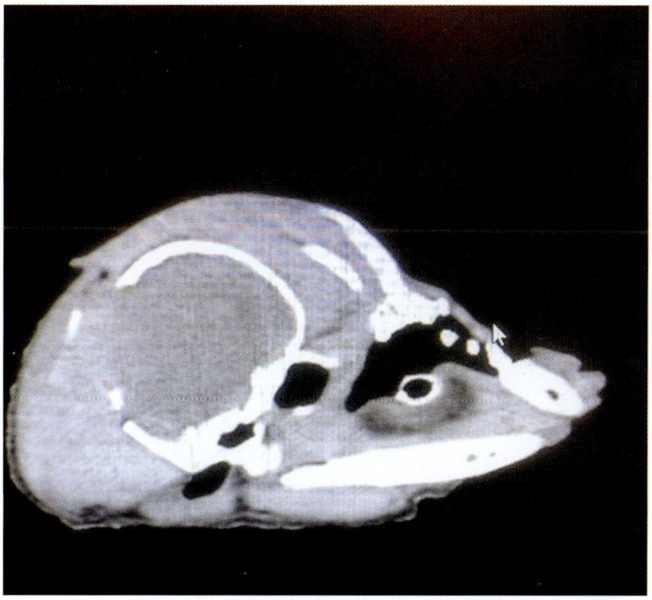

Image 17.5 Stills from a CT of a dogfight where the patient's skull was proven to not be intact, despite the dog still breathing and aware on his own. *Source:* Photos courtesy of Simone Conwell, RVT, VTS (ECC).

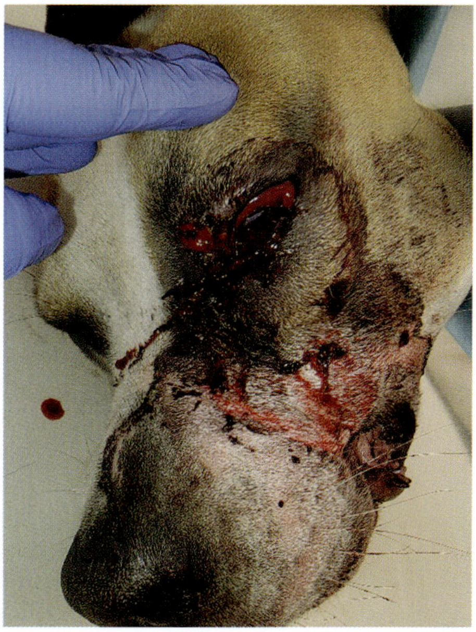

Image 17.6 Photo of a dog that was shot in the face. The suspicion is that it grazed his eye and ruptured the globe, as there was no exit wound. *Source:* Photos courtesy of Stephanie Burt, RVT.

carotids may be ligated if collateral circulation is intact. Cerebral edema has the potential to develop, though, as a result. The vertebral arteries will provide sufficient blood flow to the brain.

Esophageal damage may not be immediately observable and often doesn't reveal itself until a few days after the injury, as ingesta or water accumulates in the surrounding tissue. Once the patient is transferred, endoscopy may be necessary to sufficiently evaluate esophageal integrity (Image 17.11).

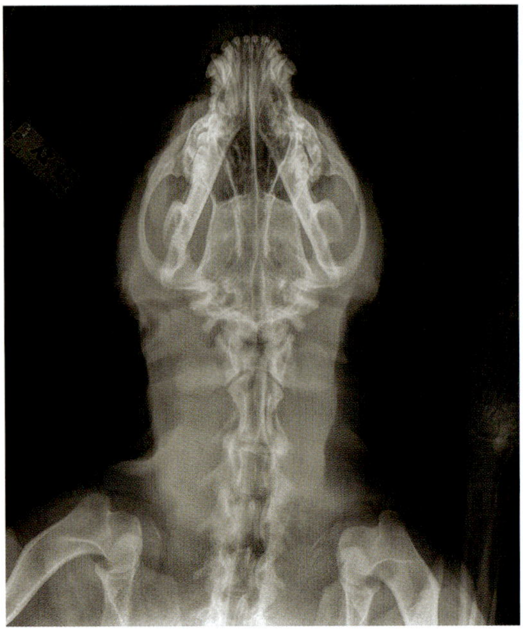

Image 17.7 VD and radiograph projections showing that the bullet did not remain in the skull. *Source:* Photos courtesy of Stephanie Burt, RVT.

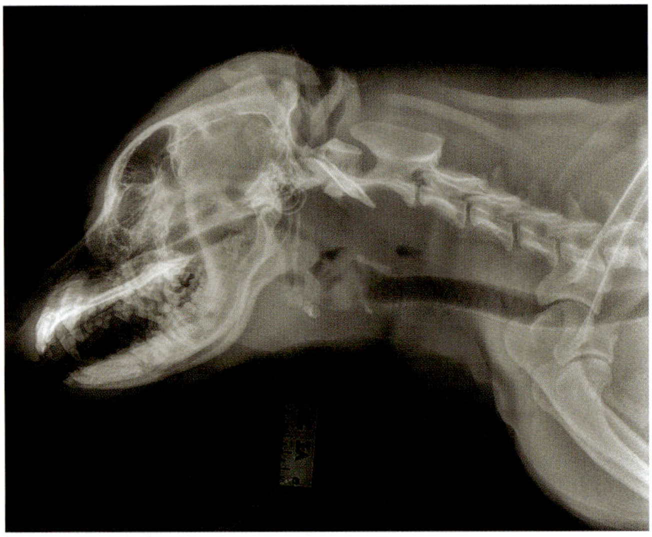

Image 17.8 Right lateral radiograph projections showing that the bullet did not remain in the skull. *Source:* Photos courtesy of Stephanie Burt, RVT.

It is very important to prepare the client for what is needed to successfully transfer the patient to a specialty care facility. They must be made aware of what to expect, and that is the job of the primary care team. Understanding that the cost of veterinary care is always increasing, your team owes it to the client to ensure that all treatments and diagnostics you complete initially are indicated, performed with proper technique, and will not contradict treatment at the transfer facility.

Radiographs must be performed with good technique. Pay close attention to collimation of the primary beam (no whole-cat or whole-dog rads), as well as penetration of the beam. In the vast majority of cases, diagnostic-quality radiographs necessitate sedation to perform safely. At the very least, adequate pain control is non-negotiable.

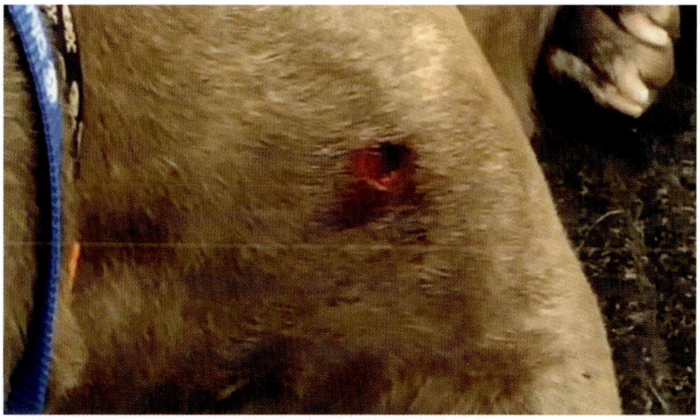

Image 17.9 Picture of a dog with a gunshot wound to the shoulder. *Source:* Photo courtesy of Simone Conwell, RVT, VTS (ECC).

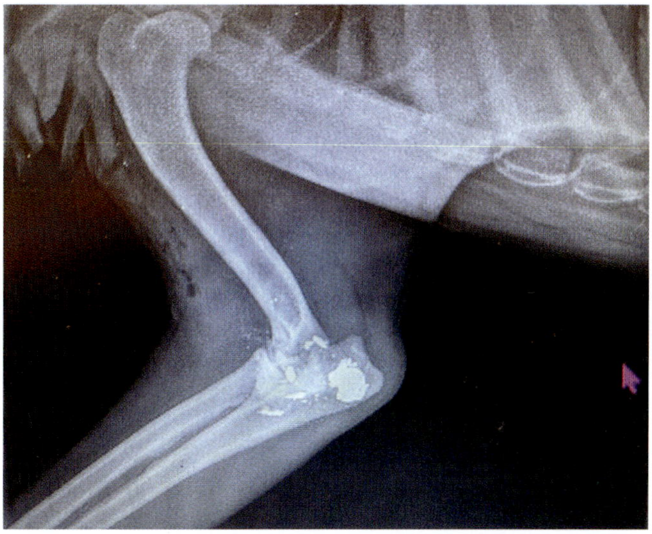

Image 17.10 Radiograph of the dog in the previous image showing the bullet was still in her. *Source:* Photo courtesy of Simone Conwell, RVT, VTS (ECC).

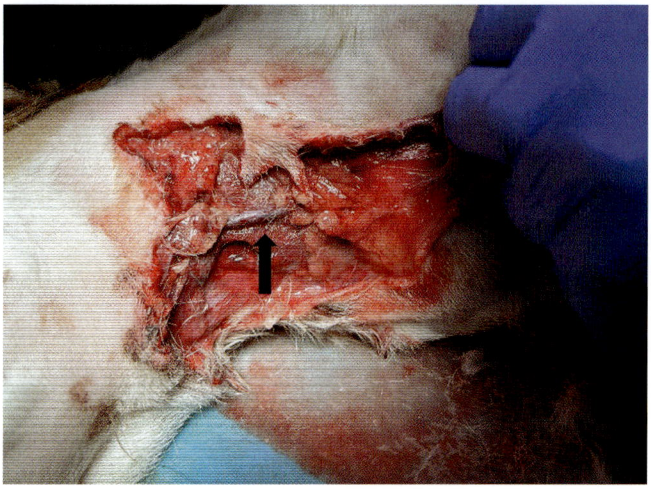

Image 17.11 The throat of the same dog from Images 17.2 and 17.3. The black arrow points to the jugular vein. *Source:* Photo courtesy of Simone Conwell, RVT, VTS (ECC).

To be clear, butorphanol and buprenorphine are inadequate for most penetrating wound emergencies. Buprenorphine has a high affinity to the mu receptor, but with its low intrinsic activity, it will displace other opioids on the mu receptor (Kumar 2025) Butorphanol will prevent higher intrinsic-activity opioids from accessing the mu receptor all together (Kumar 2025). Better choices are pure mu agonists (e.g. hydromorphone, morphine, and methadone) as they will not interfere with commonly used anesthetic protocols used in surgical specialty (Herman 2024; NRC 2009).

Another item to consider is being judicious with venipuncture. Placement of intravenous catheters is recommended. Care must be taken to ensure venous access is achieved without compromising the other easily accessible peripheral vessels, and not to place an intravenous catheter in an already compromised area. In many cases, multiple venous catheters are required during the anesthetic process to give adequate support to the patient. Vasopressors, antibiotics, blood products, etc., are routinely indicated and require a carefully placed intravenous catheter to administer. In some cases, arterial catheters are placed to more accurately monitor blood pressure under anesthesia. It is not recommended to attempt arterial catheterization prior to the patient's arrival at the transfer facility.

Lacerations

No Matter How They're Sliced, They Must Be Made Nice

Lacerations result when tissue is sliced or torn after an object has penetrated. They are common traumas seen in general practice and range in severity from very superficial to very deep. Regardless of the severity, all lacerations are treated similarly. Overall patient assessment, analgesia, and diagnostics are the first three steps.

If you expect a delay in wound treatment, a simple bandage can protect the laceration until treatment occurs. A protective layer that will not disturb the wound tissue may be placed and wrapped with cast padding or other absorbent material. Be careful not to place any bandage which may restrict blood flow to the wound. This may cause tissue necrosis, which will complicate wound resolution.

Now is a great time to consider administering antibiotics. All lacerations are to be considered contaminated and must be treated as such. Even wounds which are not visibly contaminated (bite wounds and other punctures) are very likely contaminated with bacteria. A first-generation cephalosporin like cefazolin is typically the first choice; cefazolin is commonly used in surgical specialty to prevent intraoperative infection, and is therefore the best choice when transferring your patient to the surgical facility (Shahar 1997). If intravenous antibiotics are unavailable, oral antibiotics are the next best choice. Oral amoxicillin–clavulanic acid is widely used in general practice and is therefore a fine choice to administer prior to transfer (Shahar 1997).

When addressing the wound(s), care must be taken not to disturb the healthy tissue. Removing any gross debris can be accomplished manually with gloved hands. At this stage, sterile gloves are preferred but not required. Avoid probing into and disrupting any intact tissue if it appears to have a good blood supply. Gently flushing the wound with lukewarm saline, tap water is preferred to dilute chlorhexidine. Chlorhexidine is nonselective in tissue destruction and, even in its most diluted forms, can destroy healthy tissue and prolong wound closure. It is not recommended to flush with betadine (Shahar 1997).

After the wound has been cleaned, you may replace it with a new bandage for transfer. Do not apply any ointment, sugar, manuka honey, or sterile lubricant to the wound! Apply a sterile wound

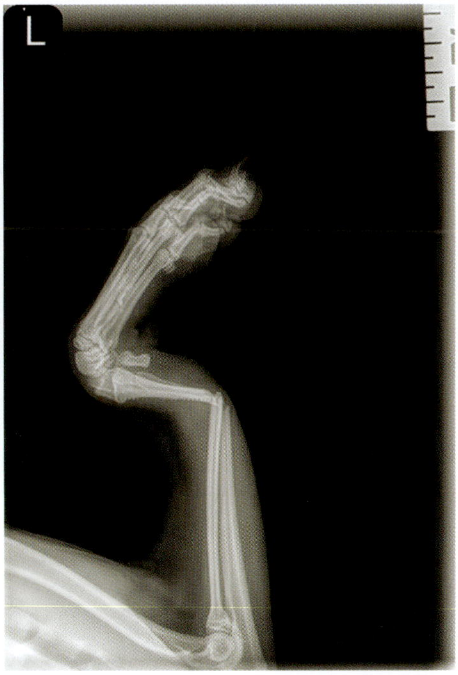

Image 17.12 A leg with a broken radius and ulna.
Source: Photo courtesy of Simone Conwell, RVT, VTS (ECC).

cover (e.g. telfa +/− adaptic) and then gently wrap the sterile dressing with cast padding and stretch gauze; do not cover with vet wrap as this material can constrict when it gets wet. Avoid placing sutures or staples on the wound prior to transfer (Image 17.12).

Fractures

Oh ... That's Definitely Broken

Generally, fractures take between 4 and 8 weeks to heal (Candela 2025). Puppies and kittens heal more quickly because they are already in the growth process; however, older animals may take 8 weeks or longer to completely heal. Even though most fractures are not life-threatening, they tend to be disproportionately fear-inducing to clients. They are painful, require a lot of strict rest, and require administering multiple medications to their pet. They are intimidating recoveries for clients in part because they also seem high stakes.

A bone can fracture in a multitude of ways, and surgeons classify them into many categories.

- Complete Fracture – this is when the full circumference of a bone is fractured into two or more pieces.
- Incomplete Fracture – this is when the bone may only in part be broken through its circumference, resulting in a bone which looks bent versus broken in pieces. Incomplete fractures are more common in young animals than in older animals.

Complete fractures are further differentiated into the following three categories: transverse (broken straight across the bone at a right angle to the length of the bone), oblique (broken at a

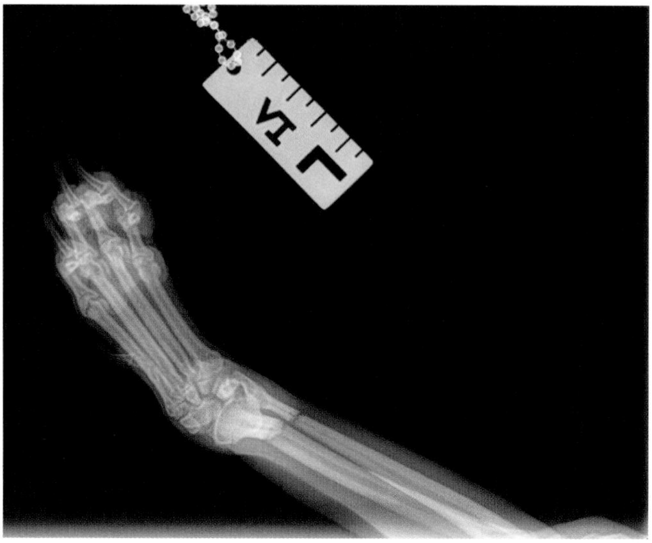

Image 17.13 Transverse fracture. *Source:* Photo courtesy of Simone Conwell, RVT, VTS (ECC).

diagonal across the bone, resulting in two fragments with sharp points), or comminuted, that is to say, broken in three or more pieces of varying shapes (Candela 2025; Gänsslen 2024) (Images 17.13–17.15).

A fracture resulting in a penetrating wound is referred to as an open fracture. Open fractures can be created when the trauma causes the bone to break and then penetrates the skin (from the inside out) or when an object penetrates the skin to fracture the bone (from the outside in). If the fracture causes no open wound, it is considered a closed fracture. Open fractures are considered more of an emergency than closed fractures due to the risk of infection.

Most fractures can be treated medically, but some must be treated surgically. If too much time has elapsed since the initial fracture trauma, the bone may become irreparable. When this is the case for limbs, amputation is necessary. There are also cases in which a very recent fracture is too severely comminuted to be repaired, and amputation is the best treatment. Some owners will opt for amputation over a surgical fix to a broken bone due to finances or if they know their pet will not be cooperative during the healing process.

It is important to set expectations with your clients about fracture recovery. The rest required is very strict; there may be multiple medications prescribed for their pets, and incisional complications may jeopardize limb recovery. The use of an Elizabethan collar is recommended to keep pets from incisional self-trauma. Stress the importance of owner compliance regarding this issue. It is possible for a pet to disturb their incision to a point where amputation is then required for treatment.

Most long bone fractures are treated with fixation or splinting/casting. However, it is strongly advised against applying a splint or bandage prior to transfer for most fractures. Applying a splint or cast without proper reduction of the fracture may compromise healing of the bone and may cause further damage to surrounding tissues. Bandages applied to stop bleeding are acceptable if the patient is immediately transferred (i.e. within the hour of presentation) (Image 17.16).

Spinal fractures are among the most devastating fractures and require careful handling. There may be several causes, though being hit by a car is among the most common. Ideally, a radiolucent backboard is used to stabilize and move the patient. Imaging should be taken under full anesthesia or heavy sedation if a spinal fracture is suspected, and care should be taken not to excessively jostle

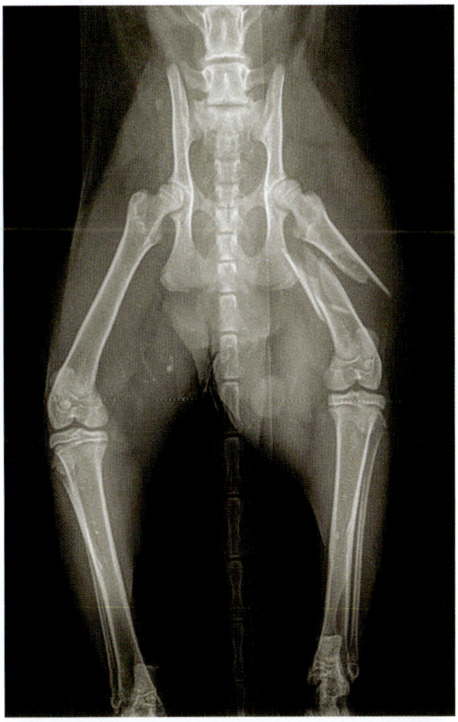

Image 17.14 Oblique fracture. *Source:* Photo courtesy of Simone Conwell, RVT, VTS (ECC).

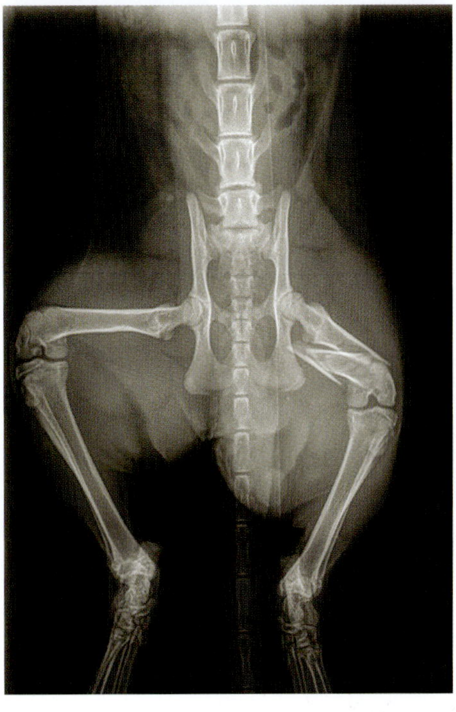

Image 17.15 Comminuted fracture. *Source:* Photo courtesy of Simone Conwell, RVT, VTS (ECC).

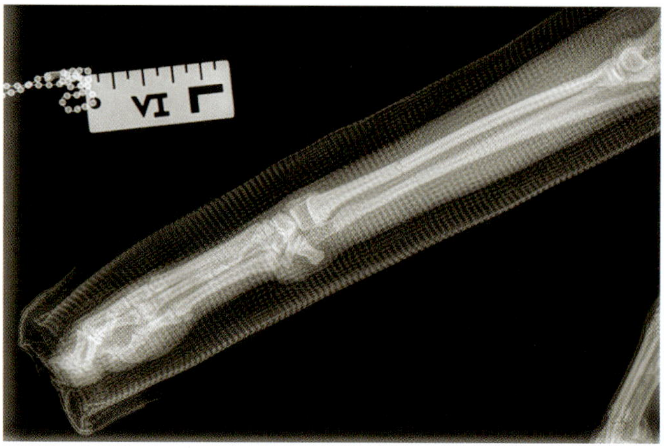

Image 17.16 A transverse fracture after splinting. *Source:* Photo courtesy of Simone Conwell, RVT, VTS (ECC).

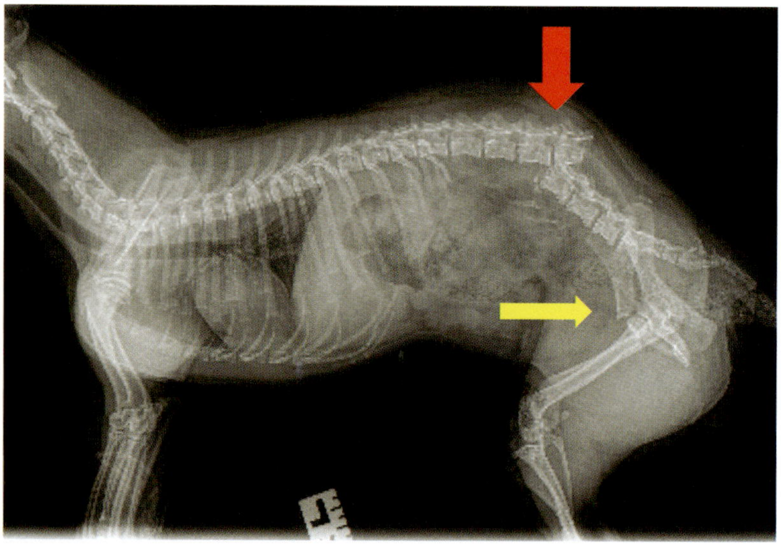

Image 17.17 Radiograph of a fractured spine (red arrow) and possibly the pelvis as well (yellow arrow). The owner elected euthanasia once seeing the spine was broken. *Source:* Photo courtesy of Simone Conwell, RVT, VTS (ECC).

the patient. Ideally, a CT is performed in cases of polytrauma to obtain a full picture with the least discomfort to the patient. Surgery or neurology is needed for a spinal fracture to determine if repair is possible (Image 17.17).

Jaw fractures can be complicated and in need of multiple specialists for evaluation. A jaw fracture may be best treated by a dentist; however, it is difficult to tell what action is needed without dental radiographs or CT imaging. Be sure to inform clients that their pet's jaw fracture may require it to be wired closed, in which case a feeding tube must be placed until adequate healing has occurred. In that case, the client will be provided with a demonstration of how to maintain and use the feeding tube (Image 17.18).

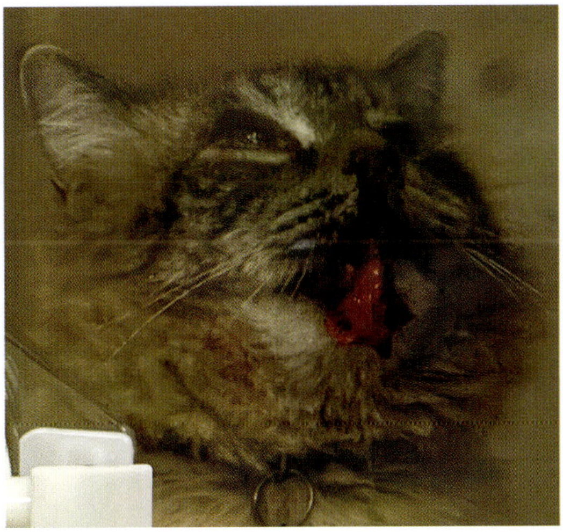

Image 17.18 A cat with a broken jaw. *Source:* Photo courtesy of Simone Conwell, RVT, VTS (ECC).

Trauma is rarely cut and dry. It truly needs emergency and often specialty evaluation as soon as possible. Adequate pain control through appropriate opioid choice, or potentially ultrasound-guided blocks, is necessary to provide adequate relief in the meantime.

Works Cited

Candela Andrade, M.P. (2025). Healing of comminuted fractures of long bones in dogs. *Animals* https://doi.org/10.3390/ani15030413.

Gänsslen, A.L. (2024). Outcomes of acetabular fractures. *Archives of Orthopaedic and Trauma Surgery* https://doi.org/10.1007/s00402-024-05596-9.

Herman, T. C. (2024). Mu receptors. *StatPearls*. Retrieved from www.ncbi.nlm.nih.gov/books/NBK551554

Kumar, R. V. (2025). Buprenorphine. *StatPearls*. Retrieved from www.ncbi.nlm.nih.gov/books/NBK459126

National Research Council (NRC) Committee on Recognition and Alleviation of Pain In Laboratory Animals (2009). *Recognition and Alleviation of Pain in Laboratory Animals*. Washington, DC: National Academies Press Retrieved from www.ncbi.nlm.nih.gov/books/NBK32661.

Shahar, R.S. (1997). A technique for management of bite wounds in teh thoracic wall in small dogs. *Veterinary* .

18

Managing Difficult Financial Discussions in Emergency Care

Ashley Salango

Practice Manager, Charm City Veterinary Hospital, 3011 Woodhome Ave, Baltimore, MD, USA

Even after over a decade as a veterinary professional, it was my own experience as an emergency room (ER) client with my pet that underscored for me that navigating financial discussions is not merely an administrative task; it is an essential aspect of veterinary care that can significantly affect the pet's treatment outcome and the owner's peace of mind. In 2017, when my pet was suffering from an unknown illness, eventually discovered to be acute lymphoblastic leukemia (ALL) of the bone marrow, we reached a point where my bill was nearly $6000. We had already performed one blood transfusion; my CareCredit was at the max, and so was my credit card. Just a mere thirty-six hours after transfusing, my dog's packed cell volume (PCV) had dropped, yet again, to below 10. He was having difficulty breathing, and his body was starting to shut down. We faced two options: to transfuse again and hope for the best or to say goodbye. This was the moment when a very kind ER doctor had a very difficult conversation with me, explaining with compassion that he had less than a 25% chance of living, and if he had what she suspected (ALL), his chance for full recovery was virtually non-existent. She told me with her words and her body language that it was ok (and kind) for me to make the hardest decision of my life. Her effective communication and the care shown during that emotional moment fostered trust, paving the way for the correct decision to be made. My story underscores the fact that when we communicate effectively, we increase compliance and trust, which ultimately improves patient care and/or helps to end animal suffering. We could go down a rabbit hole about how increasing client compliance, minimizing prolonged suffering, and providing better patient care will aid our fight against compassion fatigue, and we would fill an entire book. For now, it is important to note that professionals who work with people or animals, particularly those who are suffering, are prone to secondary traumatic stress, also known as compassion fatigue (Nu 2024). This fatigue stems from our personal feelings and emotional responses to animal suffering. Studies suggest this happens due to exposure to issues such as lack of resources, working conditions like short staffing or micromanagement, lack of patient compliance, and overwhelming guilt from feeling like you could have done more to help (Nu 2024). If not addressed, these feelings of physical and emotional exhaustion, low self-esteem, depression, and reduced personal or work satisfaction can lead to a lack of empathy for yourself and your patients (Scotney 2015). This lack of empathy occurs as a means of protecting oneself from additional secondary trauma (Scotney 2015). Beyond the mental health implications of compassion fatigue, it is also an issue because we simply cannot do our job as veterinary professionals without empathy. This is especially true for cases where difficult financial discussions and treatment options must be presented delicately. We will refer to this skill as "Veterinary Financial Advocacy" moving forward. This section of the text will break down what it means to be a financial advocate in the veterinary space and teach the skills needed to do so, such as empathy, talking with compassion, reading and using nonverbal cues, tools to assist with payments, as well as the ethics of informed consent. Additionally, we will discuss ways we can collaborate across the whole scope of care, from general practice to emergency and even specialty, to ensure that we are advocating for our patients and helping pet parents make informed decisions.

When it comes to having difficult financial discussions, a compassionate and empathetic approach is paramount. It's essential to acknowledge that pet owners often face emotional distress as they confront the health crisis of their beloved companions. Approaching these conversations with empathy and compassion while simultaneously helping to alleviate the burden of guilt or shame (for the pet owner and ourselves as veterinary professionals) is an important skill to master. By validating all the feelings surrounding the treatment plan and expressing genuine concern for a pet's welfare, veterinary professionals can foster a more collaborative atmosphere where the focus remains on finding solutions rather than dwelling on barriers. It is our job to convey treatment plans and financial considerations in an informative yet kind way, and we must be sure to provide all the information because pet parents cannot make decisions properly without it. An intriguing fact, discovered in a small, blind digital study conducted on both pet parents and veterinary professionals, was a direct correlation between owners who felt confident they understood the medical emergency occurring and veterinary professionals who felt that a high percentage of clients did not understand the gravity of the situation (Salango 2025). It is our job, however, to ensure pet parents DO understand the gravity of a given situation, and this survey suggests we can do better at that. This study was conducted via a blind digital survey, open to pet parents and veterinary professionals with two similar, yet individual, sets of questions. The goal was to determine the feelings surrounding emergency care for animals & the areas where training is truly needed to increase patient compliance, staff stress, and owner guilt (Image 18.1).

Image 18.1 shows the pet parents who answered this specific survey question, along with the number of responses in each answer category. Below, you will see the veterinary professionals surveyed. It is easy to see there is a direct correlation between pet owners who felt they understood the gravity of the situation and veterinary professionals who felt those clients did not. The numbers are very close. Simply stated, the data shows we must do better at fostering true understanding of finances, medical outcomes, and treatment options to minimize the risk of lulling clients into a false sense of security. To summarize the data collected, we must do better at ensuring pet owners truly understand (not falsely understand) what is happening with their pets. We need to more comprehensively explain treatment options because many are unsure what treatment, if any, is the best option. When we lull clients into a false sense of security, especially financial security, before an ER transfer or during emergency treatment, we are doing our field a great disservice (Image 18.2).

Why Do General Practitioners Transfer to ER?

The job of ***Veterinary Financial Advocate*** is an important role that is often overlooked in the flow of patient care from intake to discharge or end-of-life care. ***Financial Advocacy*** is the act of guiding owners through financial decisions for optimal patient care, but most importantly, it is a partnership that starts in general practice. General practitioners (GP) and their staff play a pivotal role in the initial assessment and treatment of pets. Transfers to ER are a usual occurrence in these

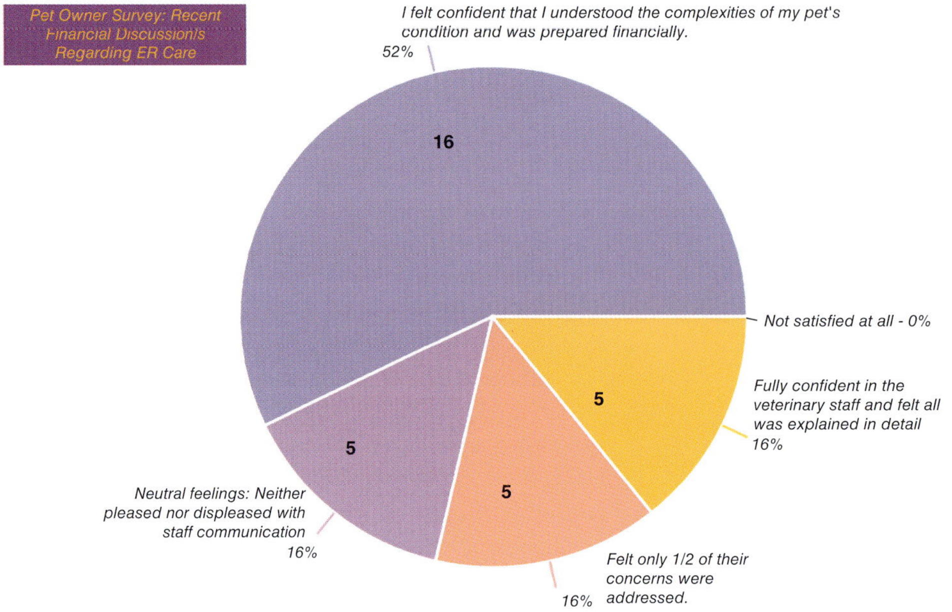

Image 18.1 Pie chart of local survey asking how financially prepared owners felt to handle their pet's illness after conversing with the ER veterinarian. *Source:* Courtesy of Ashley Salango, CVPL.

facilities, as they may not be equipped to handle the complexities of true veterinary emergencies like gastric dilatation-volvulus (GDV), disorders requiring blood product transfusion, or respiratory distress. Most general practices work on an appointment schedule, which does not allow time for the in-depth management and triage of more emergent cases. Moreover, many have set open and close hours, meaning that no staff are on duty overnight. GP clinicians may work solo or with a smaller staff, limiting their ability to coordinate proper urgent multidisciplinary care. These cases may require continued and close monitoring, along with instant action and prolonged attention, all of which do not fit into the standard GP workflow and staffing. Instead, staff at these facilities should be trained on how to stabilize a patient, prepare the owner for transfer, and then transfer the patient to the ER as expeditiously and safely as possible, because this is, in most cases, what is best for the patient. In general veterinary practice, the staff are often not well trained in emergency protocol because they simply do not handle these cases as routinely as emergency workers. They are instead trained in preventive wellness and the long-term management of chronic conditions. In contrast, emergency staff are trained in more specialized care, like life-saving measures, the safe use of life-saving drugs, and the management of more sudden and acute illnesses. Emergency and urgent care facilities are staffed with a larger number of technicians/nurses, assistants, doctors, and even specialists, all working as a unit, who work on a triage basis from the most severe cases to the least severe cases versus running on an appointment schedule. Additionally, most ER facilities have full staff all day, every day, instead of appointment times, thus ensuring continuity and vigilance in patient care that a GP often cannot provide. General practitioners should develop close professional relationships with emergency facilities and specialists close to their office locations. As a combined care team, we must trust one another to continue the care of a patient, with the ER handling the emergency care, the GP handling the transfer and follow-up care, and the specialist providing a more specialized treatment plan or input when necessary. When we coordinate care between facilities, we are better able to provide seamless and proper care. We are greatly benefiting our patients with the formation of this ***symbiotic relationship***.

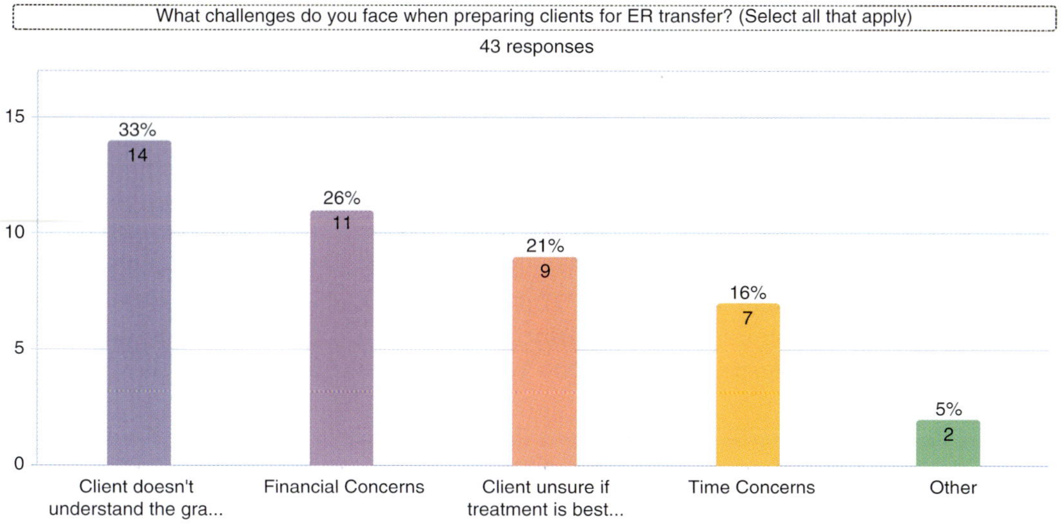

Image 18.2 Bar graph of local survey identifying challenges veterinarians face when trying to transfer sick patients to the ER. *Source:* Courtesy of Ashley Salango, CVPL.

The above-referenced survey garnered some great feedback, such as planting the seed of trust when transferring a patient to an emergency or urgent care facility from GP. This participant noted that the pet's regular veterinary office often has a lengthy relationship with the pet parents, resulting in the establishment of trust, but when the patient is transferred into the ER, this time-built trust disappears (Salango 2025). As the transferring clinicians, it is important to establish a foundation of trust for that client. We must make the client feel that we trust these ER clinicians with our own pets. When transferring patients to emergency care, it is important to start financial discussions before the transfer occurs. Frank discussions about financial considerations and the setting of treatment expectations should be a comprehensive conversation, but sadly, limited time during appointments and the urgency of care often overshadows the conversations that need to happen. General practice staff may also feel unprepared to address financial concerns due to a lack of training, insufficient resources, uncertainty about ER pricing, or personal discomfort; no one likes to talk about money. The survey placed the average confidence of veterinary staff interviewed (from a combination of ER and GP) at a 3/5 (Salango 2025). Essentially, around 60% of the professionals surveyed, some of whom are very experienced and decorated, felt they were well prepared to handle a difficult financial conversation with a pet owner. As such, it becomes critical to create an environment where we learn how to manage these conversations in a way that ensures both the pet and pet owner receive the care they need within a reasonable financial window. We must also be prepared to offer treatment alternatives based on the knowledge that affordability may play just as big of a role, if not bigger for many folks, than choosing the treatment outcome with the best odds. The Human-Animal Bond, while mutually beneficial to both species, can also intensify feelings of guilt. In her article, author Liz Munro states that pet owners will often second-guess their decisions on treatment, which can lead to guilt. The author feels this comes from the deep emotional bond shared with a pet that leads to feelings of remorse and regret. (Munro 2025). It is important, as care providers, that we do our best to help our clients to not feel they could have done more to prevent their pet's suffering while also realizing that feelings like guilt are all a part of the emotional connection they share with thier pet.

Empathetic Communication

The Importance of Empathetic Communication

Empathetic communication goes beyond merely acknowledging a pet owner's financial challenges; it requires actively listening to their concerns and demonstrating understanding. We must learn the difference between *sympathy* and *empathy*. In a 2019 issue of "Today's Veterinary Business," the author states that "expressing sympathy appears to come more naturally to most people, but expressing empathy might be more difficult because it involves being vulnerable and reaching a deeper connection with someone" (Donnelly 2019). ***Empathy*** is the ability to feel and understand another's emotions, while ***sympathy*** is simply a deep concern for those emotions and pain; it lacks the shared perspective of empathy. You see, sympathy is caring and having concern, but empathy takes it a step further by forcing you to see things from a pet owner's perspective. Empathy involves asking open-ended questions that allow pet parents to voice their worries and preferences. These questions give you more insight into how they are feeling so that you can better help them solve problems. The goal is to engage in a dialogue that not only addresses the medical necessities but also integrates the owner's emotional state. By doing this, you will foster mutual respect and cooperation throughout the treatment process. The pet parent will feel seen and understood, which leads to trust, and trust is the foundation of compliance. Recognizing emotions in pet parents and using empathy to guide you during the following conversation is a critical skill to master. The fear of losing a pet can trigger overwhelming anxiety, and this emotional state can paralyze decision-making. Our goal is to prevent decision paralysis by communicating in a manner that replaces fear with understanding. Decision paralysis is when an individual feels unable to make a choice or act due to being overwhelmed by the options, the consequences, or the emotional weight of the situation. In veterinary financial discussions, decision paralysis can arise when pet owners are presented with complex treatment options, high costs, and emotional stress, making it difficult for them to decide on the best course of action for their pet. This state of indecision can delay necessary care and increase anxiety for both the owner and the veterinary team. Veterinary professionals must be adept at identifying certain feelings from the pet owner and responding to them appropriately. By offering words of reassurance, providing information calmly and clearly, being patient, and most importantly, leading with empathy, we can help alleviate fears and empower owners to engage in the decision-making process confidently. The chart below shows how you can change five sympathetic statements into empathetic statements, which will aid you and the pet owner during your next financial discussion.

Sympathetic Statements:	Empathetic Statements:
"I'm so sorry you're going through this."	**"I can see how hard this is for you – you've given your pet so much love. I understand that deciding on your pet's treatment is very difficult and feels unfair. Please let us know if you have any questions. We are here to help!"**
Why not: There's nothing *"wrong"* with this statement. It kindly expresses sorrow, but it just doesn't invite the emotional dialogue or connection we need to foster.	***Why:*** *You are acknowledging the emotional weight the client is carrying and validating their connection to their pet. The* ***Human-Animal Bond*** *is an important thing to recognize and reference. You are also offering help and solutions for the guilt they might be feeling instead of judgment.*

Sympathetic Statements:	Empathetic Statements:
"At least they're not in pain anymore." or "At least they are / /will be no longer suffering."	**"Losing a pet is deeply personal. I know how deep your bond with NAME was. You made the right decision, but I fully understand how difficult that was for you. We are here with you through all of it."**
Why Not: While this statement is intended to show sympathy and comfort a pet parent, you risk minimizing the client's grief and loss.	***Why:*** This statement *shows presence, patience, and emotional attunement rather than just offering platitudes.*
"I'm sorry for the bad news. Let me know if you need anything."	**"It's okay to feel overwhelmed. I'd be feeling the same way in your shoes. I'm sorry you feel this way! We are here to help if there's anything you need ... "**
Why not*: Briefly shares sympathy for whatever event has befallen the pet & owner but doesn't seem as sincere in comparison to the empathic version.*	***Why***: It *shares in the emotional experience rather than just observing it, while offering a more sincere shoulder to cry on &/or ear to listen.*
"The cost is $xyz. I'm sorry, I know it's a big bill. How did you plan to pay today?"	**"The cost of the services today will be $xyz. I know that is a big number and can feel overwhelming. We offer some payment options like Care Credit or Scratch Pay that can help to break it down into smaller & more manageable payments, if you'd like to talk about those."**
Why not*: It lacks empathy and might come off as callous, like all you care about is money. Additionally, it offers no solutions to the potential problem of "How am I going to afford this?!"*	***Why****: It shares the emotional while offering genuine empathy, support, and solutions to an overwhelming financial situation.*

Now that we know and understand what empathetic communication is, we can break down the steps to practicing it. It is important to remember that this is a soft skill that will take time to master, but there's no reason you can't start practicing your craft today.

The Steps of Empathetic Communication

To make this as easy as possible to remember, we will use an engram for EMPATHY. Each step will represent a letter of the word EMPATHY. When you ponder the word and reflect on it, try to memorize, at a minimum, what each letter stands for.

E – *Emotions First*

The first step to empathetic communication is recognizing that every veterinary interaction carries an emotional context. Whether a pet is in for a routine checkup or a critical emergency, clients often arrive with varying degrees of concern. As the veterinarian, receptionist, assistant, or technician, you must remain sensitive to these emotional undercurrents, even when they are not explicitly stated. Practitioners should learn to identify nonverbal cues such as body language, facial expressions, and tone of voice. A nervous glance, hesitant posture, or cracking voice can reveal much about a client's emotional state. Simply observing and acknowledging these signs – without rushing into clinical questions – helps lay the foundation for a compassionate exchange. Use regular language when possible and ditch the fancy medical jargon, because confusing the client will only serve to further frustrate and upset them. Balancing honesty with sensitivity is key. Don't sugarcoat important information, but avoid being overly clinical or detached. Use visual aids or analogies when appropriate, and always check for understanding by asking.

M – *Make it Safe*

Create an emotionally and physically safe space. Warm greetings, a clean and calm environment, and a personal touch, like using the pet's name or correctly identifying pronouns, turn clinical encounters into comforting ones. Safety fosters vulnerability, and vulnerability builds trust. Reciprocity also builds trust. If you expect to feel safe and respected by clients, you must also reciprocate that. Empathy thrives in an environment where clients feel seen, heard, and respected. This begins with physical space: a clean, quiet, and organized clinic with minimal stressors can significantly reduce client anxiety. But beyond the physical setting, the attitude of the staff plays a critical role. Greeting clients warmly, introducing oneself clearly, treating the client with kindness, and using the pet's name show personal investment. Simple phrases like "I hear Chance had an accident today" or "How has Cinder Bear been doing since her ER visit?," both in rooms and on follow-up calls, will immediately personalize the encounter and ensure the client feels like more than a number. This subtle shift from transactional to relational interaction fosters openness and trust.

P – *Practice Active Listening*

Empathy starts with listening, not fixing. Active listening means maintaining eye contact, giving verbal affirmations of understanding, using nonverbal cues of agreement/acknowledgment, and reflecting on what's been said. This shows clients they're heard and understood, not just managed. Avoid interruptions and let clients fully express their concerns. This is one of the most powerful tools in empathetic communication leadership. ***Active listening*** is the practice of fully concentrating on, understanding, and responding thoughtfully to what a person says. This requires more than hearing words; it involves listening for emotional content and underlying concerns.

Techniques to enhance active listening include:

1) **Eye Contact**: Maintaining appropriate eye contact shows attentiveness and care. Avoid staring at the computer screen or doing other activities that make the client feel like you are only half listening. Presence is paramount to successful empathetic communication.
2) **Give Brief Affirmations of Engagement**: Using phrases like "I see" or "please go on" encourages the client to continue speaking, while nonverbal cues like nodding your head in agreement will show you are still engaged in the conversation.
3) **Mirroring (aka Paraphrasing)**: Reflect what the client says back to them by using statements like, "So it sounds like you've been worried about Lucky's appetite over the last week because he hasn't eaten." This shows that you are engaged and validating their experience. Importantly, avoid interrupting unless absolutely necessary. Let the client finish their story before offering advice or explanations. This creates a space where they feel respected and understood.
4) Clarify and summarize. At the end of the conversation, be sure to summarize or clarify any information you want to have correct. For example, you might say, "To clarify, you said that Lucky hasn't been eating well over the last week, but he has eaten a bit of wet food and treats?" This search for clarity shows that you were listening and engaged while the client was speaking.

If you want to practice your active listening skills Positive Psychology website has multiple articles and tools available for free at https://positivepsychology.com/active-listening-techniques (O'Bryan 2022).

A – *Acknowledge Without Judgment*

Validate emotions instead of dismissing or minimizing them. Avoid statements that insinuate the client should stop worrying or is overthinking an event or decision. These statements are both unkind and unhelpful. Instead, try statements that use words of validation to show you care and understand. Avoid words of comparison such as "at least." Non-judgmental acknowledgment creates a connection and helps to reduce client anxiety. One of the most critical, and often most difficult, aspects of empathetic communication is acknowledging emotions without minimizing them, correcting how someone feels, or judging them for it. Veterinary professionals may be tempted to quickly reassure clients or redirect the conversation to clinical matters, and while well-intentioned, this can invalidate the client's emotional reality.

Don't Say Vs/. Do Say:

- Don't say "don't worry, it's no big deal," instead say "It's completely understandable to be worried."
- Don't say "you are overthinking this," instead say "I can see how much you care about her."
- Don't say "at least he isn't suffering anymore," instead say "I'm sure this must be incredibly hard for you."
- Don't say "don't worry, lab work will confirm this is nothing serious," instead say "We will get the lab results back as soon as possible, I understand how worried you are, and I know waiting is stressful" their unique relationship with their pet.

T – *Transparency*

Transparency is a cornerstone of compassionate communication in veterinary medicine. When veterinary professionals are open and honest about diagnoses, treatment options, risks, and costs, it builds trust and empowers clients to make informed decisions for their pets. Transparency doesn't mean delivering information without care – it means presenting the facts clearly while also acknowledging the emotional weight clients may carry. When clients feel they are being told the full story with empathy, they are more likely to feel respected, supported, and confident in the care their pet receives.

H – *Help by Providing Treatment Alternatives*

Offering a range of treatment alternatives, from surgery to symptomatic care, is a vital part of compassionate and inclusive veterinary medicine. By presenting multiple options, clinicians help ensure that pet owners can make decisions that align not only with their medical goals but also with their financial realities. This approach acknowledges that quality care is not one-size-fits-all and that clients deserve to feel empowered, not judged, when making difficult choices. Discussing both gold-standard and more conservative treatments fosters trust, reduces guilt, and often leads to better client compliance and follow-through, ultimately improving outcomes for pets across a variety of situations.

You Are Partners

Empathy in vet med also means recognizing that clients are essential partners in the animal's care. We are partners in care. Invite them into the decision-making process rather than dictating what should be done. Offer options when appropriate and explain the benefits and drawbacks of each in a balanced way. For instance: "We have a couple of approaches we could take. One is more aggressive, involving hospitalization and testing, while the other is more supportive at home. I can walk you through both and help you decide what feels right for you and \[pet's name]." This collaborative approach not only empowers the client but also honors their unique relationship with their pet and their values and constraints, whether emotional, financial, or otherwise.

Be present, especially during difficult conversations like euthanasia or terminal diagnoses. Sit down. Use silence. Actively Listen. Don't interrupt. Foster trust and show compassion. Most importantly, make the client feel safe and understood. Allow space for grief. Balance professionalism with humanity. Follow up afterward with resources or just a check-in. These are all little ways you can let clients know you are their partner in a journey that might sometimes be difficult.

Recognizing and Responding to Emotions

In addition to learning the right things to say, a good ***Veterinary Financial Advocate*** also needs to be able to recognize and respond to emotional cues, which may sometimes be nonverbal. Nonverbal cues in communication refer to the way people express their feelings, reactions, or attitudes without using words. This includes body language, facial expressions, eye contact, gestures, posture, tone of voice, and even silence. In the context of veterinary care, nonverbal cues might manifest as a pet owner's anxious fidgeting, downcast eyes, hesitant movements, or a trembling voice. Recognizing these subtle signals allows veterinary professionals to better understand a client's emotional state, respond with greater empathy, and provide support beyond what is explicitly said. Being attentive to nonverbal cues is essential for sensitive topics to be communicated efficiently. Veterinary staff are often present during the most emotionally charged moments of a pet owner's life, and being able to recognize and respond to, sometimes subtle, emotional cues, is vital to providing compassionate & empathetic care. Pet owners can experience a range of emotions in the clinic, and subtle signals often reveal more than words. For example, anxiety or hesitation may be presented as avoiding eye contact, restless movements, or delayed responses. This typically indicates that the person feels overwhelmed or fearful about upcoming decisions. Instead of rushing through explanations, you should slow down, speak gently, and ask thoughtful questions like "Does anything feel confusing or hard to process right now?" This shows understanding, encourages the pet owner to talk openly about the things they don't understand, and creates a safe space for them. Guilt is another emotion that surfaces frequently, especially if owners feel they missed warning signs or have regret for not coming into the hospital sooner. You might notice repeated apologies or self-critical comments such as "I should've seen this sooner." In these moments, it's crucial to affirm their care and intentions without judgment. A simple statement like "It's clear you've done everything out of love" can offer reassurance and begin to ease that guilt. The ***Human-Animal Bond***, while mutually beneficial to both species, can also intensify feelings of guilt. In an article for the Munro (2025), the author states that pet owners will often second-guess their decision for pet care and treatment, which can lead to guilt. The author feels this comes from the deep emotional bond shared with a pet. It is important, as care providers, that we ensure our clients do not feel they could have done more to prevent their pet's suffering (PetDeparted). Grief can be harder to detect because it often manifests in silence, withdrawal, or difficulty speaking. Whether it's anticipatory grief or the pain of losing a companion animal, veterinary staff must resist the urge to fill the silence with platitudes. Presence matters more than words. Allowing space, offering tissues, and responding with something heartfelt like "I'm here with you, and I'm so sorry you're going through this" shows meaningful support and creates an atmosphere of emotional safety. Frustration can be misinterpreted as rudeness or hostility when, in fact, it often stems from fear, helplessness, or miscommunication. Abrupt speech or defensive body language may signal that the client is overwhelmed. The key here is not to react with defensiveness, but with curiosity and empathy. A response like "I can see this has been a tough process – let's work through it together" can de-escalate tension and redirect the interaction toward resolution. The most important thing to do is to avoid using a harsh tone yourself. Instead of trying to match the pet owner's tone, try to use a calmer one to cool down the situation. Usually, when a pet owner reaches this heightened state of emotion, the anger/frustration is not directed at you. Using empathy, place yourself in the pet owner's shoes, and ask yourself, how would you feel? Then, proceed in a manner that you would want for yourself. Recognizing these emotional cues is more than just good bedside manners. It's the foundation of trust and ultimately, the foundation of a successful client relationship. When veterinary staff respond with empathy, they reduce emotional barriers and foster collaboration in clinical decisions. Dismissing or glossing over emotions with generic comfort phrases and emotional ignorance or avoidance can make owners feel unseen and misunderstood. By demonstrating care, patience, and empathy, professionals can make the veterinary experience supportive rather than purely clinical.

Discussing Treatment Alternatives Based on Financial Considerations

Veterinary professionals also need to prioritize transparency when discussing treatment alternatives that consider financial considerations and treatment outcomes. It's essential to clearly outline all available options, including the potential conclusion/s, the costs, and the consequence/s of each choice. This not only helps pet owners feel informed but also encourages them to participate actively in their pet's care decisions. By presenting a range of options, we empower owners to choose solutions that best align with their financial capabilities, ensuring that they feel supported rather than pressured. Additionally, presenting alternatives like outpatient monitoring, referral to a specialty center, or teleconsultation with emergency clinicians (when case appropriate) allows for flexibility based on the animal's condition, the owner's financial resources, and other logistical barriers and constraints. When the case allows, a pet owner should be presented with an array of options, starting with the most ideal method to treat an ailment, which will likely also be the most expensive, moving down to options for outpatient and symptomatic care. This approach also helps reduce overcrowding in emergency rooms by diverting non-critical cases to more appropriate care pathways (BluePearl 2024). For example, if a patient were suffering from a simple (closed) fracture to a metacarpal bone in the foot, you might first offer transfer to orthopedics with a possible surgery, but if that was outside of the owner's price range, you might offer external coaptation with laser treatments or physical therapy after healing. If neither is doable financially, conservative monitoring and symptomatic treatment might be the best option for this owner's finances. It is important at each step of the way to mention the consequences and suspected outcomes of each treatment plan. Ultimately, thoughtful transfer planning and the presentation of different treatment options covering a wide array of financial responsibility, along with the coordination of care between ER, GP, and specialty providers, ensure that animals receive timely, compassionate, and effective care while minimizing stress for both the pet and the owner. It reflects a collaborative, patient-centered model that prioritizes continuity and clinical excellence.

Practicing Informed Consent in Veterinary Medicine

Informed consent is a concept commonly associated with human medicine, but it is equally vital in veterinary practice. In veterinary medicine, ***informed consent*** is the process through which we ensure pet owners are fully educated about the recommended treatments, procedures, risks, benefits, costs, and potential alternatives for their pet(s). This means providing clear, comprehensive information in a way that clients can easily understand, so they are empowered to make voluntary and knowledgeable decisions about their pet's care. We can practice informed consent by providing detailed, written estimates before beginning treatment, which allows clients to make fully informed decisions. These estimates should clearly indicate which costs are fixed and which may vary depending on the pet's response to treatment. This is often called a high/low estimate, where one column is shown for a high price and a low price. When treatments may extend beyond initial estimates, establishing financial checkpoints is essential. Rather than presenting clients with unexpectedly large bills after the fact, commit to contacting them when costs approach a predetermined threshold. This practice demonstrates respect for the client's financial boundaries and prevents the erosion of trust that occurs when bills significantly exceed expectations. A quick read through reviews of veterinary hospitals on Google or Yelp, especially emergency facilities, will reveal that unexpected costs are the primary source of dissatisfaction among pet owners. More concerning, in the survey I conducted, I found that some were hesitant to seek emergency care in the future due to their most recent experience with higher-than-expected invoices (Salango 2025). By prioritizing financial transparency, veterinary teams can prevent these negative outcomes. This should start in general practice, before the transfer, where the GP team sets realistic expectations for how much an emergency visit might cost. Informed consent also means ensuring clients understand what they're paying for. Technical language and medical jargon can obscure the value of recommended procedures. It is important to show now just the cost but also explain the value. Taking a bit of extra time to explain why specific tests or treatments are being recommended, along with what information or improvement they're expected to provide, can help clients see costs in the context of care versus cost. For example, rather than simply listing "CBC/Chemistry Panel – $180" on an estimate, you should explain why it is important. Try saying something such as "this comprehensive blood test will tell us how Bella's organs are functioning and whether or not she is suffering from an infection or if we should look a bit deeper." When you help clients understand the value of their investment and practice informed consent, you give them the ***autonomy*** to make decisions based on more than just financial considerations.

Tools to Assist Clients With Finances

We have already established that when a beloved family pet faces a medical emergency, the emotional toll can be overwhelming, but the financial burden can make an already stressful situation vastly more difficult. Emergency veterinary care often comes with high, unexpected costs that many pet owners are unprepared to handle. Fortunately, there are a variety of financial resources available to help cover urgent veterinary expenses, ranging from specialized healthcare credit cards and loans like CareCredit and Scratchpay to pet insurance, nonprofit grants, and crowdfunding. Some emergency hospitals have even started accepting Affirm for payments. Understanding these options in advance can make all the difference when time is critical and decisions must be made quickly. The guide below explores the most accessible and effective financial tools for managing the cost of emergency veterinary care, helping you plan and act confidently in a crisis. One of the most practical ways we, as the veterinary team, can support clients through financial challenges is by familiarizing them with available payment options and financial resources. Having these conversations before treatment begins allows clients to make informed decisions and may prevent the heartbreaking choice between financial stability and pet care. Third-party payment plans like CareCredit and Scratch Pay have become increasingly important in veterinary medicine. These services offer clients the ability to spread payments over time, often with deferred interest for qualifying applicants. Veterinary teams should understand the basics of these programs. Application processes and approval requirements, current promotional terms and interest rates, minimum and maximum financing amounts, and how quickly funds become available will differ based on the financing service used. By having a dedicated team member who can assist with applications to these services during emergencies, it can significantly reduce stress for clients and increase the likelihood of treatment approval. It is best to start this conversation before the emergency transfer from general practice, if there is one. Pet insurance represents another valuable tool, though its benefits are primarily preventative rather than reactive. Most pet insurance companies work on a reimbursement policy where the client must first pay, submit an invoice, and then be reimbursed. However, newer services like PumpkinNow and the Trupanion Portal now allow for more immediate approval and payment of claims while at the veterinary facility, though it should be noted that not all clinics have these options. Insurance is most beneficial when the pet it enrolled at the very first visit with the vet, before any ***"preexisting conditions"*** can develop. Discussing insurance options during emergency visits can help prepare clients for future veterinary expenses. Most general practices now provide information about various insurance options, helping clients make educated choices about coverage. Emergency assistance programs like PAWP offer another approach to managing unexpected veterinary costs. These membership-based services provide emergency funds for qualifying veterinary emergencies, typically with annual limits. Understanding which programs serve your area, their coverage limitations, and how quickly they can provide payment authorization helps teams present these options effectively. For clients facing severe financial constraints, knowledge of charitable resources can be lifesaving for their pets. Many communities have foundations that provide financial assistance for veterinary care, though these typically have specific qualification requirements and limited funds. Maintaining an updated list of local resources, including contact information, application processes, and typical response times, allows teams to quickly connect clients with potential support.

Effective Staff Training and Role Playing

Finally, it is imperative to train veterinary staff on how to handle financial discussions effectively. Engaging in role-playing scenarios can prepare staff for real-life conversations, equipping them with the skills needed to approach these discussions with confidence and empathy. A well-trained team fosters a supportive environment where financial discussions can take place without stigma, reinforcing commitment to both pet welfare and client needs. Navigating financial conversations in veterinary care is a delicate task that requires empathy, effective communication, and a commitment to transparency. By equipping staff with the right tools and training, veterinary practices can enhance the trust and support provided to pet owners, ultimately improving compliance and patient care. Moving forward, we must recognize that these conversations are not just about money; they are about the well-being of our patients and the livelihoods of their owners – an interconnected relationship that deserves our utmost attention and care.

Effective financial communication isn't an innate skill; it requires training, practice, and ongoing refinement. Investing in staff development around financial discussions yields significant returns in client satisfaction, treatment compliance, and team confidence. Exercises like worksheets to learn better active listening skills, team meetings, and role-playing are all very effective ways to develop and hone your skills. For this section, we will focus only on role-playing exercises that will develop financial communication skills. By simulating challenging financial conversations in a safe environment, team members can practice responding to various client reactions and refine their approach.

These exercises are most effective when they include realistic scenarios based on actual client interactions, rotate team members through different roles, address both verbal and nonverbal communication, and provide specific, yet constructive feedback after each scenario. Developing standardized language for common financial discussions helps ensure consistency across the team. This doesn't mean creating rigid script-authentic communication requires flexibility but rather establishing key phrases and approaches that reflect the practice's values. For example, teams might develop standard language for introducing a treatment estimate, explaining payment policies, discussing financial assistance options, or responding to clients who express an inability to pay. These standardized approaches should be regularly reviewed and refined based on client feedback and team experience. Cross-training team members on financial discussions ensure that clients receive consistent information regardless of who they speak with, from the desk to the nursing staff. While certain team members may take primary responsibility for detailed financial conversations, everyone should be able to address basic questions about costs, payment options, and financial policies. These policies will differ in each hospital, based on workflow and financial options offered. For example, Hospital A might offer in-house payment plans only, while Hospital B might offer CareCredit, Scratch Pay, and the Trupanion Payment Portal. Placing someone in charge of these training sessions, as the lead veterinary financial advocate, will be paramount to the success of these sessions. Choose a leader who can provide constructive feedback kindly and will keep your role-playing sessions on track. It is recommended to review financial offerings at your facility at least once per business quarter, as financing rates and promotional periods might change.

Summary

In this chapter, we have taken a deep dive into one of the most challenging yet essential soft skills of veterinary medicine: having compassionate, clear, and effective financial conversations in emergency care situations. These moments often occur when pet owners are overwhelmed, frightened, and emotionally vulnerable. As veterinary professionals, our ability to approach these conversations with empathy and confidence can significantly influence the pet's outcome, the owner's peace of mind, and the overall client experience.

We began with my personal story, one that many professionals will relate to on some level. Despite my professional background, I still felt the weight of uncertainty, financial strain, and emotional paralysis that so many clients endure. It was a kind and compassionate ER doctor who helped me make the most humane choice through empathetic communication. This experience set the stage for a broader conversation about how financial discussions are not just operational tasks, but instead, they are deeply human exchanges that must be handled with care and intentionality.

The chapter introduced the concept of veterinary financial advocacy, redefining financial discussions as an opportunity for partnership between the veterinary team and the pet owner. Advocacy is more than just quoting prices; it involves explaining medical options clearly, providing emotional support, and empowering pet owners to make informed decisions based on both clinical facts and personal realities. These conversations require not just medical knowledge, but also emotional intelligence, communication skills, and a commitment to transparency.

One of the key tools offered in this chapter is the EMPATHY framework, which breaks down empathetic communication into manageable, actionable steps of emotions first, making it safe, practicing active listening, acknowledging without judgment, transparency, helping with options, and a reminder that you are partners (yourself and the client).

We also examined the impact of compassion fatigue on veterinary professionals and how poor communication, especially around emotionally charged financial issues, can increase burnout.

When we fail to create space for open, empathetic conversations, we not only risk harming client relationships but also our own mental well-being. Emotional exhaustion, decision fatigue, and reduced empathy are common symptoms in our field, but by developing better communication habits, we can protect ourselves and our teams while better serving our patients.

A major theme of this chapter is clinical collaboration. General practitioners play a pivotal role in preparing clients for emergency care, and this includes initiating financial conversations early, setting realistic expectations, and building trust in the ER teams to whom they refer. When general practice, emergency, and specialty providers work as a united front, sharing information, aligning expectations, and prioritizing informed consent, our patients will benefit from a more seamless and consistent care.

We also touched on the importance of informed consent and financial transparency. This includes providing accurate estimates, explaining the value behind each service, and ensuring clients are fully aware of their options and responsibilities. The goal is to minimize surprises and support decision-making, not just from a financial standpoint, but from a position of mutual respect and understanding.

To support clients, the chapter highlighted various financial tools and resources such as CareCredit, ScratchPay, pet insurance, charitable organizations, in-clinic financing, and emergency aid programs. Knowing what options are available and taking the time to explain them can ease the burden clients feel and help ensure pets receive timely care. Equally important is staff training. Through regular team meetings, role-playing, and the development of consistent communication strategies, teams can build the confidence needed to navigate even the most difficult financial conversations.

In closing, this chapter reminds us that veterinary care doesn't end with diagnosis and treatment; rather, it includes the way we deliver information, support decision-making, and show up for our clients during their most difficult moments. When we approach financial discussions with empathy, honesty, and advocacy, we create a space where trust can flourish and where pet owners feel supported, not shamed. This emotional connection leads to better outcomes, improved compliance, and more meaningful relationships with our clients. More importantly, it reminds us why we chose this profession in the first place: not just to heal animals, but to support the people who love them.

Terms Created and/or Used for Text

***Veterinary Financial Advocacy*:** The skill of advocating for your patient's treatment, as it relates to financial discussions with pet owners, empathy with professionalism respect and in a manner that increases treatment compliance.

***Veterinary Financial Advocate*:** The actual role of being a Veterinary Financial Advocate.

***Symbiotic Relationship*:** As it pertains to the relationship between different health care providers, such as general practitioners with ER physicians or ER physicians with veterinary specialists – is a relationship built on respect, communication collaboration and a shared respect for the goal of providing excellent patient care. This relationship is rooted in mutualism, where all involved are equally benefited by the relationship, including the patient and client.

***Empathy*:** The ability to feel and understand another person's emotions. Unlike sympathy, empathy requires you to place yourself in the position of the one hurting and have a deeper connection to those feelings.

***Sympathy*:** A feeling of deep concern for someone, as it pertains to emotional events like death. It is not the same as empathy.

Active Listening: The practice of fully concentrating on, understanding, and responding thoughtfully to what a person says without interrupting.

Human–Animal Bond: The bond shared between pet owner and pet parent, that is built around the physical, physiological and environmental interactions between the two. Studies suggest this bond can increase the human life span lower blood pressure, and aid in improved mental states.

Preexisting Condition: A condition, determined by insurance claims adjustors, to have been present before an insurance policy was effective. An example would be a pet who received a tibial plateau leveling osteotomy (TPLO) before insurance enrollment, who needs another leg surgery on the same extremity. It is unlikely insurance will cover this.

Informed Consent: The process through which we ensure pet owners are fully educated about the recommended treatments, procedures, risks benefits costs and potential alternatives for their pet(s). This means providing clear comprehensive information in a way that clients can easily understand, so they are empowered to make voluntary and knowledgeable decisions. Informed consent respects the autonomy of the client, promotes trust, and supports ethical medical practice by making sure all choices are made with a full understanding of possible risk, and/or outcomes both good and bad.

Autonomy: The ability and right of an individual to make their own informed choices and decisions, free from external control or coercion. In the context of veterinary care, risks autonomy refers to empowering pet owners to decide on treatments for their animals based on a full understanding of the options and benefits, thereby respecting their values and preferences.

Works Cited

Amanda L. Donnelly, D. M. (2019, October). The value of empathy. *Today's Veterinary Business*. Retrieved from https://todaysveterinarybusiness.com/the-value-of-empathy/

Amanda O'Bryan, P. (2022, February 8). Three Worksheets to Practice Active Listening. Retrieved from Positive Psychology: https://positivepsychology.com/active-listening-techniques/#3-worksheets-to-practice-active-listening

BluePearl Veterinary Hospitals. (2024, September 4). Emergency Veterinarians: How Can They Help Your Pet? Retrieved from BluePearl Veterinary: https://bluepearlvet.com/pet-blog/emergency-veterinarians/

Munro, L. (2025). Understanding pet owner Guilt: How Vets Can Help Clients Overcome Self-Blame After Euthanasia. Roundwood Pet Hospice. (Accessed 20 March 2025).

Nu Noe, M.T. (2024). Measurement of compassion fatigue in animal health care professionals: a systemic review of available instruments and their content validity. *Frontiers in Veterinary Science* https://doi.org/10.3389/fvets.2024.1425741.

Salango, A. (2025). Thoughts and concerns of pet owners vs veterinary professionals surrounding emergency care and financial concerns. unpublished.

Scotney, R.M. (2015). A systematic review of the effects of euthanasia and occupation stress in personnel working with animals in animal shelters, veterinary clinics, and biomedical research facilities. *Journal of the American Veterinary Medical Association* https://doi.org/10.2460/javma.247.10.1121.

19

Tail-End Tactics

Talia Sundstrom

Regional Manager for Vetcor, 647 Pine Forest Dr, Brandon, FL, USA

Mission, Vision, and Values – How Can Hospital Leaders Set Their Teams Up for Success?

When faced with difficult decision-making every day, as veterinary professionals are (see the chapter on compassion fatigue), having a code of ethics to fall back on in veterinary medicine is as simple as "do no harm." Why, then, do vet med teams find themselves stuck in yet another toxic team or tolerating yet another berating clinic and feel bogged down with the weight of so many negative, mucky personal interactions? The culture of the clinic can be as imperative as having talented, knowledgeable medical team members to the clinic's success in patient outcomes. Briefly, I'll discuss the foundations of the clinic culture and how applying those concepts to everyday interactions can set the framework for a cohesive team whose biggest problem is what size intravenous catheter they can get into a hypovolemic chihuahua. I'll even throw in some templates to set clinic leadership up with the tools to create or refresh their own Mission, Vision, and Values (MVV).

Mission

A **Mission** Statement defines, broadly, what you do every day. It is the what, who, why, and how of your organization. The statement should be simple, brief, informative, and direct. Any employee who commits to it and any client who reads it should feel that they understand the statement. Let's look at some examples of well-known companies. The social media platform for networking, LinkedIn, has a mission statement reading "to connect the world's professionals to make them more productive and successful." It's easy to determine that the hope is that workers will use the site to professionally network from that statement. Google's mission is to organize the world's information and make it universally accessible and useful. Given what the phrase "Google it" means to most of us, it seems that they are fulfilling their mission. A global research and management consulting company, Gallup (2023), measures job satisfaction using 12 clearly defined factors and surveyed 64 million people to that end. One factor is whether the organization's mission makes the individual feel their job is important. This highlights how a clear, meaningful mission serves as a powerful tool to improve clinic culture. In veterinary medicine, where burnout and compassion fatigue are common, a well-communicated mission can remind team members that their work truly matters, giving purpose to even the most routine tasks (Gallup 2023). Are you doing yet another "allergies spiel," or are you bringing relief to a pet from constant discomfort? Beyond having a snapshot statement to tell people what your team does, you should also take the time to determine 3–5 core values that define how you will go about reaching that mission. A mission without values can lead to a disjointed team where the goal is clear, but the way to get there is not. Values help guide behavior, and agreeing to values as a team is a major step in building trust and employee satisfaction.

Values

Values set the tone for how a business will operate and act as a guide for decisions. "How does one act when no one is looking?" The values can be single words like "Teamwork," "Partnership," "Integrity," or "Empathy." They may even be short phrases. Vetcor (2025), a national veterinary services company, lists five core values that guide culture and communication at the company: Do the Right Thing, Provide Compassionate Care, Build Community, Pursue Learning and Growth, and Take Pride in Our Work (Vetcor 2025). These values are clear and actionable. The values shape hiring decisions, team coaching, and even client interactions. It can also help leadership hold team members accountable when their behavior does not match the team's values. For the hospital team, "Do the right thing" might mean choosing integrity, even when it might mean more work or incurring cost to the clinic. If a client declines diagnostics but the team is concerned about the pet having a leptospirosis infection, the doctor may insist on doing a patient-side lepto test at no cost to the client to protect other patients and staff from a possible zoonotic disease. "Doing the right thing" in this case would mean prioritizing safety over revenue in the moment. When clearly defined and consistently reinforced, your hospital's mission, vision, and values become more than a team-building event that is discussed once and then never mentioned again. They become a decision-making framework for every member of the team. The last piece of the culture puzzle is a vision statement; a shared goal of what your clinic wants to be in the future.

Vision

Your mission gives your team a purpose, your values offer a code of conduct, and your vision provides something to strive for. It defines the future state of your clinic. The vision is not just what you want to achieve, but who you want to become as a team. Without a clear vision, even the most well-intentioned teams can feel stuck in the daily grind. Vision brings meaning to progress and creates space for growth, innovation, and long-term alignment. Living out your mission, values, and vision takes intention and time. While the initial creation should be planned and guided by leadership, the strongest cultural alignment happens when the entire team has a voice in what makes the final cut. When everyone feels connected to the vision, communication becomes more intentional, and every interaction becomes part of something bigger. That shared framework empowers even those without a formal leadership title to make aligned, confident choices. *See guides and templates in the appendix for creating your team's mission, values, and vision statements.*

It's Important to Note

Mission, vision, and values only serve their purpose when they're consistently demonstrated by leadership. When these statements are introduced during onboarding and never referenced again, or if leadership actively contradicts them, they become empty words. This kind of disconnect actively erodes trust and contributes to disengagement. Team members may stop speaking up, stop trying to improve things, or stop believing in the culture altogether. Values must be more than framed statements. They must be modeled, reinforced, and protected by the people in charge. When mission, vision, and values are treated as mere posters, employee engagement disappears, and that isn't just bad culture; it's financially costly (Dennison 2024). Globally, disengaged employees are reported to cost $8.8 trillion annually in lost productivity (Pendell 2023). More importantly, in vet med, these losses reflect not only higher absenteeism but also poor patient care, mistakes, turnover, and burnout. One subtle but damaging form of culture misalignment is toxic positivity. This presents as pressure to appear upbeat even when real problems are being ignored. When leadership insists on keeping things positive instead of addressing issues when they arise, trust in leadership erodes. Team members learn not to speak up, not to challenge, and not to expect change. In clinics where mission, vision, and values are treated as such, toxic positivity becomes a cover for disengagement, not a cure. Real alignment requires honesty, accountability, and follow-through.

So how do you influence behavior, culture, and outcomes when you're not the one writing the schedule or giving performance reviews? The answer lies in mastering the art of **Influencing Without Authority** (Grenny 2022), a communication skill that empowers every team member, from kennel assistant to lead veterinarian, to help shape the clinic's culture. Even without a formal title, individual contributors can lean on this shared framework to make aligned, confident decisions. Communication becomes more intentional, and culture is shaped through everyday actions, not just management directives.

Influencing Without Authority

What if that framework doesn't exist or isn't clear? For those working in clinics where the mission is vague, the values are inconsistent, or the vision is never mentioned, communication and collaboration become more difficult. In these environments, influence often feels like an uphill battle. It may be that non-managerial team members are fearful of making decisions. Without a shared direction or cultural alignment, even well-intentioned efforts can be misread or dismissed. This is where the ability to influence without authority becomes critical. How can individual contributors conduct themselves and influence others if they don't have a say on their clinic's MVV? In veterinary medicine, formal titles don't always reflect where real leadership happens. You might be a client service representative who recognizes a patient in crisis, a technician trying to delegate mid-code, or a kennel assistant noticing a pattern no one else has seen for a pet in your care. These moments call for influence, not authority. Influencing without authority means guiding others toward a shared goal, even when you don't have a supervisory title or letters after your name. It's the art of being heard, respected, and followed because of *how* you show up, not just who you are on paper. According to Harvard Business School (2021), this kind of influence hinges on trust and relationship-building rather than on job titles or hierarchy.

The term "Influencer" has a new meaning in recent years, as anyone with a social media account can attest. Historically, influence is a way for folks who do not have authority to assert themselves without the benefit of formal power. In vet med, the skill of influencing is the same, but the goal is typically related to improved pet care or hospital culture as opposed to selling the latest trendy [insert trendy item]. Even if you have the title of authority, you may meet with pushback that detracts, reduces efficiency, causes bad feelings, and may lead to poor patient outcomes. Influencing others without authority is a time and effort investment.

Build Trust

The first aspect of influence, whether you are selling the latest trend or trying to persuade a veterinary assistant to practice a new skill, is trust (Harvard 2021). In vet med, trust between team members means that they believe that there is a shared sense of purpose that transcends job titles. It means that team members feel safe to share when mistakes occur and improve team performance. When trust is absent, communication breaks down, which can lead to poor patient outcomes, tension, and client dissatisfaction. Luckily, there's no grand gesture required for this step. Reasonably, if you are consistent in your actions, if you dependably do what you say you will and are reliable under pressure, you will gain the trust of your team. There may be days when earning trust seems slow or thankless, but over time, the simple act of doing what you say you're going to do creates the kind of professional credibility that can move an entire team forward.

Find Your Allies

It's important to note, when working on building your influence, that no one changes clinic culture alone. Whether you're a new technician promoting more structured rounds or a client service representative advocating for clearer communication with clients, your message will go farther if you engage the unofficial leaders first. Think about your work environment and imagine a scenario in which a new initiative is being announced. Can you picture everyone in the room turning to look at one or two people to see how they are reacting? The truth is that every team has opinion leaders. Those team members who don't necessarily hold a formal title, but who shape how others behave or feel. Observe who others watch, listen to, or follow during tough moments, and bring those individuals into the fold early. Seek their input for changes, invite them to your planning meetings, and truly listen to what they might say. They usually have the team's trust for a reason. Hopefully, you'll find that change spreads faster when it's co-owned.

Set Common Goals and Define Non-Negotiables

Realistically, even when your opinion leaders are bought in, and you've got a good foundation of trust, it does not mean that everyone will simply fall in line when decisions are being made (Heinke 2012). Influence doesn't always mean agreement; it means alignment. Even when opinions differ, progress happens when the team can rally around shared goals (Heinke 2012). Healthy teams can share differing opinions and still feel like their opinions matter and will be taken into consideration. In vet med, the ultimate common ground is patient care. When conversations center on what's best for the pet, not what's easiest or most familiar, it reframes resistance into collaboration. You just need to be clear about what can and can't be bent. Recently at my clinic, a newer-to-our-clinic technician was frustrated that the morning rounds were rushed and chaotic, often skipping updates on hospitalized patients. When she suggested formalizing rounds at 7:45 a.m. sharp, a few team members pushed back. Many didn't want to arrive and clock in earlier. Instead of arguing the details, she reframed the conversation: "Our goal is to make sure every patient gets consistent care, and no detail gets missed. The actual time of day doesn't matter. We need to agree that communication about hospitalized patients is non-negotiable." Once the focus shifted to the shared goal of patient safety, the team was more receptive. They landed on a compromise: 8:00 rounds with a rotating lead who prepared notes ahead of time. It wasn't about that technician being right and the others being wrong; it was about aligning what mattered most. That kind of alignment only happens when individuals are willing to release the need to be right, to get credit, or to have things done their way. That's where letting go of ego comes in.

Let Go of Ego

Some may find this tough to balancc, cspccially when you're trying to prove your knowledge, your value, or your place on the team. We know how much education and experience matter in vet med. But the purpose of having influence without authority is not about being right; it's about being effective. Leadership in action often means choosing progress over pride. Letting go of ego allows you to listen more fully, adjust without defensiveness, and keep the clinic's mission front and center. It's not about who gets credit for a new workflow or who came up with a patient care idea. What matters is whether the patient benefits, the team feels supported, and the culture becomes more cohesive. Ironically, the less you push for power, the more willing others are to follow your lead.

Possible Hurdles

Of course, it's not just about letting go of your own ego. Sometimes the real challenge is working alongside someone who hasn't let go of theirs. You might encounter a team member who clings to control, resists feedback, or refuses to compromise. If you're not in a position to formally hold them accountable, it can feel frustrating or even demoralizing. In these moments, it helps to remember you can't force alignment, but you can model it. Influence is about showing up consistently, not matching resistance with resistance. Over time, your example may soften that person's stance or, at the very least, reinforce trust with the rest of the team. Influence doesn't always change the loudest voice in the room, but it often empowers others who are quietly looking for someone to follow. If your clinic's mission, vision, and values are more than just lip service, ideally, those in leadership positions will step in to course correct when individual behavior threatens team cohesion. Culture is protected by accountability.

In the end, communication is both the problem and the solution to everything we experience on vet med teams. It's what connects purpose to practice, intention to impact, and people to each other. Whether your clinic has a well-defined culture or you're still trying to create one, every team member has the ability to influence the way things feel, flow, and function. Titles are helpful, but they're not required. Trust, alignment, shared goals, and humility are tools anyone can use. At the end of the day, the goal isn't to win an argument, prove a point, or protect a title. The goal is to deliver the best possible care to every patient, every time.

Appendix

*Here are **generic templates** for crafting a **Mission Statement**, **Vision Statement**, and **Core Values** for veterinary teams. These are designed to be **filled out by team members** during a meeting or workshop or completed by leadership with team input.*

MISSION STATEMENT TEMPLATE

(Why we exist – our purpose)

Prompt: What is the essential purpose of our veterinary team? Whom do we serve, and what impact do we strive to make every day?

Template:

At [Practice Name], our mission is to ______________________________

______________________________.

We provide ______________________ to ______________________,

with a focus on ____________________________ and ____________________________.

Example fill-in: "At ABC Animal Hospital, our mission is to provide compassionate, high-quality veterinary care to companion animals, while supporting pet owners with empathy, education, and trust."

VISION STATEMENT TEMPLATE

(Where we are going – our future goals)

Prompt: What do we aspire to become or accomplish long-term? How will our community, clients, or field be better because of us?

Template:

Our vision is to become ________________________________,

known for ____.

We strive to create a future where ______________________________

and ____.

Example fill-in: "Our vision is to become the most trusted and innovative veterinary team in our region, known for excellent care, progressive medicine, and a thriving work culture."

CORE VALUES TEMPLATE

(What we stand for – our guiding principles)

Prompt: What beliefs or standards guide our behaviors and decisions? How do we show up for each other, our patients, and our clients?

Instructions: List 4–6 values below, and describe what each means in action.

Value	What it looks like in action

Example: "Compassion – We treat all patients and clients as we would want our own loved ones to be treated."

Here is a **printable meeting guide** for leading a **Mission, Vision, and Values (MVV)** discussion with a veterinary team. It's designed for a 60–90-minute interactive staff meeting or retreat.

Veterinary Team MVV Meeting Guide

Purpose: Define or refine your practice's Mission, Vision, and Core Values

Recommended Duration: 60–90 minutes

Materials: Printed MVV templates, pens, whiteboard/flip chart, markers, snacks, and fidgets (optional but fun!)

Meeting Agenda

1) **Welcome and Meeting Goals (5–10 minutes)**
   - **Facilitator Says:** "Today we're working together to put into words what we already believe in: why we show up, what we strive for, and what values guide us. These statements help us align as a team and communicate our purpose to clients and new teammates."
2) **Discuss the MISSION (20–25 minutes)** *Why do we exist? What is our purpose beyond making money?*
   - **Facilitator Prompts:** What do we do really well that sets us apart? Who are we here to serve? What emotional or practical outcomes do we hope to create for our clients and patients?
   - **Activity:** Distribute **Mission Statement Templates**. Ask team members to fill them out individually or in pairs (10 minutes).
   - Then, share ideas and capture key themes on the board (10–15 minutes).

3) **Define the VISION (15–20 minutes)** *What do we want to become in 3–5 years? What are we working toward?*
   - **Facilitator Prompts:** If everything went right, what kind of clinic would we be? What would clients say about us? How do we want to grow or lead in our field or community?
   - **Activity:** Distribute **Vision Statement Templates**. Give individuals or small groups 10 minutes to write, then discuss as a team. Write strong phrases or goals on the board.
4) **Identify CORE VALUES (20–25 minutes)** *What values guide our behavior and decisions?*
   - **Facilitator Prompts:** What makes us proud to work here? What behaviors or attitudes are *non-negotiable* on this team? Think of someone on the team you admire — what do they consistently do?
   - **Activity:** Distribute **Core Values Worksheets**. Individuals brainstorm 4–6 values and their meaning in action (10 minutes), then share aloud. As a group, circle the most common or important 4–6 on the whiteboard.
5) **Close and Next Steps (5–10 minutes)**
   - **Facilitator Summary:** "Thank you all — this is a working draft and will evolve as we grow. Your input is vital in shaping how we represent ourselves." Let them know how you'll finalize the statements (e.g. leadership will draft and bring back for review at the next meeting).

Optional: Vote on a favorite phrase or word for each section to carry forward.

Works Cited

Dennison, K. (2024, July 16). Gallup says $8.8 trillion is the true scost of low employee engagement. *Forbes*. Retrieved from https://www.forbes.com/sites/karadennison/2024/07/16/gallup-says-88-trillion-is-the-true-cost-of-low-employee-engagement

Gallup, Inc. (2023). State of the Global Workplace: 2023 Report. Retrieved from https://www.gallup.com/workplace/349484/state-of-the-global-workplace-2023.aspx

Grenny, J.P. (2022). *Crucial Influence: Leadership Skills to Create Lasting Behavior Change*, 2e. New York, NY: McGraw-Hill.

Harvard Business School Online. (2021, March 16). How to Influence Without Authority. Retrieved from online.hbs.edu: online.hbs.edu/blog/post/influence-without-authority

Heinke, M. (2012). *Practice Made Perfect: A Complete Guide to Veterinary Practice*

Pendell, R. (2023, September 11). Employee Engagement Strategies: Fixing the World's $8.8 Trillion Problem. Retrieved from www.gallup.com: www.gallup.com/workplace/393497/world-trillion-workplace-problem.aspx

Vetcor. (2025). Our story. (Vetcor, Producer). Retrieved from www.vetcor.com: https://www.vetcor.com/about-us/our-story

Index

b

c

g

h

i